Metabolic Regulation

Many thanks to the authors who agreed to the use of their material in this book.

Metabolic Regulation

Edited by
Raymond S. Ochs, Richard W. Hanson,
Judith Hall

1985

Elsevier Science Publishers
Amsterdam – New York – Oxford

© 1985 Elsevier Science Publishers

ISBN: 0 444 80691 1

Published by
Elsevier Science Publishers
PO Box 1527
1000 BM Amsterdam
The Netherlands

Sole distributors worldwide (except for USA and Canada)
Elsevier Publications (Cambridge)
68 Hills Road
Cambridge CB2 1LA
United Kingdom

Sole distributors for USA and Canada
Elsevier Science Publishing Company Inc.
52 Vanderbilt Avenue
New York
NY 10017, USA

Contents

Introduction

Metabolism redux*

Raymond S. Ochs and Richard W. Hanson

'A funny thing about a chair
You hardly ever think it's there
To know a chair is really it,
You sometimes have to go and sit.'
The Chair,
from the collected poems of Theodore Roethke

Like Theodore Roethke's famous *Chair* which needs to be sat on to be experienced, metabolism has recently been taken for granted. After all, haven't all the major pathways been discovered and the last word found its way into text books? The fire seems to have gone out of this most central of all areas of biochemistry: no weekly press releases stir our imagination, no feature articles on metabolic regulation grace the pages of *Nature*. A whole generation of graduate students are coming of age who have never heard of *gluconeogenesis* and think that DNA→RNA→protein is the only new metabolic pathway worth studying.

Perhaps it is time for a metabolic *redux*, a return to vitality and a re-discovery of the many important problems in metabolic regulation which have been left unsolved. There is ample evidence of a lively debate, even in areas where the 'last word' was seemingly written decades ago. Far from weakening research in metabolic regulation, recent evidence in modern molecular and cell biology merely emphasizes the importance of asking old questions in a new and different way. Dan Koshland, when asked for his 'brilliant and far-sighted view of the future' puts it this way: 'In the case of metabolic regulation the easy reply could be that "there is no future". Large numbers of students in the modern era regard metabolic pathways as a solved problem. Science, however, has a way of providing employment to its loyal servants, so the fields of enzyme regulation and metabolic pathways, far from being dead, may be entering one of their most exciting phases'[1].

The present volume, drawn from the pages of *TIBS*, is written in the readily accessible and lively style which has become something of a trademark of that journal. Our purpose is to present the new developments and ideas of those investigators primarily concerned with metabolic regulation. In organizing this book we have grouped together classical themes such as carbohydrate and nitrogen metabolism, but the book is also sectored into areas of current interest, so that theoretical articles are separated from those dealing with specific metabolic pathways or the role of special signal molecules.

The coverage in this volume is eclectic rather than comprehensive and in many instances, we have emphasized controversies. Over the years, *TIBS* has proven to be a forum for views both *pro* and *con.* on a number of issues related to metabolism. A striking example is the claim by Williams and his colleagues that the pentose pathway in liver, a long established textbook route for the oxidation of glucose, contains several additional reactions and novel intermediates. The evidence for the traditional pentose pathway is defended by Landau and Wood, and also by Katz who present strong reservations about the interpretation of the labeling pattern supporting the new pathway proposed by Williams. For readers willing to dedicate themselves to following the metabolic fate of specific carbon atoms of glucose, these two articles make fascinating reading.

Several viewpoints are also offered on the concept of 'futile' cycling, that is, the existence in the same cell of two enzymes catalysing opposing reactions which results in the net hydrolysis of ATP. Newsholme, Challis and Crabtree review the reasons that a cell might employ such a mechanism. These authors use an abstract analogy to portray

---

* Redux (re duks) Adj. (L. fr. reducere – to bring back) Lit. lead back, indicating return to health after disease. *Webster New International Dictionary*.

control by futile cycles; a box is shown with a weak stimulus going in, and a large response coming out. How can this be? This is a trick question; there is an extra node missing from the box. This additional input in the sense of a metabolic pathway can be found in the authors' description of enzyme inter-conversion by covalent modification, or regulation by substrate ('futile') cycles. Thus, the box analogy could be extended by considering the behavior of a transistor amplifier in an electrical circuit; here the third node controls voltage or current gain precisely as modulation of one enzyme reaction in a futile cycle changes pathway flux in an opposing direction.

A more specific analysis is presented by Katz and Rognstad, who describe methods for determination of cycling in carbohydrate metabolism and its use in predicting metabolic control. Applying results from the glucokinase/glucose-6-phosphatase cycle, these authors argue against a major role for glucose-6-phosphatase in the phosphorylation of glucose. The article by Nordlie reaches just the opposite conclusion based on extensive published work from his own laboratory. As is often the case, the reader will be left to decide by evaluating two quite different experimental approaches to the same question.

Aside from its use as a model for futile cycling, the pathways of carbohydrate metabolism are the most heavily trodden both by experimenters and cells. Tejwani discusses the multiple regulators of phosphofructokinase in relation to the Pasteur effect, which represents one of the first successes in linking pathway flux (glycolysis) to the control of energy production by the cell. Phosphorylation and its relationship to allosteric modification is presented in Hardie's discussion of acetyl-CoA carboxylase. The principle of noncovalent enzyme effectors altering the ability of an enzyme to serve as a substrate for a protein kinase has also been observed with pyruvate kinase[2], and may thus be a general phenomenon. This section is concluded with two views on carbohydrate metabolism in muscle; Gould considers the possibility of ATP as a regulator, and Wilson the relative role of ATP and creatine phosphate in muscle contraction. Clearly the field of carbohydrate metabolism cannot be described as 'settled'.

Even an area as well entrenched as the regulation of acid–base balance may require a new look. Atkinson and Bourke point out

that urea synthesis removes bicarbonate and that pH controls urea synthesis. From this, they suggest that *the kidney is not involved in pH homeostasis*. This startling proposal is buoyed by the companion article by Haussinger, Gerok and Sies, suggesting that the hepatic glutamine cycle, i.e. glutaminase and glutamine synthetase, is a mechanism for such regulation. Whether the idea will cause angst for students of the kidney is an open question. There are other interpretations for some of the data. For example, the finding that NH_4^+ did not increase ureagenesis in the absence of lactate or other exogenous substrates can be predicted from the requirements for urea synthesis originally established by Krebs[3]. A source of carbon is required to provide aspartate in stoichiometric ratio to carbamoyl phosphate for the argininosuccinate synthetase reaction. Another problem of urea synthesis, control of carbamoyl phosphate synthetase, is taken up by Meijer. He addresses the question of how the enzyme's activator, *N*-acetylglutamate, is transported across the mitochondrial membrane, and its role along with arginine, ornithine, and hormones in controlling urea synthesis.

The position of phospholipid metabolism has recently moved from back seat to center stage in regulation. Interest in phosphatidylinositol has undergone a sudden rebirth from the initial studies by Hokin and Hokin[4] in the fifties, to Michell[5] in the mid-seventies, who showed its potential for involvement in hormone action not involving cyclic AMP. Recent advances are reviewed by Van Rooijen and Agranoff and by Nishizuka. Vance and Pelech present the case for CTP-choline transferase as an 'ambiquitous' enzyme, found in the cytosol or associated with membranes depending upon its phosphorylation status.

Other intracellular regulatory molecules are given their own section. Two examples of compounds involving a rare type of regulatory enzyme, a multifunctional kinase-phosphatase, are 2,3-bisphosphoglycerate of red blood cells and the recently discovered fructose 2,6-bisphosphate, which is discussed by Hers. The protein kinase which promotes cyclic AMP response itself exists in two forms in different tissues. One property distinguishing the type I protein kinase is tight nucleotide binding. This feature is also evident for adenylate cyclase. Guanine nucleotide binding proteins in particular are of current interest because of the similarities between transducin and the regulatory sub-units of adenylate cyclase. Furthermore, the product of the oncogene, *ras*, also displays this property. The recent finding of McGrath *et al.*[6], that a human c-*ras* differs from the oncogene *ras* in that only the for-mer encodes a product displaying normal GTPase activity, should heighten interest in this area.

Many investigators studying metabolic problems take the road less-travelled, and the results are often illuminating. Brown fat cells contain an unusual protein that leads to mitochondrial uncoupling. This is physio-logically useful during arousal from hiberna-tion. Nicholls reviews the information on the control of uncoupling by this protein, its hormonal regulation and direct interaction with intracellular compounds such as fatty acids and purine nucleotides. Our lack of understanding of metabolism of brown fat is underscored in the article by Cooney and Newsholme, in which they pro-pose that the contribution of this tissue to the whole animal may at present be under-estimated. The same claim is made by Masters and Holmes for peroxisomes. It is probably safe to say that anyone with a vested interest in a metabolic pathway will overestimate its contribution. The estimates for both ethanol and fatty acid oxidation by peroxisomes are at least debatable. With both substrates, significant amounts of peroxisomal oxidation are evident only when these organelles are strongly induced, so that the significance of this pathway may be pharmacological rather than physiologi-cal. Still, peroxisomes are probably involved in chain shortening of long-chain fatty acids[7], and as such play an important role in metabolism.

Ethanol metabolism has been an area of continuing interest. While the pathway itself is short, the research, discussion and contro-versy surrounding it are not. Perhaps this is because the problem is so well defined; in any event, the two major contentions of regulation by the amount of alcohol dehydrogenase *versus* the amount of NADH are both highlighted, in addition to numer-ous byways.

It is probable that even a seemingly simple pathway such as that for ethanol oxidation, as suggested by Kacser, is more complicated than is generally believed. It is suggested that this pathway is connected to others, and to really understand its regula-tion requires consideration of a wide variety of other metabolic reactions. Some of the connections made in this article may appear tenuous. It is not generally accepted, for example, that the NADH supply in the cytosol is related to ATP/ADP ratio.

Undoubtedly, a more global theoretical framework is critical for understanding the regulation of cellular energy production. One view presented by Porteous and by Gillies is that the concept of a 'rate limiting step' is artificial, and that several enzymes control pathway flux, each with their own 'control strength'. The application of control strength to oxidative phosphorylation by isolated mitochondria exemplifies this approach. Recently, Gellerick *et al.*[8] have shown that different control strengths are obtained when pyruvate kinase rather than hexokinase is used to maintain constant levels of ATP in isolated mitochondria. Thus, the specific experimental system employed markedly influences the final results.

Computer simulation of metabolic pathways is certainly an important goal. However, to date it has been only marginally useful in predicting regulation of metabolic flux in complex, multi-enzyme pathways. While it is surely important to have quantitative understanding, it is more important to have a qualitative grasp of any subject first. This represents a fundamental difference between what can be described as a model on the one hand and a simulation on the other. The difference is in detail: a computer or mathematical simulation requires exact numbers to be fitted into equations. A true model suppresses detail in order to understand the fundamental mech-anism.

It is not really possible to decide whether a model or a simulation is 'best', but an important caveat is introduced by Keech and Wallace in studies of pyruvate carboxy-lase. Previous evidence for sigmoidal initial velocity and binding-dependence of its activator, acetyl-CoA, resulted from separ-ate artifacts. These studies demonstrate the importance of careful analysis before global theory.

These problems are relevant to views on compartmentation. In the past, 'compart-mentation' gained a certain notoriety as a catch-all term often used to explain anoma-lous results. When the K_m of P-enolpyruvate carboxykinase for oxaloacetate was first reported as being 1 mM (despite the fact that the concentration of oxaloacetate in liver cells was known to be 1–10 μM), there were arguments for the compartmentation of oxaloacetate; ultimately, this inconsistency was shown to be caused by an error in the original measurement! With more recent evidence, the arguments for microenvironments become more appealing. The close organization of enzymes catalysing sequential reactions could limit substrate diffusion and allow lower intracellular concentrations of potentially reactive metabolites. This has support in the evolution of multifunctional enzymes as described by Srere. However, the wholesale packaging of entire pathways seems unlikely, since many reactions are seen to establish near equilibrium in the cell, and the concentrations of metabolites measured in cells are often near to the respective K_m values for their enzymes. In a functional sense, therefore, a cell can often be profitably viewed as a simple reaction vessel, i.e. the notorious 'bag of enzymes'.

We believe these articles demonstrate that metabolism is a most lively area of research with its own share of controversy rather than a jumble of facts presented in skeleton form as pathways on oversized wall charts. To find out if we are correct, we invite you to 'read and sit'.

References
1 Koshland, D. E. (1984) *Trends Biochem. Sci.* 9, 155–159
2 Engstrom, L. (1978) *Curr. Top. Cell Regul.* 13, 29–51
3 Krebs, H. A., Lund, P. and Stubbs, M. (1976) in *Gluconeogenesis* (Hanson, R. W. and Mehlman, M. A., eds), pp. 269–291, Wiley–Interscience
4 Hokin, M. R. and Hokin, L. E. (1953) *J. Biol. Chem.* 203, 967–977
5 Michell, R. H. (1975) *Biochim. Biophys. Acta* 415, 81–147
6 McGrath, J. P., Capon, D. J., Goeddel, D. V. and Levinson, A. D. (1984) *Nature* 310, 644–649
7 Christiansen, R. Z. (1978) *Biochim. Biophys. Acta* 530, 314–324
8 Gellerich, F. N., Bohnensack, R. and Kunz, W. (1983) *Biochim. Biophys. Acta.* 722, 381–391

RICHARD W. HANSON

Department of Biochemistry, Case Western Reserve University, Cleveland, OH 44106, USA

RAYMOND S. OCHS

Department of Biochemistry, Kansas State University, Manhattan, KA 66506, USA

Control of enzyme activity and metabolic pathways

D. E. Koshland, Jr

Large numbers of students in the modern era regard metabolic pathways as a solved problem. Science, however, has a way of providing employment to its loyal servants, so the fields of enzyme regulation and metabolic pathways, far from being dead, may be entering one of their most exciting phases.

In the first place, one must define a metabolic pathway. To some it is synonymous with 'old fashioned amino acid and carbohydrate metabolism'. But the dictionary describes metabolism as 'the chemical changes in living cells by which energy is provided and new material is synthesized'. Under such a definition gene expression, neuron processing and second messenger systems are 'metabolic pathways'. To the question 'Are they controlled in the same way as the 'old' metabolic pathways?' my answer would be 'yes, but'. Yes, because they involve discrete steps organized in an obligatory sequence and controlled by many of the devices with which we are already familiar. The 'but' is to remind us that they represent new challenges and unknown facets which may lead to new regulatory devices and molecular mechanisms.

Not only are there new horizons in terms of new pathways, but it is also clear that there are major problems in regard to understanding regulation of familiar pathways. As the major metabolic pathways of living systems become delineated, we must learn how these pathways interact. We are dealing with network systems not only within cells but also between cells. How these systems are controlled, why changes in levels of some enzymes lead to serious diseases while other changes are tolerated by the cell without difficulty remain unexplained.

A particularly interesting feature of current knowledge is that the 'less known pathways', such as the control of gene expression[1], neuronal processing[2], and second messenger systems[3] appear to be regulated by many of the same phenomena as those that control the familiar metabolic pathways. Allosteric activation and inhibition, competition for common sites, covalent regulation, sequential pathways with rate determining steps, all seem to be parts of these new pathways just as they are key features of the well worked-out metabolic pathways. There is the exciting probability that new control devices will be required to explain these new pathways but it is also likely that the added sophistication which is to be gained by studying familiar pathways in depth will be transferable to the new pathways as well. With these viewpoints in mind let us look at a few specific areas which should be of interest in the future.

Futile cycles and enzymatic perfection

One of the major problems of current metabolism is the understanding of the control of futile cycle enzymes. Futile cycles shown schematically in Fig. 1 are prevalent in nature and for an excellent reason. In any reversible situation, maximum control will be achieved if the free energy up one pathway and the free energy down its reverse are both negative. This places both pathways under

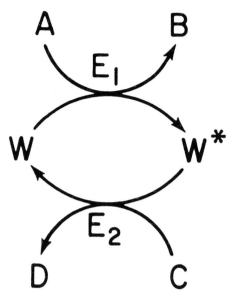

Fig. 1. Illustrative 'futile cycle' in which enzyme 1 converts protein W into a modified form W* and enzyme 2 reverses the action. Because A is converted to B in the forward step and C to D in the reverse step, both can have negative free energies at the same time. The situation in which E_1 and E_2 involve a series of steps and W is a small molecule is essentially the same.

kinetic control, allowing them to be turned on and turned off by means of regulatory molecules. The disadvantage of such a system is that unregulated enzymes would simply go around and around in 'futile cycles', dissipating energy. The conventional wisdom is that allosteric effectors or converter enzymes (which are ultimately controlled by allosteric effectors) always inhibit one pathway while activating the other. The demonstration of this mutual exclusiveness in quantitative terms is yet to be achieved in any experimental system. Because of compartmentalization problems, we do not know the concentration of the effectors in a mammalian cell in precise terms. Using averaged concentrations, the levels of the effectors which activate and inhibit enzymes *in vitro* do not seem to fluctuate sufficiently to turn off one pathway while turning on the other. So the efficiency of futile

cycles, their 'idling speed' and their quantitative relationships must be understood.

Part of this problem may be that we have not yet found all the allosteric effectors. One of the most dramatic developments in recent metabolic understanding was the discovery of fructose 2,6-bisphosphate by Hers, Hue and Van Schaftingen[4]. Phosphofructokinase was one of the most studied enzymes in control and yet possibly its most important effector had gone undiscovered for a long period of time. Thus the evaluation of futile cycles and the efficiency at which the pathways are controlled will require devices such as genetic manipulation and *in vitro–in vivo* comparisons to be sure that all the effectors are known.

In this context it is interesting to analyse the most desirable situation for a futile cycle. The system must be reversible and ultimately driven by ATP energy whether or not the specific agent is methylation, phosphorylation, or metabolite degradation. Thus a futile cycle is acting indirectly as an ATPase. If neither pathway is ever turned off completely, there will always be some waste of ATP. If that is inevitable, the enzymes in the cycle should operate very slowly to save ATP. They cannot act too slowly, however, since they must have a responsiveness appropriate to the physiological effect. Thus, in the case of phosphorylase it is important that the glucose units which are removed from glycogen be removed in seconds to promote muscular contraction and the availability of quick energy. They do not, however, have to be released in milliseconds as might be required in a neuronal pathway. Conversely they must be faster than some hormonal systems in which time scales of hours may be adequate. It would seem logical therefore that enzymes involved in futile cycles should be just fast enough to turn the switch in times that are biologically effective, i.e. milliseconds, minutes, or hours as the case may be. Then even if the cycle cannot be shut down completely the loss of ATP will be minimal. In this regard it is interesting that the turnover number of most kinases and phosphatases is very poor[5,6]; far removed from 'the enzymatic perfection' that Knowles[7] has defined for those enzymes that appear to be diffusion controlled.

A similar situation arises in bacterial chemotaxis in which the 'memory' of the bacterium is highly selected for the organism's survival[8]. The time span of this memory is in turn related to the rates of methylation and demethylation of the sensory receptors[9]. It has been found that the methylating and demethylating enzymes have extremely low turnover numbers – abysmal enzymes from the viewpoint of catalytic effectiveness. But the receptor, methylase and demethylase are produced on the same operon in approximately 3:1:1 proportions. If the enzymes were highly efficient, either the bacterium would have no memory time or the loss of ATP would be horrendous. Selecting for 'slow' enzymes will therefore probably be a common feature of futile cycles.

One might ask whether lower production of more catalytically effective molecules might not be a better biological solution to this problem. At the moment one can only guess at solutions such as 'protein–protein binding constants need minimal concentrations of each protein' or 'zero-order effects (see below) require high protein substrate levels'. The answer to this question therefore awaits future research.

Magnitude amplification in regulation

As new problems such as differentiation and neuronal control come to the forefront, the sensitivity of enzymes to regulation also becomes important. Enhancing the signal delivered by a single proton or turning on a cascade through a hormone receptor are examples in which signal amplification becomes crucial. An analysis of amplification phenomena[10] has defined two types of processes which are fundamentally different in character: 'magnitude amplification' in which a molecule of stimulus produces a larger, but linearly proportionate, output response (e.g. 1 molecule of stimulus releases 1000 molecules of response, 2 molecules release 2000) and sensitivity amplification (in which a percentage change in stimulus produces a larger percentage change in output response).

Probably the most elegant illustration of magnitude amplification is in the visual system. It is now known that the photoreceptor cell has the capacity to detect a single photon by converting the absorption of a photon into the hydrolysis of 500 000 molecules of cyclic GMP[11]. The enzymatic steps which make this possible are shown in Fig. 2. In the first step, a rhodopsin molecule (R) is activated by absorbing a photon and this activated rhodopsin (R*) binds to a transducin protein (T), which is very similar to the G protein of adenylate cyclase. The activated rhodopsin–transducin complex can catalyse the exchange of GDP for GTP producing R*.T.GTP. At this point the activated rhodopsin molecule dissociates from the transducin complex and recycles to find other transducin molecules in need of activation. It repeats this cycle approximately 500 times on average, before decaying to an inactive rhodopsin molecule. The transducin complex containing GTP is now capable of activating a phosphodiesterase (PDE) by forming at T.GTP–PDE complex. The active phosphodiesterase lasts until the transducin hydrolyses GTP to GDP. The lifetime of the transducin as a hydrolytic enzyme thus determines the number of phosphodiesterase molecules which are activated. On average, 1 000 molecules of cyclic GMP are hydrolysed before the transducin converts to the GDP complex

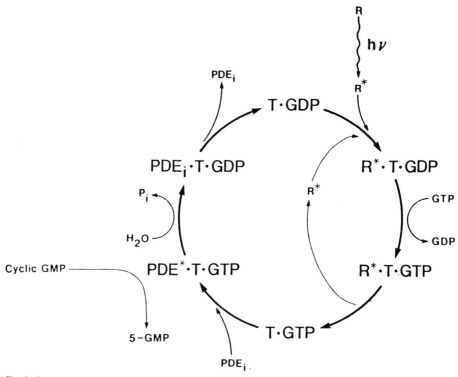

Fig. 2. Proposed light-activated amplification cycle. Information flows from photolysed rhodopsin (R*) to transducin (T·GTP) and then to the phosphodiesterase (PDE*). (Taken from Ref. 11.)

which is inactive. Thus the system has a built-in gain of 5×10^5. This number is obtained from the various rate constants in the processes of association, dissociation, and hydrolysis: quite clearly, any number either larger or smaller than this could be achieved by changing these values. For example, if GTP were hydrolysed more slowly by transducin, the PDE would stay active longer and hydrolyse more molecules of cGMP. There are many other examples: complement fixation, blood clotting, ion channels, etc. of equivalent magnitude amplification, but the light receptor case is one of the most elegantly worked out and provides a prototype for the elucidation of mechanisms by which signals are amplified in a linear relationship.

Sensitivity amplification

The devices known to produce magnitude amplification in biological systems are more extensive and better known than those to achieve sensitivity amplification[10]. Sensitivity amplification is necessary when one changes from one background level to another, i.e. not changing from zero to a finite value, but from some finite non-zero level to another finite level. One of the best known mechanisms for sensitivity amplification is allosteric cooperativity of which hemoglobin is a good example. It gives an amplification factor of 2.3 (i.e. a 23% change in response for a 10% change in stimulus). Not many proteins of higher cooperativity than hemoglobin are known, however, so we must look for more cooperative proteins or other forms of sensitivity amplification. Other mechanisms for achieving such amplification are more difficult to find and far less developed, but they may be of crucial importance in the 'new pathways'. For example, in differentiation, small changes in environment may be needed to regulate gene expression.

To clarify our understanding of this area, the term 'ultrasensitivity' has been introduced[10] to characterize all phenomena which are more sensitive to change than the Michaelis–Menten response (systems less sensitive than Michaelis–Menten are called 'subsensitive'). One potential mechanism for ultrasensitivity is the multistep effect, a process in which a single effector acts at various steps in a pathway[10,12]. For example, it is known that cyclic AMP enters in five distinct steps in the pathways of glycogen synthesis and breakdown[5]. Three of these involve the cyclic AMP-dependent phosphorylation of a protein which inhibits a phosphatase that dephosphorylates glycogen phosphorylase, phosphorylase kinase, and glycogen synthase. Two of them involve the action of cyclic AMP-dependent protein kinase which activates phosphorylase kinase and inhibits glycogen synthase. Although cyclic AMP enters in five different steps, the pathway regulation does not depend on the fifth power of the cyclic AMP concentration.

The probable reason for this is that the various steps do not have equal weight in the control of the pathway and the kinetic relationships of effectors acting at sequential steps along a pathway remain to be determined in detail in any pathway. For example, an effector working on one step in a pathway can have only a small effect on the overall flux if a subsequent step then becomes rate determing. The multiple input of an effector at many points may thus be only to activate sequential steps, so the first activation does not become rate limiting. This cannot explain all effects of the glycogen cascade, however, since in two places there is activation of one enzyme and inhibition of its reverse in a 'futile cycle'. Hence, a potential for multistep ultrasensitivity as described[10] above exists. The evaluation of this

important feature of enzymatic control deserves particular emphasis in the years ahead. Its importance is indicated by the large number of cascade processes which are now being revealed for every type of pathway ranging from lipid synthesis[13] to glutamine synthesis[12], to neuronal phosphorylation[14]. It seems logical that reversible phosphorylation cascades will be found to play a part in gene expression.

Many of these cascades seem to be more complex than would be required for the types of control described above. That many steps are needed because they provide a mechanism for rate amplification[12] and for new types of sensitivity to control are attractive possibilities.

As one examines multistep cascades, the multiplicity of effectors that control a pathway needs quantitative evaluation. If effector 1 works on step 1 and effector 2 on step 2, does the metabolic system lead to multiplicative effect or a cancelling effect? The same question arises from two effectors acting on the same enzyme. If two chemicals are always released in concert, then they could produce a sensitivity effect equivalent to an allosteric protein having a Hill coefficient of 2, and perhaps a much higher coefficient if they combined with cooperative properties of the target protein. Quantitation of multiple effectors has been evaluated for glutamine synthesis[12] but for practically no other system. The degree of ultrasensitivity would, of course, depend on the actual effector concentrations, their affinity constants for the protein, etc. These factors need to be explored, as the potential for such effects in control in complex pathways may be very important.

A new type of high sensitivity in regulatory control has been discovered to arise in covalent interconversion cycles, and has been termed 'zero-order ultrasensitivity'. It has been developed theoretically[15] and established experimentally[16] that highly enhanced sensitivity can be obtained by this mechanism, which results from a situation in which at least one of the inter-converting enzymes of a system like that shown in Fig. 1 is close to saturation, i.e. is in the zero-order region. Under these circumstances the steady-state level of protein modification can be highly sensitive to an effector binding to a converter enzyme even though that effector binds to a single protein in a Michaelis–Menten manner. The only *in vivo* case that has been discovered so far, the control of the isocitric dehydrogenase by reversible phosphorylation[16], has an ultrasensitivity slightly less than that of hemoglobin. However, the zero-order effect has the potential for much higher sensitivity and it seems likely that it will play an important role in the many covalent regulatory cascades that are found in biological systems.

Another mechanism for enhanced sensitivity, particularly in sensory systems, is adaptation. By means of adaptation, a sensory system can 'reset to zero'[10] to allow changes over background levels to be more easily detected. Thus the adaptive phenomenon which desensitizes background stimulation, increases the sensitivity to new signals. So far, the proteins identified with such adaptation in detailed studies are those involved in bacterial chemotaxis[9] and vision[17]. However, it is to be noted that a wide variety of receptors such as the acetylcholine receptor[18], the epidermal growth factor receptor[19] and the insulin receptor[20], are covalently modified and are systems which have an adaptive response. Delineating the nature of these systems and the mechanisms by which they achieve enhanced sensitivity (if that turns out to be the case) should be an extremely interesting one.

Another mechanism for reducing background noise in order to enhance sensitivity is the 'coincidence counting' device, originally delineated by Hecht *et al.*[21], which requires seven separate neurons to fire before the brain records an event, false messages are reduced and the visual system is able to record a low level of photon signal per receptor. The price is, of course, a seven-fold higher flux to initiate the event. It will be interesting to see whether coincidence circuitry can be used analogously in metabolic systems.

It is worth noting that extreme sensitivity is not needed in all systems. If a curve is very steep, i.e. a system can be turned on by very small changes in the level of the stimulus, then of course it has the concomitant feature that it is very near zero or very near 100% activity over vast ranges above and below the inflection region. Thus a less sensitive system exerts loose control over a wider range of stimulus, whereas a more sensitive system shows far tighter control over a small range. Although most enzymes are composed of multiple subunits only very few are cooperative and some are negatively cooperative, indicating that high sensitivity is not needed in all cases. Uncovering new sources of sensitivity to discover where they are applied and why those systems in which they appear are particularly in need of such sensitivity will be intriguing.

Oncogenes and overproduction

One of the most exciting areas of current research is the area of oncogenes[22]. Certain genes appear to have high relevance to uncontrolled growth and the identification of the individual genes and their mechanism of action therefore becomes not only an important problem for medical therapy but could throw a great deal of light on general understanding of metabolic control. One discovery is that overproduction of a cellular protein can cause transformation to a cancer cell and another is that a single nucleotide substitution can apparently yield the same result. What is sometimes lost in the justifiable excitement of DNA sequencing is that we must ultimately be dealing with a metabolic control problem. If a particular step in a metabolic pathway is catalysed by a low concentration of protein, overproduction of that protein may have a dramatic effect on the regulation of that pathway. It could do so by providing an added capacity for catalysis which did not exist before; it could do so by producing so much enzyme that a regulator present in limiting amounts would no longer control the pathway; it could do so by desensitizing a regulatory system without totally eliminating the regulation; it could do so by changing to or from the zero order ultrasensitivity described above. And if such were the case, a single nucleotide substitution resulting in a single amino acid substitution could be explained by its effects on the K_m and/or V_{max} of an enzyme. Effects of amino acid changes are well known and many have been identified with the onset of 'molecular diseases'[23].

Although these hypotheses are possible, we must confess that the overproduction and underproduction of enzymes is not at all well understood. Because scientists are using plasmids and utilizing recombinant DNA techniques, many enzymes are being overproduced in cells, sometimes with dramatic effects on the organism and other times with only minor effects. At times the lack of effect can be rationalized on the basis that we are overproducing a protein which is not associated with a rate-determining step but this certainly does not apply to all of the proteins that have been synthesized. In other cases, the rather minor effects of major overproduction are explained on the basis of: 'the system has feedback properties which allow it to adapt to overproduction'. But an understanding of how these feedbacks can allow the cell to adapt to a highly unnatural situation will clarify aspects of metabolic regulation.

Down's syndrome and other diseases of chromosomal aneuploidy are themselves intriguing from a metabolic point of view. In most cases the appearance of an extrachromosomal element (with demonstrated increase in protein production) has very little effect. Thus, in Down's syndrome, most metabolic systems are operating largely normally and other aneuploidy situations are similar. That the children suffer mental retardation might be explained on the basis that the brain is likely to be most sensitive to deficiencies in metabolism whereas kidney and liver work on more flexible limits. The same is true of some other aneuploidy diseases where some functions are normal while others are severely damaged. The relative health means that all the enzymes on a chromosome can be increased by 50% with little effect on most metabolic pathways of the organism. Coupled with the fact that many alleles can be eliminated from one chromosome of an individual without impairing health (the recessive trait), this means that many enzymes can undergo a concentration change by a factor of three with little effect on metabolism. Yet textbooks constantly discuss the highly efficient, highly sensitive, clever organization of biological pathways. If the system seems to operate equally well over a wide range of enzyme concentration, why is so much protein produced? If in fact it does not, why can we not detect the effects in the complex systems? The elucidation of these problems should be one of the key developments in the future of metabolic control.

Flux rate

If complex pathways are to be understood one must not only work out the parameters and the metabolic concentrations of the various metabolites and enzymes in the pathway, but one must solve the network interaction to interpret feedback and feedforward effects. A number of metabolic simulations have been made with computers[24]. These will become more sophisticated as the data to use in such complex calculations become more available. Up to now, computer simulations have been ingeniously applied on relatively meagre data, but the development of new tools means the methodology is becoming available for understanding network interactions. The steady improvement of non-invasive probes such as NMR[25] is also encouraging. So far, only metabolites present in high concentration can be observed, but interesting results have already been obtained and the instrumentation is steadily improving. The biochemistry will be difficult, but if we hope to understand ultimately how neurons integrate excitatory and inhibitory inputs or to explain how the pleiotropic effects of second messenger systems achieve their goals without causing deleterious side effects, the quantitation of the fluxes, intermediate levels of metabolites, and compartmentalization problems[26] must be solved.

Summary

Past studies on enzymes and metabolic control have revealed fundamental phenomena such as conformational changes, covalent modification, and feedback inhibition which appear repeatedly in all pathways, However, the new complex metabolic pathways pose new problems of which control of futile cycles, network interactions, and signal amplification are illustrative. Their solution may depend upon the use of new tools such as non-invasive probes and new concepts, such as new mechanisms for high sensitivity, and on the examination of the 'well understood' pathways in greater depth.

Acknowledgement

The author is grateful for financial support from the National Institutes of Health and the National Science Foundation.

References

I have used TIBS references whenever possible.

The reader should therefore use the TIBS *articles to get to primary sources in many cases.*

1 Dynan, W. and Tjian, R. (1982) *Trends Biochem. Sci.* 7, 124–125
2 Akerman, K. E. O. and Nicholls, D. G. (1983) *Trends Biochem. Sci.* 8, 63–64
3 Gillies, R. J. (1982) *Trends Biochem. Sci.* 7, 233–235
4 Hers, H. G., Hue, L. and Van Schaftingen, E. (1982) *Trends Biochem. Sci.* 7, 329–331 (see also p. 222 of this book)
5 Rosen, O. M. and Krebs, E. G. (eds) (1981) *Protein Phosphorylation*, Cold Spring Harbor
6 Fisher, E. H. and Brautigan, D. L. (1982) *Trends Biochem. Sci.* 7, 3–4
7 Knowles, J. R. (1980) *Biochemistry* 15, 5631
8 Koshland, D. E. Jr (1976) *Trends Biochem. Sci.* 1, 1–3
9 Koshland, D. E. Jr (1980) *Trends Biochem. Sci.* 5, 297–302
10 Koshland, D. E. Jr, Goldbeter, A. and Stock, J. B. (1982) *Science* 217, 220–225
11 Stryer, L., Hurley, J. B. and Fung, B. K. (1981) *Trends Biochem. Sci.* 6, 245–247
12 Stadtman, E. and Chock, P. B. (1978) *Current Topics in Cellular Regulation* 13, 53
13 Hardie, G. (1981) *Trends Biochem. Sci.* 6, 75–77 (see also p. 135 of this book)
14 Greengard, P. (1978) *Science* 199, 146
15 Goldbeter, A. and Koshland, D. E. Jr (1981) *Proc. Natl Acad. Sci. USA* 78, 6840–6844
16 LaPorte, D. C. and Koshland, D. E. Jr (1983) *Nature* 305, 286–290
17 Kuhn, H. (1974) *Nature* 250, 588
18 Teichberg, V. I., Slobel, A. and Changeux, J. P. (1977) *Nature* 267, 540
19 Cohen, S., Carpenter, G. and King, L. (1980) *J. Biol. Chem.* 255, 4834
20 Kasuga, M., Zick, Y., Blith, D. L., Karlsson, F. A., Haring, H. and Kahn, C. R. (1982) *J. Biol. Chem.* 257, 9891
21 Hecht, S., Shlaer, S. and Pirenne, M. H. (1942) *J. Gen. Physiol.* 819
22 Weinberg, R. A. (1982) *Trends Biochem. Sci.* 7, 135
23 Robinson, B. H. (1982) *Trends Biochem. Sci.* 7, 151–153
24 Garfinkel, D. (1981) *Trends Biochem. Sci.* 6, 69–71 (see also p. 20 of this book)
25 Chignell, C. F. (1983) *Trends Biochem. Sci.* 8, 74
26 Sies, H. (ed.) (1982) *Metabolic Compartmentation*, Academic Press

D. E. Koshland, Jr is at the Department of Biochemistry, University of California, Berkeley, CA 94720, USA.

How significant is homotropic cooperativity in terms of metabolic regulation?

D. Bruce Keech and John C. Wallace

This article questions the widely held belief that the sigmoidal velocity response of an enzyme to a substrate or effector molecule is necessarily attributable to the homotropic cooperative binding of that ligand. By way of an example, we show how alternative explanations are possible in the case of pyruvate carboxylase.

In recent years, allosterism has become a central theme of metabolic regulation. This phenomenon has become synonymous with sigmoidal binding (or velocity) curves and has focused attention on the models of cooperativity proposed by Monod et al.[1], and Koshland et al.[2]. Both models explained the appearance of sigmoid curves in terms of cooperative binding and subtle sub-unit interactions. So great has been the impact of these proposals that no modern textbook of biochemistry is complete without several pages of sophisticated mathematical argument proving the validity of the models. Therefore, it is not unreasonable to ask the question – just how many enzymes exhibiting sigmoidal binding or velocity profiles actually conform to one or other of the two schemes? Apart from a few enzymes such as glyceraldehyde phosphate dehydrogenase, aspartate transcarbamylase, cytidine deaminase, nucleoside diphosphatase and phosphorylase *b*, it is difficult to find other rigorously established examples. By way of contrast, Hill et al.[3] pointed out that a literature search of publications covering a 12-year period indicated that more than 800 enzymes yielded complex velocity curves. Obviously, the importance attached to the cooperative models proposed by Monod et al.[1] and Koshland et al.[2] is excessive and too little attention is given to other less aesthetically pleasing explanations.

Although Tipton[4] has listed a number of ways for distinguishing between models of cooperativity, it is not an easy task. As a result, examples exist in the literature where a sigmoidal velocity profile has been reported and assumed to be another example of homotropic cooperativity. Obviously not all, possibly very few, sigmoidal binding or velocity curves result from cooperative interactions. Many may arise as a result of artefacts of the assay procedure, or of a failure to appreciate the complexities of the system under investigation. Monod et al.[5] anticipated such events when they stated that 'the most serious objection to the concept of allosteric control is that it could be used to "explain away" almost any mysterious physiological phenomenon'.

Pyruvate carboxylase and sigmoidal curves

Pyruvate carboxylase is an example of an enzyme which exhibits non-classical binding and velocity curves under some circumstances; these can be explained without invoking cooperative binding. This biotin-dependent enzyme catalyses the following reaction:

$$\text{MgATP} + \text{HCO}_3^- + \text{pyruvate} \rightarrow \text{oxaloacetate} + \text{MgADP} + \text{P}_i \quad (1)$$

The enzyme isolated from vertebrate sources is activated by acetyl-CoA, but the manner by which this occurs is not completely understood. This is not surprising when one considers the difficulties and complexities involved in studying the overall reaction mechanism. For example, the enzyme has three substrates and three products; it has two activators, acetyl-CoA[6] and Mg^{2+} (Ref. 7) and when either pyruvate or acetyl-CoA are the variable ligands in initial velocity studies, the enzyme exhibits non-classical kinetic behaviour[6,8,9]. In addition, it is currently believed that, in common with other biotin-containing enzymes, the active site consists of two spatially distinct sub-sites with biotin acting as a mobile carboxyl carrier oscillating between the two sub-sites. However, the main point of interest here is the sigmoidal velocity profile obtained when acetyl-CoA is the variable ligand[6,8].

In the absence of any evidence to the contrary, it was assumed that this non-classical kinetic behaviour indicated that acetyl-CoA bound to the enzyme in a homotropic cooperative manner. The only support for cooperative binding has come from binding studies[10]. However, unequivocal interpretation of this data was difficult due to the fact that purified preparations of pyruvate carboxylase catalyse the deacylation of acetyl-CoA[8]. Since low enzymic concentrations and short incubation times are used in kinetic studies, this deacylase activity is of little consequence when investigating the kinetic properties of the enzyme. Binding studies, on the other hand, require high enzyme concentrations and longer time intervals. Under these conditions, the deacylase activity can have a dramatic effect on the result. This aspect has been discussed in some detail by Easterbrook-Smith et al.[11], who showed that it was difficult to assess the significance of the binding data as it stands. Perhaps a more reliable approach would

have been to use a derivative of acetyl-CoA such as ethyl-CoA which is capable of activating the enzyme and exhibits a sigmoidal response curve, but is not susceptible to deacylation.

Meanwhile, Easterbrook-Smith et al.[11] carried out a kinetic study of the deacylation reaction using acetyl-CoA as the substrate. A linear, double reciprocal plot was obtained suggesting that acetyl-CoA bound to the enzyme in a classical Michaelis–Menten manner. And so the question remained as to how the sigmoidal velocity profile arises in the carboxylation reaction.

Effect of acetyl-CoA on the kinetic response of pyruvate carboxylase to varying pyruvate concentrations

Several years ago it was demonstrated that the enzyme isolated from sheep[12] and rat[13] could catalyse an acetyl-CoA independent carboxylation of pyruvate. The assay conditions required to observe this activity in the sheep enzyme involved an increase in the concentrations of the enzyme, pyruvate and bicarbonate. By carrying out a series of parallel experiments in the presence or absence of acetyl-CoA it was shown that acetyl-CoA decreased the apparent K_m value for pyruvate 8-fold (and about the same amount for bicarbonate). This finding provided the first clue as to the origin of the sigmoid velocity profile – when acetyl-CoA is the variable ligand, the fixed concentration of pyruvate in the assay solution, although saturating at the high concentrations of acetyl-CoA, will become non-saturating as the concentration of acetyl-CoA is decreased. In other words, although only one parameter, acetyl-CoA, is varied, saturation of the enzyme is influenced by both acetyl-CoA and pyruvate.

If this explanation is correct, then changing the fixed concentration of pyruvate in the assay solution should vary the degree of sigmoidicity. This proved to be the case[11]. However, the fact that the sigmoidicity was not completely eliminated simply by increasing the pyruvate concentration (i.e. the Hill coefficient did not decrease to unity), suggested that the effect of acetyl-CoA on pyruvate saturation provided only part of the explanation and that some other factor (or factors) was involved.

Inactivation of the enzyme on dilution

Another feature of pyruvate carboxylase, first described by Ashman et al.[12] using the enzyme isolated from sheep, and since shown to be a property of the chicken enzyme, is that it undergoes irreversible inactivation on dilution. This phenomenon is also known to occur with a number of other enzymes. For example, threonine deaminase[14] isolated from *Escherichia coli* exhibits normal Michaelis–Menten kinetics provided precautions are taken to stabilize the enzyme (i.e. either a relatively high concentration of enzyme, threonine or buffer). A rapid and irreversible loss in enzymic activity occurs when the enzyme is diluted in the presence of low concentrations of threonine and buffer. Under these conditions, a sigmoid curve is obtained when the initial velocity is plotted as a function of threonine concentration. Since the sigmoid curve can be explained in terms of enzyme stability, it is not necessary to postulate more than one binding site for threonine.

Precisely the same situation prevails with pyruvate carboxylase. Acetyl-CoA stabilizes and protects quite dilute solutions of the enzyme against inactivation[12]. However, below 40 μM acetyl-CoA, a very rapid loss of enzymic activity occurs and it is not recovered on addition of more acetyl-CoA. The effect of this loss of activity on the velocity curve is that a falsely reduced rate is observed at low concentrations of acetyl-CoA.

It has been pointed out previously that, in general, if an enzyme is partially

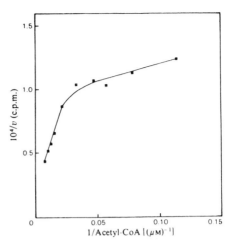

Fig. 1. Reciprocal of reaction velocity versus reciprocal acetyl-CoA concentration at saturating concentrations of all other reaction components with sheep pyruvate carboxylase. The assay contained, in a final volume of 0.5 ml (μmol): Tris chloride, pH 8.4, 40; ATP, 4; MgCl$_2$ 17; pyruvate, 36; NH$_4$Cl, 83; NaH^{14}CO$_2$ (19.86 × 10^5 cpm/ μmol), 38; 2.6 units of enzyme. The reaction time was 30 s.

inactivated during the course of the reaction velocity determination, and if the substrate (or activating ligand) influences the rate of inactivation, then a sigmoidal velocity response will be obtained[15].

Elimination of the sigmoid curve

With the effect on acetyl-CoA on the degree of pyruvate saturation and the inactivation of the enzyme on dilution in mind, Easterbrook-Smith et al.[11] carried out an experiment to determine the rate of enzymic activity at varying acetyl-CoA concentrations under conditions where these two factors no longer operated. When the data obtained under these conditions was plotted in double reciprocal form (Fig. 1), a concave downward curve was obtained indicating that the sigmoidal response to increasing concentrations of acetyl-CoA was completely eliminated.

The explanation advanced by Easterbrook-Smith et al.[11] for this result was that under these conditions, the only effect of varying the acetyl-CoA concentration would be to change the proportion of enzyme catalysing the reaction at the acetyl-CoA-dependent rate and the acetyl-CoA-independent rate. Thus, the observed reaction velocity (v) would be the sum of these two activities and given by equation:

$$V = \frac{V^{(D)}}{1 + \dfrac{K_a}{A}} + \frac{V^{(1)}}{1 + \dfrac{A}{k_a}} \qquad (2)$$

where $V^{(D)}$ and $V^{(1)}$ are the maximum velocities of the dependent and independent reactions respectively, while K_a and A are the Michaelis constant and the acetyl-CoA concentration respectively. Theoretical curves generated from this equation are shown in Fig. 2. The similarity between the double reciprocal plot of the experimental data and the double reciprocal form of equation (2) – Fig. 2 inset – implies that the explanation

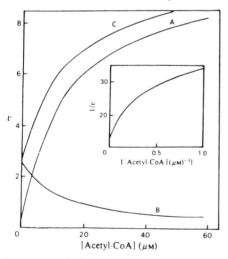

Fig. 2. Theoretical curves generated from equation (2) in the text by calculating the dependence of reaction velocity on acetyl-CoA concentration.

Curve A: the simulation of the acetyl-CoA-dependent term alone. Curve B: the simulation of the acetyl-CoA-independent term alone. Curve C: the simulation of the sum of both terms. The values of K_a $V^{(D)}$ (i.e. the maximum velocity of the acetyl CoA-dependent reaction) and $V^{(1)}$ (the maximum velocity of the acetyl-CoA-independent reaction) were 12 μM, 10.0 and 2.5 respectively. Inset: the double reciprocal plot of curve (C).

advanced by Easterbrook-Smith *et al.*[11] is a plausible model of acetyl-CoA interaction with pyruvate carboxylase. Furthermore, the concave downward curve of the Lineweaver–Burk plot eliminates explanations based on cooperative binding.

Conclusion

Although pyruvate carboxylase gave every indication of being an enzyme requiring an allosteric activator which bound to the enzyme in a homotropic cooperative manner, closer inspection now raises serious doubts concerning this interpretation. The sigmoidal binding curve[10] was probably an artefact of the technique used, while the sigmoidal initial velocity profile[6,8] can be attributed primarily to the instability of the enzyme in dilute solutions of acetyl-CoA. Perhaps as more enzymes exhibiting the non-classical binding and kinetic data are investigated, the models of allosterism based on cooperative interactions may be placed in proper perspective. Without a full explanation of how the *in vitro*, non-hyperbolic kinetic behaviour arises, it is not possible to assess the physiological significance of the observed data.

References

1 Monod, J., Wyman, J. and Changeux, J.-P. (1965) *J. Mol. Biol.* 12, 88–118
2 Koshland, D. E. Jr., Nemethy, G. and Filmer, D. (1966) *Biochemistry* 5, 365–385
3 Hill, C. M., Waight, R. D. and Bardsley, G. (1977) *Mol. Cell Biochem.* 15, 173–178
4 Tipton, K. F. (1979) in *Companion to Biochemistry*, Vol. 2 (Bull, Lagnado, Thomas and Tipton, eds), pp. 327–382, Longman
5 Monod, J., Changeux, J.-P. and Jacob, F. (1963) *J. Mol. Biol.* 6, 306–329
6 Barritt, G. J., Keech, D. B. and Ling, A. M. (1966) *Biochem. Biophys. Res. Commun.* 24, 476–481
7 Bais, R. and Keech, D. B. (1972) *J. Biol. Chem.* 247, 3255–3261
8 Scrutton, M. C. and Utter, M. F. (1967) *J. Biol. Chem.* 242, 1723–1735
9 Taylor, H., Nielsen, J. and Keech, D. B.

(1969) *Biochem. Biophys. Res. Commun.* 37, 723–728

10 Frey, W. H. and Utter, M. F. (1977) *J. Biol. Chem.* 252, 51–56

11 Easterbrook-Smith, S. B., Campbell, A. J., Keech, D. B. and Wallace, J. C. (1979) *Biochem. J.* 179, 497–502

12 Ashman, L. K., Keech, D. B., Wallace, J. C. and Nielsen, J. (1972) *J. Biol. Chem.* 247, 5818–5824

13 McClure, W. R., Lardy, H. A. and Kniefel, H. P. (1971) *J. Biol. Chem.* 246, 3569–3578

14 Harding, W. M. (1969) *Arch. Biochem. Biophys.* 129, 57–61

15 Fisher, E. and Keleti, T. (1975) *Acta Biochim. Biophys. Acad. Sci. Hung.* 10, 221–227

D. Bruce Keech and John C. Wallace are at the Department of Biochemistry, University of Adelaide, Adelaide, S.A. 5000, Australia.

Addendum

A DIALOG search of the BIOSIS preview database from 1977 through to 1983 revealed that there are still relatively few well-established examples of enzymes where the sigmoidal velocity response curve correlates to homotropic cooperative binding of substrate or effector.

One enzyme which has evidently failed to stand re-examination is serine hydroxymethyltransferase: The apparent, positive homotropic cooperativity reported previously by others for the binding of tetrahydrofolate to this enzyme has been shown by Schirch and Quahnock[16] to be an artefact of the assay procedure, attributable to the instability of tetrahydrofolate at low concentrations under the assay conditions.

Whilst there is no doubt from the careful calorimetric and equilibrium binding studies of Mateo *et al.*[17] that the two high affinity (so-called 'N') sites of the phosphorylase *b* dimer bind AMP in a cooperative manner (n_H-1.4), there is some question about the precise physiological significance of this phenomenon *in vivo* in view of the observations of Aragon *et al.*[18]. They showed that the concentration of free AMP in skeletal muscle at rest or even after various periods of exercise is nearly two orders of magnitude below the concentration required to give half maximal activation.

Indeed, as has been amply illustrated by Scrutton and Griffiths[19] in their detailed analysis of the factors known to affect pyruvate carboxylase activity *in vitro* and the possible significance of these in the control of pyruvate carboxylation *in vivo*, this can prove to be an extremely complex though valuable task. Central to their consideration was the effect of acetyl-CoA: on the one hand the isolated enzyme exhibits a high affinity ($K_A = 13$ μM) and apparently highly sigmoidal response ($n_H = 3$), while on the other hand the rate of pyruvate carboxylation by isolated chicken liver mitochondria showed a markedly less sigmoidal ($n_H = 1.5$) and lower affinity response (apparent $K_A = 320$ μM) to the matrix acetyl-CoA concentration[20]. Using an iterative procedure they computed the free concentration (of the total) of all known relevant metabolites to include in the calculation of the concentrations of enzyme–metabolite complexes. After including some 43 parameters in their simulation of the pyruvate carboxylase–acetyl-CoA interaction, they found that the value of n_H giving the best fit to the data of Barritt *et al.*[20] depended greatly on the value employed for the concentration of another acetyl-CoA binding enzyme, HMG-CoA synthase.

Thus, a rigorous analysis of any particular enzyme's regulation requires a detailed knowledge of its mechanism as well as a plethora of data gathered after careful consideration of all the possible ramifications of relevant metabolites and competing enzymes and the best way to obtain valid estimates of their interactions in the steady state *in vivo*. Not surprisingly, therefore, we may have to wait some while before a comprehensive answer can be given to our question.

References

16 Schirch, L. and Quashnock, J. (1981) *J. Biol. Chem.* 256, 6245–6249

17 Mateo, P. L., Baron, C., Lopez-Mayorga, O., Jimenez, J. S. and Cortijo, M. (1984) *J. Biol. Chem.* 259, 9384–9389

18 Aragon, J. J., Tornheim, K. and Lowenstein, J. M. (1980) *FEBS Lett.* 117, K56–64

19 Scrutton, M. C. and Griffiths, J. R. (1982) in *Short Term Regulation of Liver Metabolism* (Hur, L. and Van de Werve, eds), pp. 175–198, Elsevier/North Holland

20 Barritt, G. J., Zander, G. and Utter, M. F. (1976) in *Gluconeogenesis* (Hanson, R. W. and Mehlman, M. A., eds), pp. 3–46, John Wiley

UMP synthase: the importance of quaternary structure in channeling intermediates

Thomas W. Traut

Mammalian UMP synthases are bifunctional proteins which catalyse the conversion of orotate and phosphoribosyl pyrophosphate (PRPP) to OMP and then to UMP. Dimers of UMP synthase channel OMP from one catalytic center to another.

Enzymes are quite gregarious. Very few exist normally as fully independent molecules; in most cases they form aggregates by associating with similar molecules (homopolymers) or with other enzymes or structural proteins (heteropolymers). While the physiological significance of proteins associating to form polymers is perhaps more evident for structural proteins and allosteric enzymes, there are other functions that are derived from the quaternary structure of enzymes. Enzymes may exist as homopolymers of a single size (e.g. tetramer, hexamer); for these enzymes catalytic activity is optimum in the polymer, and in most cases exclusively associated with the polymer[1,2]. Almost all the enzymes involved in glycolysis or the citric acid cycle belong to this group[3], as do most allosteric enzymes. Another group of enzymes consists of homopolymers that may exist as mixtures of two or more polymer sizes. The salient feature of this class is that the different polymer sizes vary in their catalytic activity. In over 90% of these enzymes, catalytic activity increases, or is found exclusively, in the larger polymer. Thus subunit association generally leads to a quaternary structure with optimum catalytic activity and/or regulatory features.

UMP synthase

The dimeric form of UMP synthase offers a physiological advantage to the organism by 'channeling' an intermediate product. Defined simply, 'channeling' means that in the metabolism of compound A to form C, no significant amounts of the intermediate B diffuse away from the enzyme complex to form a free pool of B. UMP synthase from mammalian cells is a bifunctional protein containing two catalytic centers on a single polypeptide[4]: orotate phosphoribosyltransferase (EC 2.4.2.10) and orotidine-5'-monophosphate (OMP) decarboxylase (EC 4.1.1.23). UMP synthase thus catalyses the last two reactions of *de novo* pyrimidine biosynthesis:

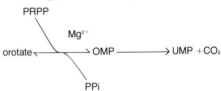

In the absence of any effector molecules, UMP synthase from mouse Ehrlich ascites cells exists as a monomer with a sedimentation coefficient ($S_{20,w}$) of 3.6. In the presence of OMP, which is a product of the first catalytic site and the substrate for the second catalytic site, the enzyme sediments with an $S_{20,w} = 5.6$ (see Fig. 1)[5,6]. At first it appeared that the association of 3.6 S subunits to form a dimer was facilitated by the binding of OMP to either or both of the catalytic sites. Further studies on the sedimentation of UMP synthase in the presence of various molecules that were known to bind to the phosphoribosyltransferase site or the decarboxylase site (i.e. substrates or competitive inhibitors) revealed that effector molecules smaller than OMP (e.g. PRPP, phosphate, and other anions), even when present at saturating concentrations produced a UMP synthase dimer with $S_{20,w} = 5.1$. This 5.1 S species can be clearly resolved from the 5.6 S species. The concentration of any effector required to convert all the UMP synthase to the 5.1 S dimer was directly related to the K_i for that effector at the decarboxylase site[6,7]. We thus concluded that formation of the 5.1 S dimer is promoted or stabilized by effectors binding at the decarboxylase site of UMP synthase (see Fig. 1).

Only pyrimidine nucleotides can promote the formation of the 5.6 S UMP synthase dimer. Since the amount of such nucleotide effectors required to convert UMP synthase to the 5.6 S species is not related to the apparent binding constants for these nucleotides at either site 1 or site 2, we concluded that a third, or regulatory site must exist on the enzyme. It is also noteworthy that OMP, the most likely physiological effector, has an apparent binding constant (determined from sedimentation studies) at site 3 of ~1 nM, which is about four magnitudes smaller than for other pyrimidine nucleotides[7].

To determine if the regulation of the quaternary structure of UMP synthase is significant, we studied the kinetics for both enzyme activities starting with UMP synthase in each of the three forms shown in Fig. 1. All forms of the enzyme had essentially the same rate of phosphoribosyltransferase

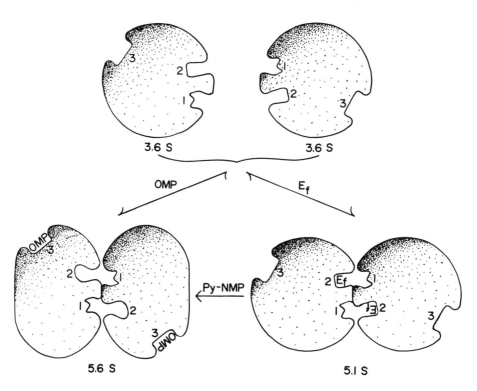

Fig. 1. Schematic representation of changes in the aggregation and conformation of UMP synthase. The subunit is the 3.6 S monomer, containing a catalytic domain for the orotate phosphoribosyltransferase activity (site 1) and for the OMP decarboxylase activity (site 2). The third site is a regulatory site distinct from sites 1 and 2. E$_f$, effectors; Py-NMP, pyrimidine nucleoside monophosphate (OMP, UMP, or azaUMP). Py-NMP is a sub-set of E$_f$. The number of sites which must be filled is unknown.

activity, but OMP decarboxylase activity was exclusively associated with the 5.6 S dimer[8].

The model in Fig. 1 can satisfactorily account for all the data. While the 5.1 S dimer is easily produced *in vitro*, we have no data to suggest that this species is an obligatory intermediate in the formation of the active 5.6 S dimer. The 5.1 S species is probably not significant *in vivo*, since the concentrations of effectors required for its formation are far above physiological levels. The 5.6 S species can be easily produced by physiological concentrations of OMP (≥ 10 nM). If pyrimidine biosynthesis were to be stopped totally, and all OMP consumed to form UMP, UMP synthase should dissociate. However, the phosphoribosyltransferase activity would still exist on the enzyme monomer, and once pyrimidine biosynthesis resumes, the formation of even a small amount of OMP would promptly promote the formation of the 5.6 S quaternary structure.

While we have no direct physical data to prove that the catalytic sites of the two monomers are juxtaposed, as in Fig. 1, such a scheme satisfactorily explains the channeling observed. Thus, OMP is synthesized at site 1, and need diffuse only a short distance to site 2 on the adjacent subunit where it is decarboxylated to UMP. Such a quaternary structure sequesters OMP, the intermediate metabolite, impeding its diffusion from the enzyme. If the monomer were the major catalytically active species, then OMP produced at site 1 would have to diffuse into the solvent before it could reach site 2, whether on the same monomer or another one.

Significance of channeling OMP

In yeast, the two catalytic activities of UMP synthase are on separate proteins; there is no channeling of OMP, and with cell homogenates OMP concentrations can reach steady-state concentrations of 40 μM. In mammalian cells, which have evolved a bifunctional protein to connect these two different catalytic domains, steady-state

concentrations of OMP are almost three magnitudes lower (50–100 nM)[6]. The most reasonable explanation for the benefit derived from channeling OMP in mammalian cells is related to the fact that mammalian cells have more active pyrimidine nucleotidases. Once OMP is degraded to orotidine, it is not readily salvaged and is therefore excreted. In general the nucleotidases have a K_m for OMP of 0.7–1 mM, and if the OMP concentration is artificially increased (100 μM), significant amounts of OMP are degraded to orotidine[9]. The recycling of orotidine to orotate (dashed arrow in Fig. 2), is not significant, and would also constitute a futile cycle. It is, therefore, the obligatory quaternary structure of this bifunctional protein that results in channeling of OMP and completely spares OMP from degradation by cellular nucleotidases[9].

How well do our data on channeling with purified UMP synthase, or cellular preparations, compare with clinical data for humans? For a 70 kg human, *de novo* pyrimidine biosynthesis produces about 4 mmoles of OMP each day[10]. During the same period only 1–5 mg of orotidine is excreted[11–13] – about 0.4% of the total OMP formed. This very low rate of excretion agrees well with our observations on the channeling of OMP. Significant orotidine production is observed only when patients are treated with certain purine or pyrimidine analogs (allopurinol for gout; azauridine or pyrazofurin for cancer); these drugs, when converted to their nucleotide derivatives *in vivo*, are potent inhibitors of OMP decarboxylase. Depending on the amount of drug used, continuous administration results in severe orotidinuria, which is offset by a substantial increase in *de novo* orotate biosynthesis. Pyrimidine biosynthesis during azauridine therapy can increase 30 fold, over 95% being excreted as orotidine or orotate[14,15] – another indication that orotidine is not readily salvaged or re-used.

The overall path of pyrimidine biosynthesis is depicted in Fig. 2. The energy content of OMP is 58 ATP equivalents. However, even during severe orotidinuria, the energy loss due to OMP degradation is only about 6% of the total energy budget* for a 70 kg person per day. In terms of energy alone, such a loss is probably quite tolerable. More significant, however, is the depletion of the phosphoribosyl pyrophosphate (PRPP) pool. Since PRPP is a vital substrate for a number of other biosynthetic and salvage enzymes, its depletion should affect the rates for all these phosphoribosyltransferases. Such perturbations would be

more significant than the energy loss itself, and thus the maintenance of a normal PRPP pool may explain the benefit derived from channeling OMP[16].

Quaternary structure and channeling in other systems

Channeling of intermediate compounds has been shown for a variety of multifunctional proteins and enzyme complexes, but this is the first example where channeling appears to be the reason for regulating the quaternary structure of a catalytic protein. Other analogous systems are sure to be found. Two enzymes that may be similar are the bifunctional tryptophan synthase[17] and the heteropolymer containing the folate trifunctional protein plus glycinamide ribotide transformylase[18].

Acknowledgements

Work in the author's laboratory has been

---

*A reasonable approximation may be derived as follows. A 70 kg human has a diet containing ~2600 nutrition cal/day (=2600 kcal or 10 870 kJ). If all the food were oxidized for ATP production with an efficiency similar to that for glucose (assuming 2 ATP from NADH and 1.3 ATP from succinate: 25.2 moles ATP/mol glu (-30.5 kJ/mol ATP) $\div -2\ 870$ kJ/mol glu = 0.27), then the energy budget = $-10\ 870$ kJ/day $\div -30.5$ kJ/mol ATP $\cdot (0.27) = 96$ moles ATP/day.

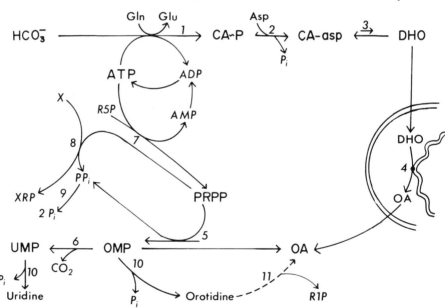

Fig. 2. Possible interactions between intermediates of the UMP biosynthetic pathway and other metabolic processes. The synthesis of UMP from HCO_3^- requires 2 ATP, L-glutamine, L-aspartate, and PRPP and proceeds in six enzymatic steps. UMP synthase contains orotate phosphoribosyltransferase and OMP decarboxylase (reactions 5 and 6). The additional reactions enumerated represent: (7) PRPP synthetase; (8) enzymes that compete for PRPP with orotate phosphoribosyltransferase of reaction 5: these include PRPP-amido transferase and the various other phosphoribosyltransferases where the acceptor X may be adenine, hypoxanthine or guanine, anthranilate, ATP, or nicotinate; (9) inorganic pyrophosphatase; (10) 5'-nucleotide phosphatase; (11) uridine phosphorylase. For reversible reactions, the longer arrow indicates the direction favored by the K_{eq} for the reaction at physiological pH[19].

supported by grants from the American Cancer Society, NIH, and the University Research Council.

References

1 Jaenicke, R. and Rudolph, R. (1980) in *Protein Folding* (Jaenicke, R., ed.), pp. 525–546, Elsevier/North-Holland Press
2 Frieden, C. (1971) *Ann. Rev. Biochem.* 40, 653–694
3 Klotz, I. M., Darnall, D. W. and Langerman, N. R. (1975) in *The Proteins*, 3rd edn (Neurath, H., Hill, R. L., eds), Vol. 1, pp. 293–410, Academic Press
4 McClard, R. W., Black, M. J., Livingstone, L. R. and Jones, M. E. (1980) *Biochemistry* 19, 4699–4706
5 Traut, T. W. and Jones, M. E. (1977) *J. Biol. Chem.* 252, 8374–8381
6 Traut, T. W. and Jones, M. E. (1979) *J. Biol. Chem.* 254, 1143–1150
7 Traut, T. W., Payne, R. C. and Jones, M. E. (1980) *Biochemistry* 19, 6062–6068
8 Traut, T. W. and Payne, R. C. (1980) *Biochemistry* 19, 6068–6074
9 Traut, T. W. (1980) *Arch. Biochem. Biophys.* 200, 590–594
10 Smith, L. H., Jr (1973) *N. Eng. J. Med.* 288, 764–771
11 Lotz, M., Fallon, H. J. and Smith, L. H. (1963) *Nature (London)* 197, 194–195
12 Fox, R. M., Royse-Smith, D. and O'Sullivan, W. J. (1970) *Science* 168, 861–862
13 Tax, W. J. M., Veerkamp, J. H. and Schretlen, E. D. A. M. (1978) *Clin. Chim. Acta* 90, 217–223
14 Cardoso, S. S., Calabresi, P. and Handschumacher, R. E. (1961) *Cancer Res.* 21, 1551–1556
15 Fallon, H. J., Lotz, M. and Smith, L. H., Jr (1962) *Blood* 20, 700–709
16 Christopherson, R. I., Traut, T. W. and Jones, M. E. (1981) *Curr. Top. Cell Reg.* 18, 59–77
17 Matchett, W. H. (1974) *J. Biol. Chem.* 249, 4041–4049
18 Smith, G. K., Mueller, W. T., Wasserman, G. F., Taylor, W. D. and Benkovic, S. J. (1980) *Biochemistry* 19, 4313–4321
19 Jones, M. E. (1980) *Ann. Rev. Biochem.* 49, 253–279

Thomas W. Traut is at the Department of Biochemistry, University of North Carolina School of Medicine, Chapel Hill, NC 27514, USA.

Addendum

The most interesting work on UMP synthase in the past 2 years used digestion with elastase or trypsin to prepare an active fragment of UMP synthase[20]. This fragment ($M_r = 28\,000$) contained the OMP decarboxylase activity, as well as the ability to form dimers. No OPRTase activity could be recovered in any of the digestion fragments. Because the isolated OMP decarboxylase domain is less stable than the same activity in the native UMP synthase, the authors suggest that formation of the multi-functional protein UMP synthase would stabilize the domain.

Since OMP is both a substrate and a positive effector, one would expect to see positive cooperativity for this enzyme. This has not been observed previously because the K_m (230 nM) is so much greater than the K_d (~1 nM) at the allosteric site. By testing at very low OMP concentrations, Floyd[21] has obtained some limited data to suggest positive cooperativity for the OMP decarboxylase domain.

References

20 Floyd, E. E. and Jones, M. E. (1984) *J. Biol. Chem.* 260 (in press)
21 Floyd, E. E. (1984) Ph.D. dissertation, Univ. of North Carolina

Computer modeling of metabolic pathways

David Garfinkel

Although computer simulation has been applied less in biochemistry than in other biological disciplines, this situation is likely to change in the near future as the cost of computers decreases sharply and as more workers become trained in their use. This article describes the present and evolving state of the subject and some of the current activities.

Introduction and history

Computer modeling is used less in biochemistry than in related fields of science such as pharmacology and physiology. However, present economic trends indicate a considerable expansion of activity in the near future.

This review is concerned with modeling the kinetic behavior of metabolic pathways and systems and of their constituent enzymes; the standard calculations of physical biochemistry, including X-ray crystallography, are well reviewed elsewhere. The experimental data to be simulated are commonly a set of concentrations measured at several different times. The basic mathematical technique used is the numerical solution of differential equations by computer.

Use of mathematical modeling in biochemistry is of considerable antiquity. An important example is the Michaelis–Menten model of 1913. Although there were sporadic attempts to use prototype computers, such as differential analysers and other analog computers, modeling in biochemistry really dates from the time when digital computers became commercially available, and some workers became established in this area, i.e. the late 50s and early 60s. Although the computers used and the general sophistication of the models have improved considerably since then, there is still no widespread agreement on techniques and standards. The same

communication problems which are common to all complex modeling efforts in all subjects are still being encountered. Perhaps the most thorough recent review is that of Heinrich, Rapoport and Rapoport[1]; there is as yet no adequate textbook.

Important current trends

Three current trends are worth noting.

(1) The cost of the computer hardware (machinery) to perform a specific calculation is decreasing rapidly, and a precipitous drop is expected within the next few years. What in the recent past has been a medium-sized computer costing hundreds of thousands of dollars may come to cost no more than a spectrophotometer or an automobile. The effects of this trend have already become evident in the laboratory, where use of devices involving computers to collect and initially process experimental data is increasing. Although the cost of the software (computer programs) to operate these cheaper computers is still high, software for biochemical simulation and related subjects is becoming more available. In particular, there is beginning to be 'friendly' software, which permits the user to communicate with the computer in his own language, to get help when it is needed, and to recover from mistakes. Specially written programs will handle routine mathematics instead of requiring the user to do so. An example of such a

program is PENNZYME, which fits steady-state kinetic data to enzymatic rate laws[2]. 'Friendly' programs cost about four times as much to operate as unfriendly ones that are able to perform the same calculations, but their use is becoming economically feasible as the cost of computer hardware decreases. The combination of cheaper hardware and friendlier software should considerably diminish some of the obstacles to the widespread use of simulation and mathematical techniques in biochemistry that have been limiting in the recent past.

(2) The number of computer models described in the biochemical literature is increasing. This trend is likely to continue because a large proportion of college students are now receiving training in computing. This increase is primarily in relatively simple models prepared by experimenters to interpret their own experimental data, rather than by persons who are primarily model-builders.

(3) There is increasing development and use of computer models in all subjects where management of complex systems is involved. Large-scale econometric models are now being used to assist with tax legislation and other aspects of national policy.

Needs for and uses of modeling

Why are models needed at all, and why must they often be computer models? These needs follow from the complex nature of the systems being studied and from the structure of the human mind. Biological systems are often complex enough that an accurate treatment is intractable mathematically. Simplification to make the mathematics tractable without a computer often leads to a result which is biologically unrealistic.

Cognitive psychologists have shown that we can simultaneously follow no more than about even simple unrelated variables[3]. Complexity reduces this number; perhaps a safe limit consists of five unrelated variables or three interacting feedback loops. Although a casual glance at any standard metabolic chart will show that most biochemical pathways exceed this limit, examination of the biochemical literature indicates a reluctance by biochemists to approach it. There is a tendency to focus on one controlling factor at a time, and then to abandon it and try another when it does not account for everything. Such behavior is not unique to biochemistry. Computer modeling allows us to exceed this complexity limit, and to obtain a deeper understanding than may be otherwise possible from a relatively few experiments on a complex subject. Increased computer power may permit us to eliminate the present requirement for mathematical competence in computer modeling, but expert knowledge of the biochemistry involved is also required, and this requirement is likely to be more permanent.

Uses of models in biochemistry include the design and interpretation of experiments, especially those generating large volumes of data, the prediction of unmeasured values in experiments, and the quantitative management of systems for therapeutic purposes. With a model, a critical experiment may be performed sooner than if there is no model.

James[4] has discussed the differences in underlying philosophy between analytic models which attempt to analyze a small set of data as simply as possible and synthetic models which combine a large volume of data from different sources in order to define the operation of a complex system. Models may be arranged along a scale between these extremes. There are presently many simple models and few complex ones.

As discussed at some length elsewhere[5] a model need not be universally valid or free of all defects to be valuable. Perhaps the most famous, and probably the most valuable, quantitative model in biochemistry is the Michaelis–Menten model of enzyme kinetics; nevertheless it appears that for most enzymes, conditions exist where it does not apply or is inaccurate.[6]

Techniques

Simulation is a technique with a considerable literature which has been applied to a wide variety of subjects. Models fall into two classes: discrete event models, where a succession of separate events is considered; and continuous models, where system behavior is followed as a function of time. Most biochemical models fall into the second class. These models are commonly expressed as a set of differential equations which require solution by computer since they are too complex to be solved analytically with pencil and paper. Strictly speaking, the Michaelis–Menten equation is a simplification of this type of model. Both general-purpose and simulation languages specialized for biochemical problems[7] have been developed to handle these systems of equations. As is common with most natural systems, the differential equations representing a biochemical model are often 'stiff' because processes occurring at widely differing rates are represented. Unreasonably large amounts of computer time are required for their solution unless special procedures are used. These have been reviewed by Garfinkel et al[8].

The procedures and goals of simulation are still evolving. An important technique involves determining, by formal optimization, which of a series of possible models most closely fits the experimental data being examined, and whether the model parameters are well determined by the data and have reasonable values. Research continues on sensitivity analysis, the response of a model to changes in its numerical values. It is often more practical to perform such analysis with a computer model than to perform the corresponding experiments[9].

Examples of models

There is relatively little interaction between workers in this field, and attempts to discuss their work on the basis of the techniques employed would be of little interest to most readers interested in the biological subject matter. Work is therefore described in terms of the types of problems being studied and results being obtained, arranged approximately in order of increasing complexity.

A simple example where it was possible to obtain useful results with pencil and paper is the study of Wombacher[10] involving the enzyme pathway that degrades cyclic AMP in the adrenal cortex. He showed that a sequential organization among the enzymes reduces the diffusion time between them, probably by some kind of association with a formed element of the cell. Welch and Gaertner[11] obtained similar results using an analog computer model to study an enzyme complex that synthesizes aromatic amino acids in Neurospora. Another simple example is the model developed by James[4] for a specific set of experimental measurements of gluconeogenesis in hepatocytes. He derived relationships between glucose production and substrate availability and determined regulatory properties of the redox potential.

Two other biochemical models which deserve mention are:

(1) A model of the Calvin cycle of photosynthesis in isolated chloroplasts in terms of 17 differential equations by Milstein and Bremermann[12]. They were able to obtain at least preliminary values for the rates of the 17 reactions, do an error analysis, and design additional experiments to obtain better values.

(2) The model of glycolysis in the red blood cell of Rapoport et al.[13], which is simplified down to the irreversible kinases and the enzymes handling 2,3-bisphosphoglycerate. All reversible en-

zymes in the pathway were assumed to be fast enough to be near equilibrium and not controlling. Here there was a sensitivity analysis and a study of the effect of the important natural restriction that certain masses (e.g., NADH and NAD) are conserved. It was found that 2,3-bisphosphoglycerate could act as a temporary energy source and that the pathway involving it could act as an energy buffer.

Some workers carry on programs of research which involve (and require) both simulation and experiment, as well as active interaction between the two. In some instances this is directed at understanding the metabolism of one particular organism. An important example is the work of J. J. Blum, which is concerned with the protozooan *Tetrahymena pyriformis*. It assumes that this organism is in a metabolic steady state, but it is recognized that this may not always be valid. A model representing glycolysis, the Krebs cycle, fatty acid metabolism and the pentose shunt in terms of 39 highly interconnected reactions has been evolved and developed to the point where it can represent experimental results under different growth conditions[14]. It is strongly concerned with intracellular compartmentation and enzyme content, e.g. there are three distinct acetyl-CoA pools. An experimental design has been developed for use with the modeling techniques; it is based on measurements of radioactivity at 20-min intervals for an hour. This model has been able to follow the changes in metabolic fluxes under varying conditions, and in particular to evaluate the appreciable amount of 'futile cycling' and the way it changes with conditions.

A similar effort involving the slime mold *Dictyostelium discoides* has been carried on by B. E. Wright and her collaborators. A recent version of the resulting model involved representations of 19 enzymes[15], but its goal is still more nearly analytical than synthetic. Here the concern is with the way in which this organism metabolizes such complex polysaccharides as cellulose and glycogen and with some of the detailed intermediate reactions during its growth and differentiation cycle. Predictions regarding compartmentation of metabolites and permeability of the cells to them, as well as the amounts of complex sugars produced under particular circumstances, have been made and verified. The effects of perturbations on the metabolism have been examined both experimentally and theoretically (by sensitivity analysis).

J. H. Ottaway has recently been concerned with examination of the control of the Krebs cycle and its constituent enzymes by a combination of simulation and experiment. He has been able to use simulation to guide experimental investigation, especially to focus on what is inadequately understood, because this causes difficulty in modeling. He has been particularly concerned with the effects of conservation of coenzymes on control of succinate thiokinase, finding the partition of CoA among its various thioesters particularly important[16,17]. A recent model of control of the Krebs cycle in heart mitochondria including sensitivity analysis indicates that there is no single control point for the cycle at high oxidation rates[17].

One of the largest groups using simulation in their research is the Max Planck Institute in Dortmund, headed by B. Hess. They have primarily been concerned over the years with the behavior of the glycolytic system and glycolytic enzymes, mostly in yeast. Much of their work has emphasized glycolytic oscillations and their control; this has been reviewed by Hess and Boiteux[18]. Their more recent work has emphasized the use of progress curves to study enzyme kinetics and depends heavily on concurrent simulation and elaborate computer control of the experiments. It is particularly valuable in the case of complex regulatory enzymes where the enzyme exists in several allosteric conformations which interact with several ligands, typically more than four. In such a case a given ligand may either activate or inhibit depending on conditions, thus an enormous number of measurements of initial velocities are required for a complete study[19]. In a recent investigation of pyruvate kinase, Markus *et al.*[20] found two equally well-fitting models of the Monod–Wyman–Changeux type for the enzyme from *E. coli*. They then used these models to find the experimental conditions under which their behavior differed the most and then performed the experiments to distinguish between them. On examining pyruvate kinase from other species, they found that the number of allosteric conformations may differ between species[19].

Simulation techniques can be used to simulate the distribution of radioactivity in complex metabolic systems. Such studies of the Krebs cycle were carried out in liver and kidney[21] and brain[22]. Heath and Threlfall[21] showed that the relationship between the Krebs cycle and gluconeogenesis differed in liver and kidney. Garfinkel[22] found that the Krebs cycle in brain as then understood could not transform radioactively labeled substrates at the observed rate. It was therefore necessary to compartment the Krebs cycle into a large slow cycle and a small fast one; this finding was subsequently confirmed experimentally.

The most complex metabolic model now in existence is the author's model of the energy metabolism (the Krebs cycle, glycolysis, and associated metabolism) in the heart (e.g. Achs and Garfinkel[23]). This synthetic model draws information from many sources. The published versions involve about 65 enzymes and membrane transport mechanisms; recent unpublished work has added 15 more enzymes of the pathway that oxidizes fatty acids. Summarizing the findings from so large a model is impossible here. Under physiological conditions it indicates behavior which is not intuitively obvious, or which was not noticed by the experimenters involved.

The principal reason for building so large a model is to determine what manipulation of this metabolism might be possible to alleviate the effects of ischemia, a major component of heart disease. The role of membrane transport in this disease has been found to be more important than had been appreciated. In particular, it is difficult for accumulated lactate to be transported out of myocytes and into the extracellular space when the circulation is inadequate.

Acknowledgements

Preparation of this article was supported by NIH Grants HL15622 ad GM16501.

References

1 Heinrich, R., Rapoport, S. M. and Rapoport, T. A. (1977) *Prog. Biophys. Molec. Biol.* 32, 1–82

2 Kohn, M. C., Menten, L. and Garfinkel, D. (1979) *Computers and Biomedical Research* 12, 461–469

3 Miller, G. A. (1956) *Psychol. Rev.* 63, 81–97

4 James, A. T. (1980) *J. Theoret. Biol.* 83, 623–646

5 Garfinkel, D. (1980) *Am. J. Physiol.* 239, R1–R6

6 Hill, C. M., Waight, R. D. and Bardsley, W. G. (1977) *Mol. Cell. Biochem.* 15, 173–178

7 Roman, G.-C. and Garfinkel, D. (1978) *Computers and Biomedical Research* 11, 3–15

8 Garfinkel, D., Marbach, C. B. and Shapiro, N. Z. (1977) *Ann. Rev. Biophys. Bioeng.* 6, 525–543

9 Wright, B. E. and Park, D. J. (1975) *J. Biol. Chem.* 250, 2219–2226

10 Wombacher, H. (1980) *Arch. Biochem. Biophys.* 201, 8–19

11 Welch, G. R. and Gaertner, F. H. (1975) *Proc. Natl. Acad. Sci. U.S.A.* 72, 4218–4222

12 Milstein, J. and Bremermann, H. J. (1979) *J. Math. Biol.* 7, 99–116

13 Rapoport, T. A., Heinrich, R. and Rapoport, S. M. (1976) *Biochem. J.* 154, 449–469

14 Stein, R. B. and Blum, J. J. (1979–80) *J. Biol. Chem.* 254, 10385–10395; 255, 4198–4205

15 Wright, B. E., Tai, A. and Killick, K. A. (1977) *Eur. J. Biochem.* 74, 217–225

16 Ottaway, J. H. (1979) *Biochem. Soc. Trans.* 7, 1161–1167

17 Ottaway, J. H. and McMinn, C. L. (1980) in *Enzyme Regulation and Mechanism of Action* (Mildner, P. and Ries, B., eds), pp. 69–82, Pergamon Press, Oxford

18 Hess, B. and Boiteux, A. (1971) *Ann. Rev. Biochem.* 40, 237–258

19 Boiteux, A., Markus, M., Plesser, T. and Hess, B.

(1980) in *Kinetic Data Analysis: Design and Analysis of Enzyme and Pharmacokinetic Data* (Endrenyi, L., ed.), Plenum

20 Markus, M., Plesser, T., Boiteux, A., Hess, B. and Malcovati, M. (1980) *Biochem. J.* 189, 421–433

21 Heath, D. F. and Threlfall, C. J. (1968) *Biochem. J.* 110, 337–362

22 Garfinkel, D. (1966) *J. Biol. Chem.* 241, 3918–3929

23 Achs, M. J. and Garfinkel, D. (1977) *Am. J. Physiol.* 232, R164–R174, R175–R184

David Garfinkel is at the Department of Computer and Information Science Moore School of Electrical Engineering D/2 University of Pennsylvania, Philadelphia, Pennsylvania 19104, USA.

Addendum

Within the last three years the number of small metabolic models, published with the relevant experimental work, has increased faster than the number of larger models, often published independently of the experimental work. The larger models have tended to be concentrated in such areas as blood clotting, molecular biology of protein synthesis, and cardiac metabolism. At the present time, developments in computing and techniques which are relevant to this type of modeling particularly require mention.

A recent development in computing which is particularly important for small-scale metabolic modeling is the advent and widespread distribution of the microcomputer and of personal computers based on it. Many relatively simple models which nevertheless have biological significance can be implemented on microcomputers, even though they typically have smaller memories and less capable software than larger computers. Examples exist where a model of a system being studied experimentally has been implemented on a microcomputer in the laboratory. Experimental results can be entered into such a model as soon as they are obtained, followed by the calculation of the optimal experiment to be performed next. Even large models can be handled by microcomputers. This author and colleagues are now building a revised version of the models described in Ref. 23. It now contains about 65 enzymes and transport mechanisms and represents about ten experimental conditions from several laboratories; it is written in BASIC on an IBM Personal Computer. BASIC is a common computational language on microcomputers, and may have to be used for modeling (which can be fairly sophisticated) although it is not a very powerful language, and differs in detail from one microcomputer to another. Although microcomputer languages are usually less powerful than their large-computer counterparts, this may be compensated for by operating the small computer connected to a larger one. Additional program packages which can be used for modeling, especially on microcomputers, are also becoming available.

At the present time it seems probable that developments such as the use of 'natural language' inputs to computers and the application of artificial intelligence techniques to modeling (within the last year it has become fashionable to have artificial intelligence sessions at modeling meetings) will result in techniques which are both easier to use and more powerful.

Regardless of the programs and

computers used, it is important to have adequate knowledge of the biological subject matter and data and, in particular, to understand the assumptions and conventions underlying one's techniques. We recently encountered a case in which two groups of experimenters obtained quite different results from essentially identical experimental data[24]. We found that the difference lay in the simulation of the experiments. One of the groups of experimenters had used, without reconciliation, three different operational definitions of chelation equilibria involving ATP and metal ions. (In particular, biochemists and physiologists often have different conventions and definitions for this subject.)

Reference

24 Garfinkel, L. and Garfinkel, D. (1984) *Biochemistry* 23, 3547–3552

Understanding pathway control (without the aid of computers)

R. J. Gillies

Over the years, investigation of metabolic pathways has led to the inevitable definition of some enzymes as being 'rate limiting' or 'controlling'. Most often, these enzymes are thus distinguished by the useful and time-honored crossover theorem, introduced in 1955 by Chance and Williams[1]. However, it has become clear that simple distinctions such as 'rate limiting step' and 'controlling enzyme' are not adequate to explain empirical observations.

One of the first investigators to impose a more rigorous analysis of pathway flux was Higgins who, in 1965, introduced the concept of 'control strength' (C_x) (Ref 2). C_x for an enzyme (E_x) in a pathway is defined as the fractional change in pathway flux induced by a fractional change in the activity of E_x. The sum of all C in a pathway is defined as unity. In most cases, however, Higgins' treatment was too theoretical to be of practical use to experimentalists.

The next major step in these analyses was taken in 1973 by Kacser and Burns who published an elaboration of Higgins' methods, supported by empirical observations of the ornithine–arginine and the phenylalanine–melanin pathways[3]. However, once again, the treatment was extremely theoretical and seemingly applied to only simple systems. At about the same time as Kacser and Burns, a trio of reports emerged from the laboratories of Heinrich, Rapoport and Rapoport in Berlin[4-6]. In the first of these[4], the authors present their analyses which introduce three cardinal terms to describe enzyme systems: control strength (flux), control matrix (metabolite concentrations) and effector strength (dependence of an enzyme's velocity on effector concentration). In their second paper, they demonstrate that certain effector conditions can produce 'pseudo-'

or 'half-crossovers', which would lead to erroneous conclusions if one used the crossover theorum alone. These conditions include effectors with more than one site of action, the influx and efflux of metabolites and internal pathway rearrangements secondary to an effector's actions. The final paper in the series is an analysis of erythrocyte glycolysis[6]. The proposed model was shown to agree with experimental observations in the resting state and was tested under a number of varying conditions, such as pH, inorganic phosphate, ammonium or temperature. In all cases, their model quantitatively described the complicated patterns of changes which took place. The startling prediction to come from their analyses is that the entire control of glycolytic flux in erythrocytes can be described in terms of hexokinase and phosphofructokinase activities alone. Metabolite concentrations (control matrix), on the other hand, are controlled by pyruvate kinase.

Although the analyses of Kacser and Burns, and Hienrich and Rapoport are useful it was not until recently that these methods have begun to be used by experimentalists. A good case in point is the work of Groen et al.[7], who studied the controls of State 3 respiration in rat-liver mitochondria. This work was prompted by the controversy over whether State 3 respiration is regulated by extra-mitochondrial ATP/ADP ratios via the adenine nucleotide translocator or by the cytoplasmic phosphate potential, mitochondrial redox state and the activity of oxygen. Analysis of the control strengths in different parts of this system has proved very fruitful.

First, oxygen consumption was determined at different respiratory rates (induced by hexokinase) in the presence of different concentrations of carboxyatractyloside, an irreversible inhibitor of the adenine nucleotide translocator. Control strength of the translocator, estimated from the initial slopes, was shown to vary with rates of respiration, reaching a maximum of 0.3 at 80% of State 3 respiration. Note that the C_i of proton leak, extrapolated to zero unity, indicates the presence of other controlling steps at all respiratory rates.

In an attempt to identify these other steps, the C_i of proton permeability was then analysed by titrating mitochondria with uncoupler (FCCP) in the presence of oligomycin (to block oxidative phosphorylation). The authors found a linear relation between O_2 consumption and amount of uncoupler, the slope of which is related to the C_i of proton leak. Extrapolating to zero respiration gives the amount of uncoupler that stoichiometrically compensates for the proton permeability. C_i for proton leak was determined by titrating with uncoupler at different rates of respiration induced by various hexokinase concentrations.

In addition to the two systems mentioned above, the authors have also determined C_i of hexokinase itself (by titrating with enzyme), the dicarboxylate carrier (using the competitive inhibitor phenylsuccinate), cytochrome oxidase (by titrating with azide) and of the cytochrome bc_1 complex (by using the non-competitive inhibitor hydroquinoline-N-oxide). These data have been summarized as a function of respiration. In the resting state, as expected, oxygen consumption is almost totally a function of proton permeability. In going from State 4 to State 3, the C_i of proton-permeability decreases monotonically and the C_i values of the dicarboxylate carrier and the adenine nucleotide translocator increase. The control strength of hexokinase is maximal (0.5) at about half-maximal respiration, being near zero during the resting state and in State 3.

During State 3 respiration, the greatest amount of control is exerted equally by the adenine nucleotide translocator ($C_i = 0.29$) and the dicarboxylate carrier (0.33).

Cytochrome c oxidase also exerts substantial control ($C_i \pm 0.17$) whereas variations in the proton leak, the bc_1 complex and hexokinase do not significantly alter respiratory rates.

Although the results of this study are not entirely new, their treatment within the theoretical framework of control strength has introduced new concepts to this well-studied field. Not only do different enzymes play key roles at different rates of pathway flux, but, at any given flux, control is exercised at a variety of steps working in concert. The methods of Kacser and Burns, and Heinrich and Rapoport not only provide a theoretical framework for the interpretation of data but they also suggest experimental protocols for the gathering of such data. Use of these methods in the study of other pathways may prove equally fruitful. The beauty of such a treatment is that it makes the quantification of pathway control less esoteric and more accessible to biochemists in general.

References

1 Chance, B. and Williams, G. R. (1955) *J. Biol. Chem.* 217, 409–427
2 Higgins, J. J. (1965) in *Control of Energy Metabolism* (Chance, B., Estabrook, R. W. and Williamson, J. R. eds), pp. 13–48, Academic Press
3 Kacser, H. and Burns, J. A. (1973) in *Rate Control of Biological Processes* (Davies, D. D. ed.), pp. 65–104, Cambridge University Press
4 Heinrich, R. and Rapoport, T. A. (1974) *Eur. J. Biochem.* 42, 89–95
5 Heinrich, R. and Rapoport, T. A. (1974) *Eur. J. Biochem.* 42, 97–105
6 Rapoport, T. A., Heinrich, R., Jacobasch, G. and Rapoport, S. (1974) *Eur. J. Biochem.* 42, 107–120
7 Groen, A. K., Wanders, R. J. A., Westerhoff, H. V., van der Meer, R. and Tager, J. M. (1982) *J. Biol. Chem.* 257, 2754–2757
8 Porteous, J. W. *Control and Constraint in Metabolism* (in press) Cambridge

R. J. Gillies is at The Department of Biochemistry, Colorado State University, Fort Collins, CO 80523, USA.

Sound practice follows from sound theory – the control analysis of Kacser and Burns evaluated

John W. Porteous

Dr Gillies has drawn most welcome attention (see p. 27) to important new approaches to the experimental investigation of the regulation of metabolic fluxes in growing or non-growing cells, or in suspensions of isolated subcellular organelles such as mitochondria. This new approach is as yet confined to a select band of biochemists. The need for a general and substantial change in our attitude to this topic – and for a consequential change in our experimental approach to the investigation of 'control' phenomena – can be simply illustrated.

Biochemistry claims to be one of the quantitative sciences. But, until very recently, no quantitative measure of 'control' was available. Our vocabulary was strictly limited to qualitative terms such as those commonly embodied in statements about 'rate-limiting' or 'bottle-neck' or 'pacemaker' or 'key' enzymes. By how much these enzymes could, or did, 'control' flux through metabolic systems was never stated; nor was it ever clear what relative quantitative importance should be attached to each of several allegedly 'key' enzymes in a metabolic sequence of facilitated translocations or catalysed reactions. Furthermore, it was not clear under what quantitatively-specified conditions these enzymes operated *in vivo*, when scores of authors made (often conflicting) claims to have discovered the crucial 'controlling step' in a metabolic pathway. Analogous qualitative statements that a particular effector, or coenzyme-ratio, 'controlled' the activity or synthesis of a 'key enzyme' similarly failed to substantiate the claim

that biochemistry was a quantitative science with something useful to say about the molecular activities of intact living systems. It is clear, at least in hindsight, that we biochemists had fallen into the habit of talking and writing in metaphors and had failed to apply the rigorous analysis to this problem, which we were trained to apply in other aspects of our science. For these reasons, Dr Gillies' article has performed a timely service in drawing attention to recent important changes in the experimental examination of the control of metabolic fluxes.

However, I make here a strong plea for a re-evaluation of Dr Gillies' statement that the pioneering paper by Kacser and Burns[1] 'was extremely theoretical and seemingly applied only to simple systems'. It is true that this original paper[1] was concerned primarily with a comprehensive and stimulating theoretical treatment of the parameters and variables involved in determining the fixed or changing flux through a metabolic system. But the objective of the theoretical exposition was to enable us henceforth to perform and interpret useful (i.e. quantitative) experiments. As Kacser and Burns[1] stated: 'We have suggested what new types of experiments might be done – and what experiments we could do without. Our theory generates its own methodology and the technique of modulation . . . (makes) it possible to match operational and algebraic procedures.' Preliminary experimental results, reported in the same paper, substantiated the theory.

The Kacser and Burns treatment[1,2,3] is no

more, and no less, 'theoretical' than is the familiar Michaelis–Menten–Henri treatment of the kinetics of reactions catalysed by an isolated enzyme[4]. In fact, their theory takes this equation seriously by applying it in a very simple way to any succession of porters or enzymes in an intact metabolic sequence; such a system possesses additional, systemic, properties which are not exhibited by the isolated enzymes or porters. A remarkable collection of 'Properties of Enzyme Systems' is revealed by the Kacser and Burns treatment, so bridging the experimental and theoretical gap between the classical enzymology of single enzymes and the biochemistry of intact metabolizing systems. A consequence of the theory is that it requires us to employ a new modulation methodology[1,2,3]; one of the most important predictions of the theory – repeatedly confirmed by experiment – is that control is shared among many if not all steps in a pathway[1,2,3]. Experimental determination of the magnitude of appropriate coefficients then tells us, unambiguously, the existing quantitative apportionment of control amongst various steps in the pathway, under specified conditions of experimentation, as illustrated briefly below.

The initial assertions[1] about the applicability of the new 'control' theory have been borne out by published work from Kacser's laboratory on metabolism in *Neurospora*[5,6], in mice[7] and in *Drosophila*[8]; and Tager's laboratory[9,10] has exploited brilliantly the Kacser and Burns theory, especially by applying their 'Response Coefficient' and 'Connectivity Property' to a study of the control of mitochondrial respiration.

If others now follow the lead, we can look forward to the rapid abandonment of qualitatively evocative, but quantitatively meaningless and misleading, terms such as 'pacemaker' or 'key' enzyme; because the great strength of the Kacser and Burns theoretical approach[1,2,3] is that it is entirely general. It applies to any linear, branched or cyclic succession of solute translocations

and chemical transformations in any subcellular organelle, cell, tissue or organisms of any complexity. It applies to growing or non-growing systems; in the former case, Kacser and colleagues[5,6] have identified and measured the fluxes to expansion which are necessary to sustain a growing system – yet another illustration of the utility of the original theoretical paper[1]. This is exactly what we have needed for so long: a general but rigorous theoretical framework permitting (and encouraging) experiments which lead to *quantitative* results and *precise* interpretations.

A further remarkable feature of the original Kacser and Burns paper[1], was the care taken to invent and define new terms to describe the quantifiable coefficients which they proposed it should henceforth be our aim to measure. They deliberately avoided attaching the adjective 'control' to any coefficient, perhaps because it had come to mean all things to all biochemists. To what they term 'global' coefficients, they assigned appropriate Roman letters (R = response coefficient, Z = sensitivity coefficient); to 'local' coefficients they assigned Greek letters (κ = controllability coefficient; ϵ = elasticity coefficient). Of central importance in the Kacser and Burns treatment[1,2,3], and unique to it, is the relationship:

$$dF/F = Z\,\kappa\,\frac{dP}{P}$$

Interpreting, we can say that the fractional change in the observed flux (dF/F) is determined quantitatively by the product of the two coefficients Z and κ and the fractional change in an appropriate external parametric effector (dP/P). There are as many sensitivity coefficients (Z) and controllability coefficients (κ) as there are enzymes and effector interactions in a given pathway. It follows that a highly controllable enzyme E_i (κ is large) does not necessarily have a marked effect on flux through the pathway (even when dP/P is significant) if flux through the pathway happens to be insensitive to changes in the activity of this particular enzyme E_i ($Z_i \approx 0$ for this enzyme embedded in the metabolic pathway). In contrast, a pronounced change in the observed flux could be brought about at a step catalysed by an enzyme E_i possessing a relatively small value of (κ) if it so happened that flux through the pathway was peculiarly sensitive to small changes in the activity of that particular enzyme E_i ($dP/P \neq 0$; $Z_i \approx 1.0$). The significant point is that the two preceding sentences, though they describe part of the Kacser and Burns treatment, become redundant once the theory is understood. Given an understanding of the theory, it is possible to determine experimentally the value of any or all of the coefficients mentioned; these quantitative values then express all that it is necessary to know about the control of flux at any chosen point in any pathway and the need for long qualitative descriptions disappears. This is one aspect of the Kacser and Burns theory so fruitfully exploited by Tager and his colleagues[9,10].

Since it is certain[1,2,3] that the sum of all the sensitivity coefficients attached to any pathway cannot exceed unity ($\sum_{i=1}^{n} {}^{j}_{i} = 1.0$), and any enzyme E_i can only be regarded as 'fully controlling' when $Z_i \to 1$, it is unlikely, in general, that 'control' of flux resides only at one enzyme-catalysed or porter-facilitated step in a metabolic pathway. The Kacser and Burns theory[1,2,3] contains two other Summation Properties, one of which (the Connectivity Property) links the local effects at individual enzyme-catalysed steps to the global response of the whole system of steps in a metabolic pathway. The generality, simplicity, elegance and precision of the Kacser and Burns treatment, in theory and in practice, is immediately appealing to undergraduate students and is well within their intellectual grasp.

Dr Gillies paid particular and deserved attention to the work of Heinrich and Rapoport[11,12,13]. Their explicit solution of the problem of control of glycolysis through the glycolytic pathway in erythro-cytes is a model combination of sound theory and astute experimentation[14,15]. The astonishing fact is that the Edinburgh and Berlin teams arrived independently and almost simultaneously at the identification of two quantifiable parameters which are relevant to the autoregulation of flux in intact metabolic systems. Not surprisingly, different nomenclatures were chosen, each for good reasons, but anyone familiar with the work of one team can immediately understand the papers of the other (control strength in Berlin = sensitivity coefficient in Edinburgh; elasticity coefficient in Edinburgh = effector strength in Berlin). The two laboratories are in complete accord about the theoretical foundations and treatment of the problem of control of flux through intact metabolic systems (though the metabolic systems in which they are each interested are quite different). The differences in the two published systems of nomenclature are trivial; the concepts behind them are identical. Concerted efforts are now in progress to devise a unified and expanded nomenclature; several laboratories are involved in these efforts.

Kacser and Burns have subsequently published a quite outstanding paper which provides the first credible (and simple) explanation for dominance/recessivity since Mendel's observation of the phenomenon in 1866. This later paper[16] is a profound theoretical treatment – a direct descendant of the original paper[1] – and, like it, is immediately supported by experimental evidence from a variety of biological systems. It is a remarkable tribute to the insight gained from the Kacser and Burns theoretical treatment of flux through intact metabolic pathways[1,16] that it leads not only to a simple explanation for dominance/recessivity, but also explains the occurrence of epistasis and pleiotropy; and further, explains why pairs of alleles which otherwise display all the attributes of Mendelian inheritance do not always exhibit either dominance or recessivity.

My purpose here has been to draw attention to the potency of sound theoretical expositions; without such expositions we are lost. The more general and rigorous the theoretical treatment, the greater is the benefit to experimental work. To quote Kacser and Burns again[2]: 'We have presented a conceptual framework, a theoretical analysis and an experimental approach to enzyme systems in terms of modulation *in vivo*. . . . Our analysis makes possible the experimental determination of the relevant control coefficients.' Garfinkel[17] has pointed out that we biologists are strangely different from physicists in at least one respect. We are trained to regard theory with suspicion whereas physicists theorize and experiment alternately, or alternatively, and with equal regard for both activities! I believe Kacser and Burns may have been overlooked, even consciously disregarded by most biochemists, simply because the first in a series of papers from Kacser's laboratory was primarily a general (but rigorous) theoretical consideration of flux control in any intact metabolizing system.

References

1 Kacser, H. and Burns, J. A. (1973) *Symp. Soc. Exp. Biol.* 32, 65–104

2 Kacser, H. and Burns, J. A. (1979) *Biochem. Soc. Trans.* 7, 1149–1160

3 Kacser, H. (1983) *Biochem. Soc. Trans.* 11, 35–40

4 Porteous, J. W. (1983) *Biochem. Soc. Trans.* 11, 29–31

5 Flint, H. J., Porteous, D. J. and Kacser, H. (1980) *Biochem. J.* 190, 1–15

6 Flint, H. J., Tateson, R. W., Barthelmess, I. B., Porteous, D. J., Donachie, W. D. and Kacser, H. (1981) *Biochem. J.* 200, 231–246

7 Kacser, H., Bulfield, G. and Wright, A. (1979) in *Models for the Study of Inborn Errors of Metabolism* (Hommes, F. A., ed.), Elsevier

8 Middleton, R. J. and Kacser, H. (1983) *Genetics* 105, 633–650

9 Groen, A. K., Wanders, R. J. A., Westerhoff, H. V., van der Meer, R. and Tager, J. M. (1982) *J. Biol. Chem.* 257, 2754–2757

10 Tager, J. M., Groen, A. K., Wanders, R. J. A., Duszynski, J., Westerhoff, H. V. and Vervoorn, R. C. (1983) *Biochem. Soc. Trans.* 11, 40–43

11 Heinrich, R. and Rapoport, T. A. (1974) *Eur. J. Biochem.* 42, 89–95

12 Heinrich, R. and Rapoport, T. A. (1974) *Eur. J. Biochem.* 42, 97–105

13 Rapoport, T. A., Heinrich, R., Jacobasch, G. and Rapoport, S. (1974) *Eur. J. Biochem.* 42, 107–120

14 Heinrich, R. and Rapoport, S. (1983) *Biochem. Soc. Trans.* 11, 31–35

15 Rapoport, T. A., Heinrich, R. and Rapoport, S. M. (1981) *Biochem. J.* 154, 449–469

16 Kacser, H. and Burns, J. A. (1981) *Genetics* 97, 639–666

17 Garfinkel, D. (1980) *Amer. J. Physiol.* 239, R1–R6

John W. Porteous is at the Department of Biochemistry, Marischal College, University of Aberdeen AB9 1AS, UK.

Metabolic regulation and the microenvironment

C. J. Masters

Research into cellular regulation engenders a basic dilemma: although analytical accuracy may be improved by using purified components, such approaches often proceed at the cost of physiological credibility. Some of the classical concepts of control require re-examination in the light of the realities of the microenvironment.

In the last two decades, much of the emphasis in acute intrinsic metabolic control has centred on the self-regulating properties of enzyme systems, and in particular the interaction of regulating metabolites (variously termed effectors, modifiers and modulators) with key enzymes. A 'classical' view of metabolic regulation by appropriate regulatory circuits has emerged, with such circuits being typically composed of an allosteric enzyme located at the initial unique step in a pathway and interacting with an end product by means of feedback regulation. This visualization has provided an extremely elegant picture of control possibilities, and has satisfied many of the initial questions which arise in relation to the fine control and coordination of metabolism[1-6].

In assessing the significance of such models, however, it must be recognized that many of the conditions commonly employed in classical enzymology are biologically abnormal and bear little relation to the conditions under which the enzymes act *in vivo*. Most laboratory studies, for example, use dilute aqueous solutions of enzymes, because these are the conditions that are most manageable experimentally. In such *in vitro* studies, it is common for the molarity of the substrates to be 10^6 times that of the enzyme, whereas it is becoming increasingly clear that, in fact, the concentrations of enzymes, substrates and effectors in the cell are comparable for

major metabolic pathways[7]. Model analytical systems also usually take little notice of the biphasic nature of much of the microenvironment, the modifications of the kinetic characteristics of enzymes in such gel-like conditions, or the influence of concentration effects on the interactions between metabolites and macromolecules. In consequence, most of our accumulated knowledge on the behaviour of enzyme systems is confined to conditions that cannot occur in living cells.

Requirements for new concepts and considerations

Because of the vast differences between the usual conditions for the *in vitro* examination of control enzymes, and the conditions in the cellular microenvironment, there is a clear need for biological scientists to examine the 'classical' concepts of intrinsic metabolic regulation in the light of the realities of biological function.

Many reviews, for example, have stressed the importance of phosphofructokinase as a control point in glycolysis, the irreversible nature of the reaction catalysed by this enzyme and the influence of modulators on the typical sigmoidal kinetics[8-10]. Indeed, this point of control has probably been cited as an example more times than any other. However, neither the elegance of much of this work, nor the plausibility of the *in vitro / in vivo* correlations, should lead us to accept that irreversibility or other characteristics of this enzyme are universal properties of control enzymes. Failure to observe allosteric effects with an enzyme *in vitro*, for example, does not necessarily preclude this form of control in biological systems. It has been demonstrated that enzymes that catalyse reversible reactions, such as aldolase, may occur in cellular systems largely in a form reversibly adsorbed to membranes, and that this association may be disrupted by physiological increases in substrate concentration. The kinetics of such a system may display allosteric characteristics and provide a feedback system in which the available activity of the enzyme may be regulated in response to cellular conditions: or in other words, under cellular conditions enzymes catalysing reversible reactions may provide a biphasic analogy of the type of uniphasic variations commonly observed in *in vitro* studies of regulatory enzymes[11,12].

Dimensions of maximal velocity

Another characteristic of control enzymes that is widely recognized by classical analogy is the 'bottleneck' positioning of these components in the activity of profiles of relevant pathways[13,14]. The significance of this regulatory property comes from knowing that the most effective point at which control might be applied in a pathway is the point of minimum flux. However, two points deserve wider consideration:

(1) Although the majority of metabolic studies have been concentrated in liver, where phosphofructokinase is well known to be inhibiting, a wider survey of the catalytic components in major mammalian tissues reveals that the potential bottlenecks in glycolysis/gluconeogenesis, as indicated by the dimensions of maximal velocity, are not restricted to unidirectional reactions. A number of the enzymes common to both pathways also have relatively low maximal capacities (e.g. aldolase and enolase).

(2) The amount of enzymatic activity available in the cell may be very much less than that commonly deduced from *in vitro* assays, because of the tendency of some enzymes to bind to particulate structures. As we have already noted, aldolase may occur mainly as the bound form in some tissues, with binding to membranes occurring via the active site. The total activity available in the cellular microenvironment may thus be very much less than that extractable in soluble form under the common *in vitro* conditions. Hence, a more realistic representation of such adsorption in pathway profiles may widen considerably the number of instances where enzymes are present in limiting concentrations.

End-product regulation

Another appealing feature of the classical models of metabolic control is provided by the possibilities of self-regulation and the interrelationship of various aspects of metabolism that are inherent in the concept of end-product inhibition. Perhaps the most highly

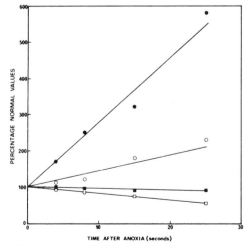

Fig. 1. Sequential alterations in the relative concentration of glycolytic metabolites in rat brain following anoxia. ●, *fructose 1,6-bisphosphate:* ○, *ATP:* ■, *glucose:* □, *glycogen.*

developed theoretical extension of such possibilities is the energy-charge concept[8-15]. Elegant schemes for the regulation of all major aspects of metabolism in response to the concentrations of adenine nucleotides in the cell have been advanced on this basis[16].

Attractive as such unifying concepts are, however, it is suggested that they should still be viewed in the cellular context, as well as in the light of the information gained from test-tube reactions. In one pioneering, oft-quoted example of glycolytic control, for example, Lowry and co-workers have studied the sequential changes in cellular metabolites that occur in mammalian brain after metabolic perturbation[17]. In relation to the reality of cellular signals, it is noteworthy that only a small percentage change occurred in adenine nucleotide levels within 30 s of anoxic perturbation. This degree of response can hardly be viewed as the dramatic fluctuation one might expect on the basis of the general role proposed for this metabolite system in cellular regulation. Furthermore, it may be noted that in the same experiment, the maximal change in the concentration of a particular metabolite occurred at the level of fructose 1,6-bisphosphate, where the levels changed by a factor nearly two orders of magnitude greater than that of ATP, in identical time periods (Fig. 1). Again, a response that may give rise to serious reservations on the nature of the primary regulatory messenger.

Sandwich situations, and signalling via median metabolites

What are the reasons for the particular localization of metabolite variation that was noted in the last paragraph and why do these results not agree with the predictions of classical end-product inhibition? Is this positioning of metabolic response indicative of the functioning of control circuits *in vivo* which are different in composition and localization to these ascribed on the basis of *in vitro*

experiments? It is suggested that these questions are worthy of serious contemplation by those interested in cellular regulation, and the proposition is advanced that a possible solution may lie in the resultants of an opposite conjunction of two adjacent regulatory enzymes in a metabolic sequence. Such a sandwich-type system could explain the positioning of such effects, and conceivably provide a more rapid and effective means of a metabolite signalling than end-product regulation.

In the case of fructose 1,6-bisphosphate, for example, it is evident that fluctuations in concentration might be contributed to either by the enzyme controlling synthesis of this metabolite (phosphofructokinase), or by the enzyme governing the conversion of fructose 1,6-bisphosphate to triosephosphate (aldolase), or both of these activities simultaneously.

Another possibility of such a sandwiching influence is the pairing of aldolase and fructose bisphosphatase. Different tissue and metabolic localization would of course be expected for these different pairings. Both phosphofructokinase and fructose bisphosphatase are widely recognized as control enzymes, and the control possibilities of aldolase are referred to here. It should also be mentioned that each of these enzymes exists as several multiple forms in different cell types, and each of these forms may exhibit individual characteristics in catalysis, membrane binding and other pertinent properties[18]. Consequently, the scope for a subtle variation in the combined operation of these control components is considerable, and well tailored to meet the diverse metabolic situations in the many separate tissue, cellular and subcellular compartments.

Molecular interactions in the cell

Another important influence that is commonly neglected in *in vitro* studies of metabolic control is the contribution of molecular interactions to metabolism under cellular conditions. The high concentrations of protein (usually about 10%) in the cell are known to influence the localization of free metabolites, for example, and may exert potent effects on metabolism via such concentrations rather than by virtue of their other specific biological functions. For example, fructose bisphosphate concentrations are markedly influenced by adsorption to aldolase, and this enzyme may bind up to 90% of cellular fructose bisphosphate in this manner[19]. Hence, the ability of this metabolite to move freely within the cell and function as a regulatory signal is influenced by the concentration, subunit character and metabolic status of the aldolase present in the cell.

Again, weak protein–protein interactions may exert a considerable influence on cellular metabolism. For the enzymes of the glycolytic sequence, for example, the possible existence of a glycolytic complex and its inherent metabolic advantages have been widely canvassed over many years[11,20]. Despite the biological importance of these concepts, however, it is only recently that definitive proof has been provided for the existence of such an association. It is of interest that the stability of this association of glycolytic enzymes is markedly influenced by fructose bisphosphate, ATP and other function-dependent metabolites, and that in consequence metabolic flux in this pathway is subject to influences which may be obscured under the common conditions of enzymatic assay.

Areas of metabolism influenced by fructose bisphosphate

Hopefully, the arguments advanced so far will have been accepted as suggesting a rapid alteration in the cellular concentration of median metabolites such as fructose bisphosphate, and as providing some indication of the pos-

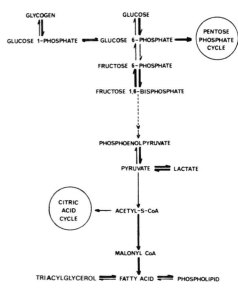

Fig. 2. Established areas of influence (broad arrows) of the metabolite, fructose 1,6-bisphosphate, in relation to carbohydrate and lipid metabolism.

sible effects of such variation on enzyme interaction and control. To conclude any consideration of the significance of these effects, however, evidence should be provided for the influence of the metabolites on areas of metabolism.

The influences of fructose bisphosphate on carbohydrate metabolism are well documented and relevant here. This metabolite is known to be able to influence glycolysis by activating phosphofructokinase, and to affect gluconeogenesis by inhibition of fructose bisphosphatase[30]. It also exerts important influences on this area of metabolism by modulating the activities of pyruvate kinase[21] and lactate dehydrogenase[22]. In addition, fructose bisphosphate can affect such diverse areas as the glucose 6-phosphate crossroads by inhibition of hexokinase[23], the pentose phosphate pathway via 6-phosphogluconate dehydrogenase[24], glycogenolysis, fatty acid synthesis (by stimulating the fatty acid synthetase)[25], the synthesis of phospholipids, lipolysis[27] and the regulation of photosynthetic CO_2 assimilation[28].

Finally, it may be noted that fructose bisphosphate concentrations have been shown to play a significant role in the regulation of adenyl cyclase activities, and it would appear from these results that a reciprocal control system involving glycolytic intermediates may exist that regulates both adenyl cyclase and glycolysis[29].

Although aldolase does not qualify as a control enzyme by the application of the 'classical' control criteria[5,6], there are abundant indications in the literature of localization of regulation at this point. Nonequilibrium of the aldolase-catalysed steps has been noted in brain and other tissues under a variety of metabolic conditions[30], and negative crossover at this enzyme has been demonstrated during studies of glycolysis in insect flight muscle[31]. Also, in developmental studies of rat neonatal tissues, accelerated synthesis of phosphofructokinase and aldolase has been described, an ontogenetic behaviour that is consistent with both of these enzymes functioning as major points of regulation of the glycolytic flux[32]. There is also an increasing interest in the metabolic significance of 'futile' cycling of ATP at the phosphofructokinase/fructose bisphosphatase steps in glycolysis, and the attendant realization that aldolase and fructose bisphosphate play limiting roles in this system[33].

In summary, it may be seen that considerable scope exists for the possible interaction of median metabolites such as fructose bisphosphate with broad areas of metabolism, and for the inclusion of aldolase as a regulatory enzyme. These relationships would appear to justify continued and increased consideration of similar control combinations in the cell. Undoubtedly many similar and significant 'non-classical' points of control remain to be researched.

In retrospect, the concepts of end-product feedback have dominated considerations of metabolic control in cells and tissues in recent years, and have markedly advanced our ability to comprehend the nature of self-regulation and the strategic positioning and complex inter-relationships of cellular control systems. Indeed, this marriage of *in vitro* attributes of control with *in vivo* potentialities for regulation is deserving of its frequent nomination as a triumphant example of the analytical approach in biology.

One of the intentions of this article, however, is to draw attention to the fact that as with many major advances, a subsequent tendency towards over-generalization and over-dependence on these concepts may be found in many current treatments of cellular regulation. The need for a continuing critical appraisal of regulatory requirements in the light of conditions which prevail in the cellular microenvironment is stressed, and attention drawn to several aspects of the subject that would appear to be worthy of greater attention; the realities of enzyme and metabolic concentrations in tissues, the feasibility of reversible reactions contributing to control, the concept of 'sandwiching' of regulatory metabolites between controlled enzymes, and the importance of interactions between macro- and micromolecular components[34]. For our concepts of metabolic regulation to be meaningful, they must be firmly based on the physiological realities of the microenvironment.

References

1 Umbarger, H. W. (1961) *Cold Spring Harbor Symp. Quant. Biol.* 26, 301–312
2 Monod, J., Changeux, J. P. and Jacob, F. (1963) *J. Mol. Biol.* 6, 306–329
3 Stadtman, E. R. (1966) *Adv. Enzymol.* 28, 41–154
4 Koshland, D. E. (1968) *Adv. Enz. Regul.* 6, 291–304
5 Krebs, H. A. (1963) *Adv. Enz. Regul.* 1, 385–400
6 Weber, G., Singhal, R. L., Stamm, N. B., Fisher, E. A. and Mentendick, M. A. (1964)

Adv. Enz. Regul. 2, 1–38

7 Srere, P. A. (1967) Science 158, 936–937

8 Atkinson, D. E. (1968) Biochemistry 7, 4030–4034

9 Underwood, A. H. and Newsholme, E. A. (1965) Biochem. J. 95, 868–875

10 Aschroft, S. J. H., Capito, K. and Hedeskov, C. J. (1973) Diabetologia 9, 299–302

11 Clark, F. M. and Masters, C. J. (1976) Int. J. Biochem. 7, 359–365

12 Masters, C. J., Sheedy, R. J., Winzor, D. J. and Nichol. L. W. (1969) Biochem. J. 112, 806–808

13 Gumaa, K. A. and Maclean, P. (1969) Biochem. J. 115, 1009–1029

14 Ashworth, J. M. (1975) in Cell Differentiation, p. 58, Chapman and Hall, London

15 Shen, L. C. and Atkinson, D. E. (1970) J. Biol. Chem. 245, 3996–4000

16 Larner, J. (1971) in Intermediary Metabolism and its Regulation, p. 226, Prentice-Hall, New Jersey

17 Lowry, O. H. and Passoneau, J. V. (1964) J. Biol. Chem. 239, 31–42

18 Masters, C. J. and Holmes, R. S. (1975) in Haemoglobin, Isoenzymes and Tissue Differentiation, North-Holland, Amsterdam

19 Sols, A. and Mario, R. (1970) Curr. Top. Cell Regul. 2, 227–273

20 Green, D. E., Murer, E., Hulthin, H. O., Richardson, S. H., Salmon, B., Brierley, G. R. and Baum, H. (1965) Arch. Biochem. Biophys. 112, 635–647

21 Hess, B., Haeckel, R. and Brand, K. (1966) Biochem. Biophys. Res. Commun. 24, 824–831

22 Brown, A. T. and Wittenberger, C. L. (1972) J. Bacteriol. 110, 604–615

23 Wakil, S. J., Goldman, J. K. and Williamson, I. P. (1966) Proc. Natl Acad. Sci. USA 55, 880–887

24 Kumar, S. and Porter, J. W. (1971) J. Biol. Chem. 246, 7780–7789

25 Volpe, J. J. and Vagelos, P. R. (1973) Annu. Rev. Biochem. 42, 21–60

26 Williams, M. L. and Bygrave, F. L. (1970) Eur. J. Biochem. 17, 32–38

27 Bornstein, J. (1972) Israel J. Med. Sci. 8, 407–412

28 Joint, I. R., Morris, I. and Fuller, R. C. (1972) Biochim. Biophys. Acta 276, 333–337

29 Khandelwal, R. L. and Hamilton, I. R. (1972) Arch. Biochem. Biophys. 151, 75–84

30 Rolleston, F. S. and Newsholme, E. A. (1967) Biochem. J. 104. 524–533

31 Ford, W. L. L. and Candy, D. J. (1972) Biochem. J. 130, 1101–1112

32 Baquer, N. Z., Maclean, P. and Greenbaum, A. L. (1973) Biochem. Biophys. Res. Commun. 53, 1282–1288

33 Clark, M. G., Kneer, N. M., Bosch, A. L. and Lardy, H. A. (1974) J. Biol. Chem. 249, 5695–5703

34 Masters, C. J. (1976) Curr. Top. Cell Regul. 12, 75–105

C. J. Masters is at the School of Science, Griffith University, Nathan, Queensland, 4111, Australia.

Why are enzymes so big?

Paul A. Srere

The size of enzymes may be related to their need to have sufficient surface area to contain specific binding sites for their localization in a cell and for their integration into metabolic complexes.

Two communications in *TIBS*[1,2] have addressed the question: why are enzymes so big? Kell[1] discussed the problem from the view that additional free energy necessary for the activation energy may come from spatiotemporal ordering[3] of the fluctuations of parts of the protein away from the active site. Payens[2] pointed out that random, nonspecific binding of the substrate to additional sites on the enzyme surface may serve to trap substrates[2] and enhance rates of diffusion to the active site. Electrostatic interactions may also contribute to the rate of the enzyme reaction[2].

I will consider two other possibilities that may be important in determining the size of enzymes. First, it is accepted that to form catalysts with high activity and specificity many amino acid residues with precise spatial relationships are required (active sites). A long polypeptide chain may be needed to ensure that the required site is formed and that protein structural requirements are met (hydrophobic residues in the interior and the hydrophilic residues on the exterior of the protein).

Second, it is known that the outside surfaces of proteins help to locate the enzyme in the cell and to specify its

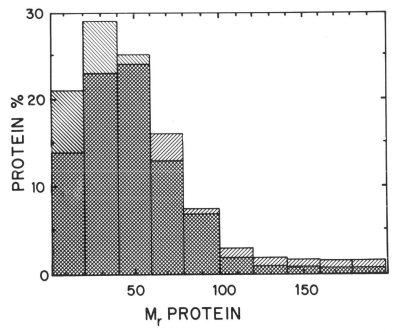

Fig. 1. The distribution of polypeptide molecular weights in HeLa cells (▨) and in E. coli (▧). (Redrawn from data of Kiehn and Holland[16].)

interactions with other related enzymes (Refs 4–8 and refs therein). Thus, these multiple interactions require proteins to be large.

These hypotheses are not mutually exclusive or all inclusive; all may be important in the action of enzymes and in the determination of their sizes.

The size of proteins

The distribution of sizes of polypeptide chains synthesized by different living cells is remarkably similar. Kiehn and Holland[9] have shown that there exists only a small difference in the molecular weight distribution of polypeptides from *E. coli* and from HeLa cells (Fig. 1). Polypeptides between 30 000 and 50 000 mol. wt make up 50–55% of the total proteins, whereas only 3 to 5% of the total have molecular weights greater than 80 000. The size of an average *E. coli* polypeptide is 25 000, while that of an average HeLa cell polypeptide is 31 700.

These results suggest that there are inherent limits to the size of polypeptides. It is clear that, although most polypeptides are in the 30 000 to 50 000 range, the cell can (and does) make both very large and very small proteins. Generally, the small proteins (consisting of single polypeptides) ($< 20\,000$ mol. wt) are secreted proteins, hormones or extracellular proteases, and the very large proteins ($> 80\,000$ containing very large polypeptide chains) are either structural proteins or enzymes which catalyse a complex overall reaction (multifunctional enzymes).

Wetlaufer[10] has concluded that a polypeptide chain of about 20–40 amino acids is sufficiently long to have a unique secondary structure (a stable folded structure) and could thus be viewed as the size of a 'unit' domain of a protein. Although there are functional proteins of this size, I know of no naturally occurring enzymes that are this small. The molecular weights of certain bacterial ribonucleases, cytochromes and ferri-doxins are about 10 000 and the subunits of a few enzymes seem to be in the 10–15 000 range. Some rubredoxins are in the 5 000 range of molecular sizes. Blake[11] has noted that exon-encoded units have an average length of about 40–45 residues (4 400–5 000 mol. wt).

The size of catalysts

Is it necessary to have a large number (5–20) of amino acid residues in a specific spatial configuration in order to obtain the full catalytic power and specificity exhibited by enzymes? How long a polypeptide chain is needed to place the amino acid residues in the active site in the correct positions?

The number of amino acid residues necessary in an active site may be quite large. For example, Remington *et al.*[12] list eight amino acid residues of citrate synthase which form hydrogen bonds to citrate and eight amino acid residues which form hydrogen bonds to Coenzyme A. The amino acid residues range from number 46 to number 421. In addition, it was shown that both subunits of citrate synthase contribute residues to each binding site.

We cannot yet determine how long a polypeptide chain is necessary to bring the 16 required amino acid residues of citrate synthase into the appropriate spatial configuration. The fact that yet another subunit contributes some of the binding residues indicates that all or most of the 437 amino acids may be required. In light of data on the fluctuations in proteins, the concept of an active site as a rigid entity is no longer tenable. The residues need only be brought into a space such that normal protein fluctuations will produce the fixed active site that is seen by X-ray crystallography as one of the possible conformations. This flexibility may facilitate active site formation.

The serine proteases offer an example of the variation in size of a group of enzymes with identical active site struc-

Table I. Comparison of serine proteases

Enzyme	Source	Amino acid residues in active enzyme
Protease B	*Streptomyces griseus*	185
α-Lytic Protease	*Myxobacter*	198
Trypsin	*S. griseus*	221
Trypsin	Bovine	223
Kallikrein (tissue)	Rat	237
Elastase	Pig	240
Chymotrypsin	Bovine	245
Factor X	Bovine	396
Thrombin	Bovine	308
Factor XII	Bovine	700
Plasmin	Human	714
Kallikrein (plasma)	Bovine	800

All contain His, Asp and Ser in a close relative relationship.
(Partially from *Atlas of Protein Sequence and Structure*, M. O. Dayhoff 5, suppl. 3 1978, pp. 86, 87.)

tures. The size of serine proteases varies from about 20 000–90 000 mol. wt (Table I). These large differences are most easily interpreted by assigning specific recognition functions to the other portions of the protein surfaces present in the larger proteases. The proteases with the highest substrate specificity, the blood clotting factors, are the largest.

Recent work in catalysis (see review by Maugh[13]) has shown that some chiral catalysts can match both the specificity and activity of enzymes for some synthetic reactions. Thus, the biomimetic capabilities of these small (mol. wt 500) catalysts seem to indicate that it may not

be necessary to have such large molecules with so many chemical groups for efficient catalysis. This does not rule out the proposition that large active sites require a long polypeptide chain. However, the existence of these small, selective non-biological catalysts does cause one to question explanations of an enzyme's specificity and efficiency based solely upon its large size.

Surface area of proteins and protein–protein interactions

The surface-to-volume ratio of a protein depends upon its shape. For compact symmetric molecules, the minimum ratio of the surface area to volume is $3/r$ (for a sphere of radius, r). Thus, as the radius increases, proportionately less surface becomes available. More surface can be obtained by changing the axial ratio from one (sphere) to something larger than one (though this effect is not large, see below) or by making the surface irregular.

Rose and Wetlaufer[14] have pointed out that the surface-to-volume ratio for most proteins is constant and about the same for spheres and both oblate and prolate ellipsoids. Thus, the volume of the sphere occupied by a 40 amino acid polypeptide would be 5400 $Å^3$ and its surface area would be 1415 $Å^2$. The surface area necessary for a protein which participates in multiple interactions can be estimated by assuming that, aside from the active site, three sites are necessary. One site is necessary for location on a membrane or on a structural component of the cell (Fig. 2), and at

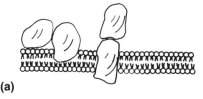

(a)　　　　　　　　　　　　　　**(b)**

Fig. 2. Enzymes binding to structural elements in cells. (a) Binding to either a protein of the membrane (left) or to the membrane itself (right). (b) Binding to structural proteins in the cell.

least two sites for interaction with metabolically related enzymes. The area required for such interactions may vary greatly depending upon their strength.

It is difficult to estimate the surface area necessary for protein–protein interactions, but two examples may help with the estimate. From crystallographic studies we know that in the tight interaction of citrate synthase subunits (no dissociation has been seen in aqueous nondenaturing buffers) 1670 $Å^2$ of a total surface of 5800 $Å^2$ are involved in the interaction[12]. Matthew, Weber, Salemme and Richards[15] have shown that for the ionic strength sensitive (K_{assoc} 10^5–10^7 from I = 0.16 to 0.01) interaction, between positively charged flavodoxin and negatively charged cytochrome c, approximately 40–60% (my estimate from their figure) of the surface of each is involved in the oriented electrostatic fields. For proteins of this size (~10 000 mol. wt), the surface can be calculated to be about 2400 $Å^2$ (assuming spherical protein molecules). Thus, for the weaker ionic interaction, about 1000 $Å^2$ may be necessary for the interaction.

It would appear, therefore, that at least 1000 $Å^2$ surface is necessary for weak interactions and that small proteins (< 10 000 mol. wt) with a surface area of around 1500 $Å^2$ would therefore have a limited capacity for multiple interactions with other proteins or membranes. On the other hand, a spherical protein of 50 000 mol. wt would have a surface of 7500 $Å^2$, allowing more than sufficient surface for additional interactions. These considerations indicate that larger proteins have enough surface for multiple interactions with other cellular components. Since further increases in size would give much larger mass increments than surface area increments, this may set the upper limit for the size of polypeptides.

For a series of proteins ranging in molecular weight from 6 100 to 36 000 accessible surface areas of 3500 to 17 000 $Å^2$ were calculated[16]. When buried surface areas were calculated for protein dimers in the same series of proteins, values from 1400 to 5000 $Å^2$ were obtained[16]. These values are 1.7 times the area of smooth inertial ellipsoids of the proteins[17], because of the roughness of the surface. When proteins bind to each other their surfaces probably do not interdigitate as closely as the accessible surface would indicate. Thus, the estimates we have made above are probably acceptable.

Interactions of sequential metabolic enzymes

Multienzyme complexes and multifunctional enzymes

Protein–protein interactions are the rule rather than the exception, since most proteins are composed of subunits which readily interact. A large number of multienzyme complexes are known and the binding of enzymes to structural elements of cells has been described. Regulatory significance has been postulated for the binding or release of enzymes to structural elements.

The range of sequential active site interactions is large (Fig. 3). The most effective of such interactions are in multifunctional proteins where active sites are covalently linked. There are numerous examples of these systems, including animal fatty acid synthetase, animal and yeast tryptophan synthetase, and animal UMP synthetase. It is interesting to note that all of these systems have multienzyme counterparts in lower life forms.

Welch and DeMoss[18] have pointed out that the enzymes of both the polyaromatic pathway and tryptophan pathway in microorganisms and higher plants show an increasing organizational tightness when the most primitive organisms are compared to the most advanced.

Manney[19] has a mutant of yeast in which the two individual activities of tryptophan synthetase exist on separate proteins rather than on a single polypeptide chain, as in the wild-type yeast. It is possible that *in situ* the two separate polypeptides still function as a single interacting unit, but even if they do, it is clear that the channeling of the indole intermediate is more efficient when the two sites are covalently linked. The metabolic disadvantage to the mutant is reflected in an increased lag phase during the growth of the yeast. During the lag phase the indole concentration in the mutant increases to a critical level before growth commences. This high indole concentration is not necessary for growth in the wild-type yeast.

Interactions of 'soluble' enzymes

Among the first experimental reports that there may be no free enzymes in cells were those of Kempner and Miller[20] using *Euglena* cells and Zalokar[21] using *Neurospora* in which it was demonstrated that all enzymes in these cells sedimented as high molecular weight complexes. There has been a great deal of discussion about the possibility of *in vivo* organization of apparently soluble metabolically sequential enzymes. Mitchell[7] discussed integrational amino acid residues on proteins, Munkres and Woodward[8] presented evidence on locational specificity, Srere and Mosbach[4] presented evidence of microenvironments, and theoretical discussions are found in reviews by Welch[5] and Welch and Keleti[6].

Unequivocal evidence exists that clearly demonstrates the presence and the kinetic advantage of interactions between sequential enzymes in a metabolic pathway[5]. As noted above, the optimal situation apparently occurs when such active sites are covalently linked. Not only are there kinetic advantages, but by eliminating the need of a large pool for free intermediates, the limited solvent capacity of the cell is not taxed.

The evidence for interactions between sequential enzymes in a metabolic pathway takes a variety of forms, from channeling studies to studies which present physical evidence for the interaction of enzymes. I have listed some of the pathways for which evidence of interaction of sequential enzymes has been presented (Table II).

For example, in recent years the following metabolically significant interactions have been demonstrated between TCA cycle enzymes–citrate synthase: malate dehydrogenase[22], pyruvate dehydrogenase complex–citrate synthase[23], succinate thiokinase–α ketoglutarate dehydrogenase complex[24], fumarase–malate dehydrogenase[25]. Additional interactions between transaminases and glutamate dehydrogenase and malate dehydrogenases have been demonstrated by Fahien and others[26].

Not only have interactions between the related TCA cycle enzymes been demonstrated, but many of these enzymes interact with proteins in inner membranes of mitochondria[27]. Recently, we have extended these membrane

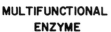

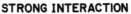

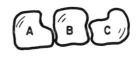

Fig. 3. Sequential metabolic complexes. The multienzyme complexes are designated strong or weak, depending upon their dissociation constants in aqueous media at low total protein concentrations. A, B and C represent the individual sequential enzyme activities of a metabolic pathway.

Table II. Sequential metabolic interactions

Pathway	Type of evidence
Glycolysis	A, B, C, D, E
Tricarboxylic acid cycle	B, C, D
Fatty acid oxidation	A, B, C, D
Fatty acid synthesis	C
Protein synthesis	B, C, D
Nucleic acid synthesis	A, B, C, E
Aromatic amino acid synthesis	A, B, D, E
Purine synthesis	A, E
Pyrimidine synthesis	A, B
Cyclic AMP degradation	A, D, E
Urea cycle	B, D

A = channeling;
B = specific protein–protein interactions;
C = specific protein membrane interactions;
D = kinetic effects;
E = isolation. For references see Refs 5, 30.

studies to show that the enzymes for β-oxidation of fatty acids also bind to the inner surface of the mitochondrial inner membrane.

All of these interactions have been shown to be specific for the particular enzymes and membrane or structural element involved. Some of them are shown to be affected by 'physiological' concentrations of their substrates, so that it is possible to propose regulatory behavior based upon complex formation and dissolution of complexes. On the other hand, many of these weak interactions are not seen at 'physiological' ionic strength. However, it should be remembered that: (1) we do not have an accurate assessment of ionic strength within the cell; (2) cellular protein concentrations are quite high (20–50%) and molecular crowding[28] can markedly affect these weak protein interactions; and (3) the interactions are specific for enzymes of sequential metabolic reactions.

Evolutionary considerations

McConkey[29], labeled the proteins of HeLa cells (human) with [^{14}C]leucine and the proteins of CHO cells (hamster) with [^{3}H]leucine, combined the extracts and performed two-dimensional gel electrophoresis on the mixture of polypeptides. By differential exposure techniques, the polypeptides of each cell line could be detected and polypeptides which behaved identically in the gels could be visualized. The surprising result was that, despite the length of time between the appearance of the two organisms in evolution, the number of 'identities' was much higher than predicted using the expected mutation rate. McConkey[29] hypothesizes that the strong conservation of cellular proteins indicates that much more of a protein than its active site is conserved and that binding sites on the exterior of proteins are also conserved. There may be genetic defects which cause diminished interactions between sequential enzymes and are expressed only under certain stress conditions.

Acknowledgement

I am indebted to my colleagues for their interest and discussions. I thank Dr Welch for preprints. I am also indebted to Penny Perkins for secretarial assistance. Supported by the Veterans' Administration, USPHS, NSF and the Welch Foundation.

Note added in proof

After the submission of this manuscript, another letter appeared (Wombacher H. (1984) *Trends Biochem. Sci.* 9, 93) which briefly discusses the problem of metabolic enzyme interaction and the size of enzymes.

References

1 Kell, D. G. (1982) *Trends Biochem. Sci.* 7, 1
2 Payens, T. A. J. (1983) *Trends Biochem. Sci.* 8, 46
3 Welch, G., Somogyi, B. and Damjanovich, S. (1982) *Prog. Biophys. Molec. Biol.* 39, 109–146
4 Srere, P. A. and Mosbach, K. (1974) *Ann. Rev. Micro.* 28, 61–83
5 Welch, G. (1977) *Prog. Biophys. Molec.*

Biol. 32, 103–191

6 Welch, G. and Keleti, T. (1981) *J. Theor. Biol.* 93, 701–735

7 Mitchell, P. (1959) *Annu. Rev. Microbiol.* 13, 407–440

8 Munkres, K. D. and Woodward, D. O. (1966) *Proc. Natl Acad. Sci. USA* 55, 1217–1224

9 Kiehn, E. D. and Holland, J. J. (1970) *Nature* 226, 544–545

10 Wetlaufer, D. B. (1981) *Adv. Prot. Chem.* 34, 61–92

11 Blake, C. (1983) *Nature* 306, 535–537

12 Remington, S., Wiegand, G. and Huber, R. (1982) *J. Mol. Biol.* 158, 111–152

13 Maugh, T. H. (1983) *Science* 221, 351–354

14 Rose, G. D. and Wetlaufer, D. B. (1977) *Nature* 268, 769-770

15 Matthew, J. B., Weber, P. C., Salemme, F. R. and Richards, F. M. (1983) *Nature* 301,169–171

16 Wodak, S. J. and Janin, J. (1980) *Proc. Natl Acad. Sci. USA* 77, 1736–1740

17 Richards, F. M. (1977) *Annu. Rev. Biophys. Bioeng.* 6, 151–176

18 Welch, G. R. and DeMoss, J. A. (1978) in *Microenvironments and Metabolic Compartmentation* (Srere, P. A. and Estabrook, R. W., eds), pp. 323–344, Academic Press

19 Manney, T. R. (1970) *J. Bacteriol.* 102, 483–488

20 Kempner, E. S. and Miller, J. H. (1968) *Exptl Cell Res.* 51, 150–156

21 Zalokar, M. (1960) *Exptl Cell Res.* 19, 114–132

22 Halper, L. H. and Srere, P. A. (1977) *Arch. Biochem. Biophys.* 184, 529–534

23 Sumegi, B., Gyocsi, L. and Alkonyi, I. *Biochim. Biophys. Acta* (in press)

24 Porpaczy, Z., Sumegi, B. and Alkonyi, I. (1983) *Biochim. Biophys. Acta* 749, 172–179

25 Beeckmans, S. and Kanarek, L. (1982) *Eur. J. Biochem.* 117, 527–535

26 Fahien, L. A. and Kmiotek, E. (1983) *Arch. Biochem. Biophys.* 220, 386–397

27 D'Souza, S. F. and Srere, P. A. (1983) *J. Biol. Chem.* 258, 4706–4709

28 Minton, A. P. (1981) *Biopolymers* 20, 2093–2120

29 McConkey, E. H. (1982) *Proc. Natl Acad. Sci. USA* 79, 3236–3240

30 Srere, P. A. and Estabrook, R. (eds) (1978) *Microenvironments and Metabolic Compartmentation*, Academic Press

Paul A. Srere is at the Pre-Clinical Science Unit, Veterans' Administration Medical Center, Dallas, TX 75216 and the Department of Biochemistry, The University of Texas Health Science Center at Dallas, 5323 Harry Hines Boulevard, Dallas, TX 75235, USA.

The role of phosphofructokinase in the Pasteur effect

Gopi A. Tejwani

The inhibition of glycolysis in the presence of oxygen is mediated through the changes in the concentrations of metabolites which regulate the activity of phosphofructo-kinase. Certain tissues which lack this control of glycolysis by respiration exhibit high aerobic glycolysis which is needed for the very survival of these tissues.

In 1861, Louis Pasteur observed that the rate of fermentation of sugar by yeast was higher in the absence of oxygen than when oxygen was present[1]. Sixty years later, Pasteur's original observation was confirmed by Warburg and Meyerhof, who independently observed that the production of lactic acid from glucose in various animal tissues was increased in the absence of oxygen. The term 'Pasteur effect' was introduced by Warburg and since then this phenomenon has been observed in a number of systems including skeletal muscle, heart, brain, kidney cortex, liver, Novikoff hepatoma, adeno-carcinoma, yeast and bacteria (see Ref. 2 for details).

The biochemical basis of the Pasteur effect is still unclear, although a number of possible explanations have been presented[3-6]. Some of the earlier theories were advanced by pioneer scientists like Warburg, Meyerhof, Burk, Lynen, and Lipmann, when little was known of complexity of allosteric regulation, and yet these theories are still valid[3]. For example, in 1941, Lynen[7] and Johnson[8] independently suggested that P_i was responsible for the enhanced glycolytic rate in the absence of oxygen. They observed that when oxygen is present, P_i is preferentially utilized for respiration and is not available for glycolysis. The involvement of P_i in the Pasteur effect was also supported by Loomis and Lipmann[9], who suggested that in the presence of oxygen, ATP was responsible for inhibition of glycolysis. They reported that nitrophenols uncouple phosphorylation from respiration and prevent the formation of ATP, which results in the increased rate of glycolysis in these cells.

The experimental evidence

In 1943, Engelhardt and Sakov[10] for the first time suggested that phospho-fructokinase which catalyses the phosphorylation of fructose 6-phosphate to fructose 1,6-bisphosphate in the presence of ATP, could be the site of the Pasteur effect. They reasoned that hexokinase could not be inhibited in the presence of oxygen because glucose 6-phosphate which is the product of hexokinase reaction was required in the oxidative shunt pathway of glucose degradation and therefore the formation of glucose 6-phosphate could not be inhibited under aerobic conditions. Furthermore, since fructose 1,6-bisphosphate was readily fermented in the presence of oxygen, which inhibited glucose fermentation, none of the reactions involved in the fermentation of fructose 1,6-bisphosphate could be the site of inhibition by oxygen. Thus by eliminating other stages they concluded that phosphofructokinase must be the site of the Pasteur effect.

Their hypothesis was supported by the experiments of Aisenberg and Potter[11] who, in 1957, observed that addition of a respiring mitochondrial preparation to the brain cytosol inhibited the conversion of glucose to lactate in brain cytosol. They postulated that an intermediate in oxidative phosphorylation, probably ATP, was responsible for this inhibition. It is noteworthy that about a year earlier Lardy and Parks[12] had observed the inhibition of partially purified rabbit skeletal muscle phosphofructokinase by ATP. This was conclusively proved by the studies of Lynen et al.[13] who observed a decrease in ATP and increase in P_i and fructose 1,6-bisphosphate concentrations upon transition from aerobic to anaerobic conditions in yeast, thus supporting the idea that a decrease in the concentration of ATP was largely responsible for the increased activity at the phosphofructokinase step.

Abrahams and Younathan[27] suggested that the concentration of NH_4^+, which is a powerful activator of phosphofructokinase, rises in certain tissues under anoxia. Cyclic AMP is shown to be an activator of phosphofructokinase and

recently it has been shown that cyclic GMP inhibits this enzyme[28]. In this context, it is interesting to note that recently Kobayashi et al.[29], observed a 5- to 13-fold increase in the concentration of cyclic AMP, and a 5-fold decrease in the concentration of cyclic GMP in brain during ischemia. A high concentration of NH_4^+ and a high ratio of cyclic AMP to cyclic GMP would increase the activity of phosphofructokinase, implicating this enzyme further in the mechanism of the Pasteur effect.

Regulation of phosphofructokinase activity by its allosteric effectors

Soon after the report of inhibition of phosphofructokinase by ATP yet another product of respiration was shown to be involved in the inhibition of this enzyme. Passonneau and Lowry observed that ATP[14] and citrate[21] inhibited the activity of phosphofructokinase and this inhibition was reversed by AMP, ADP and P_i. Salas et al.[15] identified citrate as the mitochondrial product that increases in aerobic conditions and

Table I. Effectors of phosphofructokinase[a]

Inhibitors	Activators[b]	Deinhibitors[c] of ATP, citrate, or Mg2+
ATP	$NH_4^{+\ d}$	3',5'-cyclic AMP
Citrate		5'-AMP
Mg^{2+}	$K^{+\ d}$	ADP
Ca^{2+}	P_i	Fructose 6-P
P-creatine		P_i
3-P-glycerate	5'-AMP	
P-enolpyruvate	3',5'-cyclic AMP	
2-P-glycerate	ADP	Fructose-1,6-bis-P
2,3-bis-P-glycerate	Fructose-1,6-bis-P	Glucose-1,6-bis-P
Oleate or Palmitate	peptide stabilizing	Mannose-1,6-bis-P
Fructose 1,6-bis-	factor	
phosphatase		
3',5'-cyclic GMP		

[a] Modified from Ref. 4.

[b] Activators increase the velocity of the phosphofructokinase reaction at noninhibitory concentrations of ATP.

[c] Deinhibitors increase the velocity of phosphofructokinase reaction at inhibitory concentrations of ATP.

[d] NH_4^+ and K^+ also increase the maximum velocity of enzyme.

inhibits phosphofructokinase in yeast. Since then, the number of metabolites which are known to regulate the activity of phosphofructokinase has increased to about 20 (Table I) and their action on this enzyme may serve as a mechanism by which glycolysis can be regulated *in vivo*. Thus the activity of phosphofructo-kinase is inhibited by one of its sub-strates, ATP, which also binds at an allosteric site resulting in the inhibition of enzyme.

The control of phosphofructokinase activity by ATP is visualized by Atkinson[16] in terms of the 'energy charge' of the adenylate system

$$[(ATP + \tfrac{1}{2}ADP)/(ATP + ADP + AMP)]$$

and it is defined as the fundamental metabolic control parameter that inver-sely alters phosphofructokinase activity. The energy charge of living systems is about 0.8–0.9. The inhibition of phos-phofructokinase activity by ATP, citrate or phosphoenolpyruvate is overcome by increasing the concentrations of positive effectors, such as, fructose 1,6-bisphosphate, fructose 6-phosphate, and P_i. A decrease in the energy charge facilitates the reaction of this enzyme by a decrease in the concentration of ATP and increase in concentrations of ADP and AMP. In 1966, Stadtman[17] had also suggested that activation of the phos-phofructokinase reaction under anaer-obic conditions is effected by a decrease in ATP concentrations of ADP, AMP and P_i, all positive effectors of enzyme in the cell[17]. Facilitation of phosphofructo-kinase reaction during anoxia has been demonstrated in almost all the tissues in which the Pasteur effect is observed[27].

Phosphofructokinase links with hexokinase and pyruvate kinase

One of the reasons why phospho-fructokinase activity is the limiting step in glycolysis is that regulation of activity of this enzyme in turn affects the activities of hexokinase and pyruvate kinase. In 1964, Lowry et al.[18] reported that the glycolytic flux was increased by about 6-fold in mouse brain during ischemia (anaerobic conditions). This effect was associated with a decrease in the intracellular concentrations of glu-cose, glucose 6-phosphate and fructose 6-phosphate, and by increase of all sub-strates from fructose 1,6-bisphosphate to lactate, indicating that the activity of phosphofructokinase is increased during ischemia (Table II). Activation of phos-phofructokinase under anaerobic con-ditions is also coupled to activation of hexokinase, because the decrease in the concentration of fructose 6-phosphate resulting from the activation of phos-phofructokinase leads to a decrease in the concentration of glucose 6-phos-phate (Table II). A decrease in the con-centration of glucose 6-phosphate which is a potent inhibitor of hexokinase results in the activation of hexokinase[22]. In addition, P_i and K^+ increase the activity of hexokinase as well as that of phosphofructokinase.

The activation of phosphofructo-kinase is also associated with activation of pyruvate kinase which is inhibited by alanine and ATP[23]. This inhibition of pyruvate kinase is overcome by fructose 1,6-bisphosphate, the concentrations of which increase during activation of phosphofructokinase (Table II).

Mechanisms of action of effectors

When glucose is a main source of energy, undergoing either oxidation or fermentation, the concentrations of ATP, ADP, AMP and P_i are ideal sig-nals for the control of glucose degrada-tion. In this situation, the maintenance of a high concentration of ATP by resynthesis from ADP and P_i is the physiological reason for glucose degra-dation. Phosphofructokinase from all mammalian tissues and various other sources is inhibited with higher con-centration of ATP and this inhibition is

Table II. Substrate levels in mouse brain after 25 seconds of ischemia[a]. All values are recorded as micromoles per kg wet weight

| Substrate | Concentrations | | Change as a result of ischemia (%) |
	Initial	Ischemia	
Glucose	2560	1930	−25
Glucose-6-P	224	91	−59
Fructose-6-P	50	27	−46
Fructose-1,6-bis-P	27	153	+467
Dihydroxyacetone-P	13	39	+200
Glyceraldehyde-P	0.9	3.3[b]	+267
1,3-bis-P-glycerate	<1	<1	0
3-P-glycerate	25	85	+240
2,3-bis-P-glycerate	29	29	0
2-P-glycerate	2.8	8.8	+214
P-pyruvate	3.5	8.5	+151
Pyruvate	39	72	+85
Lactate	770	1820	+136

[a]Data taken from Ref. 18.
[b] Sixty seconds after decapitation.

overcome by increasing the concentrations of AMP, ADP and P_i in the cell during anaerobic conditions. For example, as shown in Table III, the activity of mucosal phosphofructokinase with 0.2 mM fructose 6-phosphate is zero with ATP concentrations of 0.2 mM or 1.6 mM. In the presence of any single positive effector the activity of the enzyme with 0.2 mM ATP is a small fraction of maximum activity and in the presence of 1.6 mM ATP, it is only 0–3% of maximum activity. However, in the presence of AMP, ADP, P_i and NH_4^+ together, the maximum activity of enzyme is obtained with 0.2 mM ATP or 1.6 mM ATP. Such synergism among the positive effectors in deinhibiting the phosphofructokinase from skeletal muscle[19] and various other tissues has also been reported[26].

Inhibition of phosphofructokinase by ATP at the allosteric site results in an increase in the $(F6P)_{0.5}$ value, that is, the concentration of fructose 6-phosphate required for half-maximal activity of enzyme. AMP, ADP, P_i, NH_4^+, SO_4^{2-} increase the activity of enzyme by decreasing its $(F6P)_{0.5}$ value (Table IV).

These effectors decrease the $(F6P)_{0.5}$ value of phosphofructokinase in a synergistic manner, by 13-fold with non-inhibitory concentration of ATP (Table IV) and more than 20-fold with inhibitory concentration of ATP[20].

Physiological significance

Anaerobic glycolysis is a primitive mode of life and probably evolved when the atmosphere was devoid of oxygen. In anaerobic glycolysis much of the chemical energy of sugar is wasted by the cell with carbon by-products such as lactate or ethanol. Lactate formation can decrease the cellular pH leading to toxic effects and ethanol can have narcotic effects. Combustion of one mole of glucose, under anaerobic conditions, produces 2 moles of ATP, compared to 36 moles of ATP produced in the presence of oxygen. The existence of the Pasteur effect in most of the systems, therefore, means that whenever oxygen is available respiration plays a major role as a more economical and potentially less harmful mechanism for the synthesis of ATP. This is confirmed again by the fact that under anaerobic conditions, the rate of consumption of sugar by cells is six to eight times faster than under aerobic conditions[6].

There are certain tissues in which the rate of conversion of glucose to lactate is not affected by the presence of oxygen and therefore they normally have a high rate of aerobic glycolysis. These systems include striated muscle, intestinal mucosa or jejunum, renal medulla, erythrocytes, fetal tissues during parturition, malignant tumors, retina and leukocytes, etc. However, not much is known about the mechanisms(s) which can explain the high aerobic glycolysis in these tissues[3-5].

Phosphofructokinase from jejunal mucosa

Our efforts to explain the lack of the Pasteur effect in terms of properties of phosphofructokinase led us to partially purify this enzyme from rat-jejunal mucosa[2]. We also measured the concentrations of various effectors of this enzyme in the jejunum[20]. The jejunal phosphofructokinase, like the enzyme from many other sources, is inhibited by higher concentrations of ATP and this inhibition is reversed by the positive effectors such as AMP, ADP, P_i and NH_4^+ (Table III). However, the concentrations of NH_4^+ in the jejunum is very high and it is about 4, 5 and 150 times higher than the concentration of NH_4^+ in the brain, liver and resting skeletal muscle respectively[20]. A high concentration of NH_4^+ deinhibits the enzyme by acting synergistically with other positive effectors and maintains a high aerobic glycolytic rate. In fact, the assay of jejunal phosphofructokinase with its effectors maintained at physiological concentrations resulted in maximal activity of the enzyme, which was not increased further by increasing the concentrations of positive effectors[20].

Thus it appears that phosphofructokinase in jejunal mucosa is maximally active. However, the enzyme activity in vivo can be still regulated. The phosphofructokinase activity and the glycolytic rate in intestinal mucosa is mainly controlled by the concentration of fructose 6-phosphate, which is a substrate and a positive effector of phosphofructokinase[20]. In jejunum as much as 50% of the absorbed fructose is immediately phosphorylated and ultimately appears as lactate. It is noteworthy that glycolytic enzymes are adaptive in this tissue. The activities of hexokinase, glucokinase, fructokinase, phosphofructokinase and pyruvate kinase in rat jejunum decrease on fasting and increase on feeding glucose or fructose[24].

Table III. Effect of positive effectors, separately and in combination, on the activity of phosphofructokinase[a]

| | | | | Relative activity | |
AMP (mM)	ADP (mM)	P_i (mM)	NH_4^+ (mM)	ATP (0.2 mM)	ATP (1.6 mM)
0	0	0	0	0	0
0.20	0	0	0	8	0
0	0.80	0	0	6	3
0	0	1.0	0	16	3
0	0	0	2.0	6	0
0.20	0	1.0	2.0	97	74
0.20	0.80	1.0	2.0	100	93

[a] Modified from Ref. 2.
0.2 mM fructose 6-phosphate was used in assay system. For details of assay system see Ref. 2.

Table IV. Effect of positive effectors separately and in combination on the $(F6P)_{0.5}$ value of phospho-fructokinase[a]

AMP (mM)	ADP (mM)	P_i (mM)	NH_4^+ (mM)	SO_4^{2-} (mM)	$(F6P)_{0.5}$ value[b] relative to control
0	0	0	0	0	1.0
0	0	0	0.30	0	1.0
0	0.76	0	0	0	0.46
0	0	0	0	0.50	0.40
0	0	0.50	0	0	0.32
1.0	0	0	0	0	0.28
0	0	0	0.30	0.50	0.32
0	0	0.50	0.30	0	0.22
1.0	0	0.50	0	0	0.16
0	0.95	0.50	0.30	0	0.09
1.0	0	0.50	0.30	0	0.08

[a] Data taken from Ref. 2. The enzyme was assayed with varying concentrations of fructose-6-P and 0.2 mM ATP.

[b] $(F6P)_{0.5}$ value refers to the concentration of fructose 6-phosphate required for half-maximal activity of enzyme.

Tissues lacking the Pasteur effect

In most of the tissues, the function of glycolysis is to provide ATP and other intermediates required for the biosynthetic pathways, which is then stringently controlled to suit the immediate demands of the cell. However, there are many other tissues where the Pasteur effect is not observed. Although no single mechanism can satisfactorily explain the lack of the Pasteur effect in all cases, it appears that high aerobic glycolysis is needed for the immediate survival of these tissues.

For example, in the intestinal mucosa, the glycolytic pathway serves the additional function of converting glucose and other sugars to lactate, an obligatory step in their transport from the intestine to liver[25]. During severe exercise the oxidation of glycose via the tricarboxylic acid cycle is not sufficient to provide ATP at a rate required for contraction of muscle and is therefore supplemented by aerobic glycolysis in striated muscle.

Retina has a sparse population of mitochondria which is correlated with the absence of blood vessels and therefore most of the ATP is produced through aerobic glycolysis. If respiration were to be the major source of ATP in retina, light absorption by the red blood cells, and decrease in transparency of retina by light scattering caused by mitochondria would interfere with visual perception[3].

Large glycogen reserves accumulate in fetal tissues towards the end of term. In the liver the glycogen reserves can rise to 10% of the wet weight. This is matched by a high glycolytic capacity of fetal tissues and the organs of the new-born. The fact that new-born babies can survive anaerobiosis for 30 min is no doubt connected with the high glycolytic capacity of the new-born. Lastly, the proportion of energy derived from glycolysis is very high in neoplastic tissue which contributes to their uncontrolled growth[3,5].

In summary

The inhibition of glycolysis in the presence of oxygen, that is, the Pasteur effect, remained unexplained until recently when the properties of key glycolytic enzymes were studied in detail. It is fair to conclude that the allosteric properties of phosphofructo-kinase can account for most aspects of the Pasteur effect. The glycolysis is regulated mainly by alteration in the concentrations of numerous effectors of phosphofructokinase in the cell. Although no single mechanism can satisfactorily explain the lack of Pasteur effect, that is, high aerobic glycolysis observed in many tissues, it appears that the high aerobic glycolysis is needed for the very survival of these tissues. In the intestinal mucosa, high aerobic glycolysis may be the result of high activity of phosphofructokinase maintained by the favorable ratio of positive to negative effectors of this enzyme.

References

1 Pasteur, L. (1861) *C.R. Acad. Sci.* 52, 1260–1264
2 Tejwani, G. A. and Ramaiah, A. (1971) *Biochem. J.* 125, 507–514
3 Krebs, H. A. (1972) *Essays Biochem.* 8, 1–35
4 Tejwani, G. A. (1973) *Ph.D. Thesis* submitted to All-India Institute of Medical Sciences, New Delhi
5 Ramaiah, A. (1974) *Curr. Top. Cell. Regul.* 8, 297–345
6 Sols, A. (1976) in *Reflections on Biochemistry* (Kornberg, A., Horecker, B. L., Cornudella, L. and Oro, J., eds), pp. 199–206, Pergamon Press, New York
7 Lynen F. (1941) *Justus Liebigs Ann. Chem.* 546, 120–141
8 Johnson, M. (1941) *Science* 94, 200–202
9 Loomis, W. F. and Lipmann, F. (1948) *J. Biol. Chem.* 173, 807–808
10 Engelhardt, V. A. and Sakov, N. E. (1943) *Biokhimiya* 8, 9–36
11 Aisenberg, A. C. and Potter, V. R. (1957) *J. Biol. Chem.* 224, 1115–1127
12 Lardy, H. A. and Parks, R. E., Jr (1956) in *Enzymes: Units of Biological Structure and Function* (Gaebler, O. H., ed.), pp. 584–587, Academic Press, New York
13 Lynen, F., Hartman, G., Netter, K. F. and Schuegraf, A. (1959) in *Ciba Foundation Symposium on Regulation of Cell Metabolism* (Wolstenholme, G. E. W. and O'Connor, C. M., eds), pp. 256–273, J. and A. Churchill, Ltd, London
14 Possonneau, J. V. and Lowry, O. H. (1962) *Biochem. Biophys. Res. Commun.* 7, 10–15
15 Salas, M. L., Vinuela, E., Salas, M. and Sols, A. (1965) *Biochem. Biophys. Res. Commun.* 19, 371–376
16 Atkinson, D. E. (1968) *Biochemistry* 7, 4030–4034
17 Stadtman, E. R. (1966) *Adv. Enzymol.* 28, 41–154
18 Lowry, O. H., Passonneau, J. V., Hasselberger, F. X. and Schulz, D. W. (1964) *J. Biol. Chem.* 239, 18–30
19 Tejwani, G. A., Ramaiah, A. and Ananthanarayanan, M. (1973) *Arch. Biochem. Biophys.* 158, 195–199
20 Tejwani, G. A., Kaur, J., Ananthananayanan, M. and Ramaiah, A. (1974) *Biochim. Biophys. Acta* 370, 120–129
21 Possonneau, J. V. and Lowry, O. H. (1963) *Biochem. Biophys. Res. Commun.* 13, 372–379
22 Walker, D. G. (1966) *Essays Biochem.* 2, 33–67
23 Seubert, W. and Schoner, W. (1971) *Curr. Top. Cell Regul.* 3, 237–267
24 Stifel, F. B., Rosensweig, N. S., Zakim, D. and Herman, R. H. (1968) *Biochim. Biophys, Acta* 170, 221–227
25 Wiseman, G. (1964) *Absorption from the Intestine*, Academic Press
26 Bloxham, D. P. and Lardy, H. A. (1973) in *The Enzyme* (Boyer, P. D., ed.), pp. 239–278, Academic Press, Inc., New York
27 Abrahams, S. L. and Younathan, E. S. (1971) *J. Biol. Chem.* 246, 2464–2467
28 Beitner, R., Haberman, S. and Cycowitz, T. (1977) *Biochim. Biophys. Acta* 482, 330–340
29 Kobayashi, M., Lust, W. D. and Passonneau, J. V. (1977) *J. Neurochem.* 29, 53–59

G. A. Tejwani is at the Department of Pharmacology and Radiology, College of Medicine, The Ohio State University, Colombus, OH 43210, USA.

Addendum

During the last few years, major discoveries have been made which further support the sensitive role played by phosphofructokinase in regulation of glucose metabolism.

Regulation by fructose 2,6-bisphosphate

Fructose 2,6-bisphosphate is the most potent activator of phosphofructokinase discovered so far. It stimulates the activity of phosphofructokinase from all the mammalian species studied, as well as the enzyme from yeast. In many systems, the activity of phosphofructokinase is negligible in the presence of physiological concentration of substrates, especially in the presence of its negative effector, ATP. Fructose 2,6-bisphosphate overcomes the inhibition of phosphofructokinase by ATP and acts synergistically with AMP to increase the activity of the enzyme. It is also an inhibitor of fructose-1,6-bisphosphatase. Fructose 2,6-bisphosphate is formed from fructose 6-phosphate and ATP by fructose-6-P,2-kinase and hydrolysed by fructose-2,6-phosphatase. The stimulation of glycolysis by glucose is now explained by the accumulation of fructose 2,6-bisphosphate which allows phosphofructokinase to work even in the presence of inhibitory concentrations of ATP. However, the concentration of fructose 2,6-bisphosphate is not elevated in anoxia or during muscular contraction, and therefore it may not be involved in the facilitation of phosphofructokinase reaction during anaerobic conditions.

It has been proposed that fructose 2,6-bisphosphate stimulates glycolysis mainly for anabolic purposes such as lipogenesis[30-34].

Critical role of ammonium and inorganic phosphate in yeast

Recent studies done on *Saccharomyces cerevisiae* have indicated that the Pasteur effect is not characteristic of growing yeast, but takes place in special conditions like resting yeast cells or cultures in chemostat with limited sugar. The lack of Pasteur effect in growing yeast cells has been ascribed to a high concentration of NH_4^+ (5.5 mM) in these cells, which keeps phosphofructokinase stimulated. In contrast, the NH_4^+ concentration in the resting cells is 0.5 mM which results in the reduced rate of fermentation[35]. In the growing yeast cells which *do* exhibit the Pasteur effect, measurements of the metabolite levels show that a crossover exists at the level of phosphofructokinase. The concentrations of hexose monophosphates decrease in anaerobic conditions and the concentration of fructose 1,6-bisphosphate increases. An increase in the P_i concentration observed during these conditions is the main stimulus for phosphofructokinase activity in yeast during anaerobiosis[36].

Pasteur effect regulates enzyme content

Until a few years ago, regulation of glycolysis under anaerobic conditions was thought to occur primarily at the level of enhanced glycolytic flux, mediated by changes in the activity of the key enzymes without affecting their total contents. However, recent studies indicate that this regulation also occurs at the level of enzyme content[37-39]. Chronic hypoxia stimulates the activity of all the glycolytic enzymes and is associated with an increase in glycolytic capacity in the rat skeletal muscle cells (L8). Phosphofructokinase[37] and pyruvate kinase[38] concentrations per cell are more than doubled in cultures maintained under chronic hypoxic conditions compared to cultures under normoxic conditions. These studies have been confirmed in L2 lung cells, WI-38 fibroblasts and mouse lung macrophages[38,39].

References

30 Hers, H. G. and Hue, L. (1938) *Annu. Rev. Biochem.* 52, 617–653

31 Hue, L. (1983) *Biochem. Soc. Trans.* 11, 246–247

32 Pilkis, S. J., El-Maghrabi, M. R., McGrane, M., Pilkis, J., Fox, E. and Clause, T. H. (1982) *Mol. Cell. Endocrinol.* 25, 245–266

33 Uyeda, K., Furuya, E., Richard, C. S. and Yokoyama, M. (1982) *Mol. Cell. Biochem.* 48, 97–120

34 Tejwani, G. A. (1983) *Advan. Enzymol. Relat. Areas Mol. Biol.* 54, 121–193

35 Lagunas, R., Dominguez, C., Busturia, A. and Saez. M. J. (1982) *J. Bacteriol.* 152, 19–25

36 Lagunas, R. and Gancedo, C. (1983) *Eur. J. Biochem.* 137, 479–483

37 Ptashne, K. A., Theodore, J. and Robin, E. D. (1983) *Biochim. Biophys. Acta* 763, 169–174

38 Hance, A. J., Robin, E. D., Simon, L. M., Alexander, S., Herzenberg, L. A. and Theodore, J. (1980) *J. Clin. Invest.* 66, 1258–1261

39 Robin, E. D., Murphy, B. J. and Theodore, J. (1984) *J. Cell Physiol.* 118, 287–290

Cyclic AMP and the synthesis of phosphoenolpyruvate carboxykinase (GTP) mRNA

Herman Meisner, Wouter H. Lamers and Richard W. Hanson

The regulation of cytosolic phosphoenolpyruvate carboxykinase RNA by cyclic-AMP-dependent hormones is discussed, with special emphasis on transcriptional control in isolated nuclei. A model is proposed to account for stimulation of phosphoenolpyruvate carboxykinase RNA synthesis by cyclic AMP.

Effect of hormones on concentrations of PEPCK enzyme and its mRNA

The response of the cytosolic form of phosphoenolpyruvate carboxykinase (GTP) (EC 4.1.1.32) (PEPCK) in rat liver and kidney to a variety of hormones has been intensively studied. In liver, the synthesis of the enzyme is regulated by the relative· concentration of glucagon and insulin[1], and by catecholamines. Injection of glucagon increases intracellular cAMP concentration and stimulates the synthesis of PEPCK[2], while a fall in glucagon or an increase in the insulin/glucagon ratio reduces enzyme synthesis[1]. Stimulation of the sympathetic nervous system *in vivo* or adding catecholamines to primary cultures of hepatocytes increases the concentration of intracellular cAMP and stimulates the synthesis of PEPCK[3]. The central role of cAMP in the hormonal regulation of PEPCK is underscored by the fact that administration of dibutyryl cyclic AMP (Bt$_2$cAMP) to rats re-fed with glucose stimulates enzyme synthesis eight-fold within 90 min[4].

We have measured hormone-dependent changes in the concentration of mRNA coding for PEPCK by *in vitro* RNA transla· tion, and RNA–DNA hybridization using a cDNA to PEPCK mRNA[5]. Glucose re-feeding of starved rats, a process that inhibits hepatic gluconeogenesis and PEPCK synthesis, results in a reduction of both cytosolic and nuclear mRNA for PEPCK. This process has a half-life of about 20 min. Similar turnover times of the cytosolic PEPCK mRNA in starved rats have been obtained by administering cordycepin, an inhibitor of mRNA processing, and α-amanitin, a polymerase II inhibitor, and measuring the disappearance of mRNA[6]. The molecular basis for this rapid turnover rate is not understood, although work in other systems has suggested that size of the mature mRNA and length of the poly(A) segment may be important considerations[7,8].

Cyclic AMP and transcription of the PEPCK gene

The mechanism by which cAMP-dependent hormones control the synthesis of hepatic enzymes is controversial. Earlier work had suggested that cAMP regulated both PEPCK[9] and tyrosine aminotransferase enzymes at the level of translation[10,11]. This conclusion was based, in large part, on the induction of PEPCK activity by Bt$_2$cAMP in animals or Reuber H-35 cells treated with actinomycin D, an inhibitor of RNA synthesis[12,13]. More recent studies using DNA–RNA hybridization techniques have shown that injection of Bt$_2$cAMP into rats re-fed with glucose causes an eight-fold increase in the concentration of PEPCK mRNA within 1 hour[14,15], suggesting that cAMP acts transcriptionally. However, recently Noguchi *et al.*[11] have presented evidence that Bt$_2$cAMP increases the level of translatable mRNA for tyrosine amino-transferase in livers of adrenalectomized rats by altering the rate of template translation so that it is possible that the cyclic nucleotide acts at several sites during enzyme induction.

To test directly whether cAMP acts on RNA synthesis, we isolated hepatic nuclei from rats in different nutritional and hormonal conditions, and measured the incorporation of $\alpha[^{32}P]UTP$ into hybridizable RNA for PEPCK[16]. Under these conditions most of the labeled RNA is derived from elongation of nascent molecules synthesized from the engaged DNA-dependent RNA polymerases in the transcriptional apparatus, and therefore reflects rates of synthesis at the moment of nuclear isolation. The basal rate of transcription of PEPCK mRNA by hepatic nuclei from rats re-fed with glucose was found to be 400 p.p.m., or 0.04%. Adrenalectomy, which reduces the circulating glucocorticoid level, did not lower this synthesis rate further. By contrast, in nuclei isolated from livers of starved rats, the rate of gene transcription increases to 3 500 p.p.m. When rats re-fed with glucose were injected with Bt2cAMP, the rate of hepatic PEPCK RNA synthesis increased approximately seven-fold within 15 min. Similarly, glucose re-feeding of starved rats reduced the rate of transcription of PEPCK RNA over 90% in 2 hours, with a half-time of about 30 min. However, we could find no effect of Bt2cAMP on the transcription of the albumin gene, suggesting that the effect of the cyclic nucleotide is specific and not due to a general activation of RNA polymerase II.

Using PEPCK cDNA as a hybridization probe, we also demonstrated a number of putative nuclear RNA precursors ranging in length from 6.5 kb to about 3.0 kb, as well as three nuclear RNA species shorter than the 2.8 kb length of mature, cytosolic PEPCK mRNA[14] (Fig. 1). All of these nuclear RNA species contain a poly(A) tract and are found only in the nucleus. The sequence abundance of these nuclear RNAs changes dramatically upon glucose re-

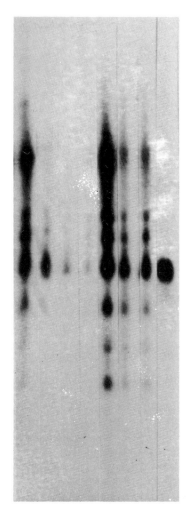

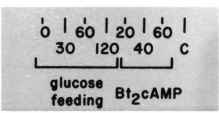

Fig. 1. Effect of glucose and dibutyryl cyclic AMP on P-enolpyruvate carboxykinase mRNA level in rat liver nuclei. Starved and adrenalectomized rats were refed glucose at 0 min, and injected with Bt2cAMP at 120 min[16]. Nuclear RNA was isolated from livers at the indicated times, electrophoresed, and after transfer to nitrocellulose, hybridized to a [^{32}P]cDNA for P-enolpyruvate carboxykinase. The line marked C represents cytosolic P-enolpyruvate carboxykinase mRNA (2.8 kilobases).

feeding or after the administration of Bt₂cAMP (see Fig. 1) in a manner that directly parallels the change in the transcription rate of the PEPCK gene. Preliminary studies using specific intron probes suggest that these precursors represent processing intermediates in the maturation of the primary transcript of the PEPCK gene, which is approximately 6 kb in length (Yoo-Warren et al., unpublished observations).

We conclude from these studies that cAMP stimulates the synthesis of PEPCK by specifically increasing the rate of transcription of the gene for the enzyme, and that a decrease in cAMP, which occurs with glucose re-feeding due to a reduced glucagon/insulin ratio, acutely depresses transcription. To our knowledge, the only other direct example of a cAMP-dependent effect on gene transcription in higher eukaryotes is the report by Maurer[17] that the synthesis of prolactin mRNA in cells from the anterior pituitary gland of rats treated with ergotamine is restored to normal by Bt₂cAMP.

In Table I, we compare the rate of synthesis of the PEPCK gene with other genes that have been transcribed using this same technique. It is rather striking that the synthesis rate of PEPCK in the de-induced state is comparable to the rates found for several considerably more abundant mRNAs such as prolactin[17], growth hormone and albumin, while in the induced state the rate is as great as that found for the heat-shock genes of Drosophila[18,19] or estrogen-activated ovalbumin synthesis in chick oviducts[22,23]. The synthesis rate of the gene for the major heat-shock protein (3 000 p.p.m.) is unusually high, in part because most of the RNA normally transcribed by polymerase II is inhibited[18]. Table I also shows that the sequence abundance for PEPCK mRNA in the induced state is about 1% of the poly(A)⁺ RNA, which is considerably less than that determined for other species of mRNA synthes-

Table I. Transcription rate and steady-state concentration of polymerase-II-dependent RNA from various sources

Gene	Source	Total cell mRNA(%)	Transcription rate (p.p.m.)	Refs
Heat-shock (87°C)	Heat-shocked Drosophila	–	3 000[a]	18
α_{2u}-Globulin	Rat liver	0.002	50	21
Prolactin	Bovine anterior pituitary	18	400–650	17, 20
Growth hormone	Bovine anterior pituitary	13	270	20; Meisner unpublished
Ovalbumin	DES[b]-stimulated chick oviducts	50	1 540	22, 23
Conalbumin	DES-stimulated chick oviducts	10	800	22, 24
P-enolpyruvate carboxykinase	Rats re-fed with glucose	0.2	400	16
	Starved or cAMP stimulated rat liver	1.0	3 500	16
Metallothionine	Steroid-treated rat liver	0.7	260	25
Albumin	Rat liver	10	300	25; Meisner, unpublished

[a] Rate of synthesis/gene, based on six copies/cell[18].

[b] DES = diethylstilbesterol.

ized at a comparable rate. The high turnover rate of PEPCK mRNA is responsible for its relatively low intracellular steady-state level, and the response of the gene to cAMP appears to be the result of a rapid increase in the rate of its transcription.

Mechanism of action of cAMP on transcription of PEPCK genes

Our current hypothesis for the regulation of hepatic PEPCK mRNA synthesis is that cAMP-dependent hormones generate a cytosolic factor, perhaps a phosphoprotein, which diffuses into the nucleus and mediates the induction of the PEPCK gene. Glucose blocks the synthesis of PEPCK mRNA by stimulating insulin secretion which lowers the concentration of the putative transcription effector via a cAMP-independent mechanism. The proposed cAMP-generated factor has not been isolated as yet. However, using isolated nuclei, marked stimulation of transcription of the heat-shock genes in *Drosophila*[26] and the β-casein gene in mammary tissues[27] by cellular extracts from the respective tissue has been described. Kelly *et al.*[28] have partially purified the β-casein gene effector from mammary tissue and found it to be a protein with a mol. wt of about 1 500.

The cAMP-generated factor is pictured as binding to a control region near the PEPCK gene, thereby enhancing transcription by allowing greater contact between RNA polymerase II and the TATA sequence located 5' to the initiation start site. The region on the DNA to which this putative effector binds may be an upstream control region that several groups have shown modulates the efficiency of transcription *in vivo*[29-31]. A clear example of the interaction of a protein with the upstream control region is the binding of T-antigen to a sequence of SV40 DNA close to the TATA box, and the subsequent inhibition of early SV40 virus transcription[32]. Interestingly, the T-antigen, which is a phosphoprotein, acts by blocking initiation of transcription, rather than by retarding the movement of RNA polymerase along the DNA. If the putative cAMP-generated factor affects PEPCK transcription in an analogous manner, only newly initiated RNA molecules should be affected.

In summary, the rapidity and magnitude by which the gene coding for cytoplasmic PEPCK in hepatic tissue responds to intracellular cyclic AMP concentration provides an excellent model to examine various molecular aspects of cAMP-dependent hormone action. A nearly full length cDNA as well as the entire genomic DNA of PEPCK were recently isolated in our laboratory, and these probes are being used to answer questions such as the nature of cytosolic factor(s) involved in gene expression, nuclear processing of PEPCK hnRNA, and DNA sequences necessary for expression in the region around the transcription start site.

References

1 Tilghman, S., Gunn, M., Fisher, L., Hanson, R. W., Reshef, L. and Ballard, J. (1975) *J. Biol. Chem.* 250, 3322–3329
2 Wicks, W. D., Lewis, W. and McKibbin, J. (1972) *Biochim. Biophys. Acta* 264, 177–185
3 Wolfle, D., Hartmann, H. and Jungermann, K. (1981) *Biochem. Biophys. Res. Commun.* 98, 1084–1090
4 Iynedjian, P. and Hanson, R. W. (1977) *J. Biol. Chem.* 252, 655–662
5 Yoo-Warren, H., Cimbala, M., Felz, K., Monahan, J., Leis, J. and Hanson, R. W. (1981) *J. Biol. Chem.* 256, 10225–10227
6 Nelson, K., Cimbala, M. and Hanson, R. W. (1980) *J. Biol. Chem.* 255, 8509–8515
7 Meyuhas, O. and Perry, R. (1979) *Cell* 16, 139–148
8 Nudel, U., Soveq, H., Littauer, U., Marbaix, G., Huez, G., LeClercq, M., Hubert, E. and Chantrenne, H. (1976) *Eur. J. Biochem.* 64, 115–125
9 Wicks, W. and McKibbin, J. (1972) *Biochem. Biophys. Res. Commun.* 48, 205–211
10 Roper, M. and Wicks, W. (1978) *Proc. Natl Acad. Sci. USA* 75, 140–144
11 Noguchi, T., Diesterhaft, M. and Grammer, D. (1982) *J. Biol. Chem.* 257, 2386–2390
12 Wicks, W. (1974) *Adv. Cyclic Nucleotide Res.* 4, 335–438
13 Tilghman, S. M., Hanson, R. W. and Ballard, F. J. (1976) in *Gluconeogenesis: Its Regulation in Mammalian Species* (Hanson, R. W. and Mehlman, M. A., eds), pp. 47–87, John Wiley

and Sons, New York

14 Cimbala, M., Lamers, W., Nelson, K., Monahan, Y., Yoo-Warren, H. and Hanson, R. W. (1982) *J. Biol. Chem.* 257, 7629–7636

15 Beale, E., Hartley, J. and Granner, D. (1982) *J. Biol. Chem.* 257, 2022–2028

16 Lamers, W., Hanson, R. W. and Meisner, H. (1982) *Proc. Natl Acad. Sci. USA* 79, 5137–5143

17 Maurer, R. (1981) *Nature (London)* 294, 94–97

18 Ashburner, M. and Bonner, J. (1979) *Cell* 17, 241–254

19 Craine, B. and Kornberg, T. (1981) *Cell* 25, 671–681

20 Miller, W., Martial, J. and Baxter, J. (1980) *J. Biol. Chem.* 255, 7521–7524

21 Chan, K.-M., Kurtz, D. and Feigelson, P. (1978) *Biochemistry* 17, 3092–3096

22 Palmiter, R. (1975) *Cell* 4, 189–197

23 McKnight, S. and Palmiter, R. (1979) *J. Biol. Chem.* 254, 9050–9058

24 Palmiter, R., Mulvihill, E., McKnight, G. and Senear, A. (1978) *Cold Spring Harbor Symp. Quant. Biol.* 42, 639–649

25 Hager, L. and Palmiter, R. (1981) *Nature (London)* 291, 340–342

26 Craine, B. and Kornberg, T. (1981) *Biochemistry* 20, 6584–6589

27 Teyssot, B., Houdebine, L.-M. and Djiane, J. (1981) *Proc. Natl Acad. Sci. USA* 78, 6729–6733

28 Kelly, P., Djiane, J., Houdebine, L. and Teyssot, B. (1982) *J. Cell Biochem., Suppl.* 6, 175

29 McKnight, S. and Kingsbury, R. (1982) *Science* 217, 316–324

30 Breathnach, R. and Chambon, P. (1981) *Annu. Rev. Biochem.* 50, 349–385

31 Grosschedl, R. and Birnstiel, M. (1980) *Proc. Natl Acad. Sci. USA* 77, 1432–1440

32 Tjian, R. (1981) *Cell* 26, 1–2

Herman Meisner and Richard W. Hanson are at the Department of Pharmacology (H.M) and Biochemistry (R.W.H.), School of Medicine, Case Western Reserve University, Cleveland, OH 44106, USA. Wouter H. Lamers is at the Department of Anatomy and Embryology, University of Amsterdam, Amsterdam, The Netherlands.

Fine tuning of blood glucose concentrations

Robert C. Nordlie

Blood glucose homeostasis is maintained by the correct balance between phosphoryl-ation of glucose and hydrolysis of glucose 6-phosphate in the liver. The enzyme glucose-6-phosphatase can synthesize glucose 6-phosphate as well as degrade it, and its synthetic activity therefore acts as an adjunct to glucokinase activity. The ratio of this phosphotransferase activity of glucose-6-phosphatase to the activity of gluco-kinase may adjust to maintain the steady-state blood glucose concentration as the physiological circumstances demand.

The most important factors affecting blood glucose concentration are:

(1) The rate of consumption of dietary carbohydrate.

(2) The rate of intestinal absorption of dietary carbohydrates.

(3) The rate of utilization of glucose by peripheral tissues.

(4) The rate of loss of glucose through the kidney tubule.

(5) The rate of removal of glucose from the blood by the liver.

(6) The rate and extent of release of glucose from liver via glycogenolysis plus gluconeogenesis[1].

The predominant mechanisms for controlling these factors, and therefore maintaining blood glucose homeostasis, occur in the liver, and are shown in Fig. 1.

The liver is essentially an energy reservoir, being capable of taking up and storing (as glycogen) glucose in times of plenty (after a meal) and of releasing this stored potential chemical energy in times of need (in brief fasting glycogenolysis). In addition, the liver can manufacture and release glucose in situations of pronounced need, as in starvation or untreated diabetes mellitus (gluconeogenesis). There are two major reactions in this hepatic machinery for hexose-sugar homeostasis: (1) the enzyme-catalysed phosphorylation of glucose (reaction B, Fig. 1) and (2) the release of glucose *via* hydrolysis of glucose 6-phosphate (reaction A, Fig. 1). The hepatocyte, unlike most cells, is freely permeable to glucose but not to charged glucose 6-phosphate molecules which, once formed, are effectively trapped within the liver cell. Therefore, the direction and net rate of flux of glucose between the hepatic cell and the blood is ultimately determined by the relative rates of glucose phosphorylation and opposing glucose 6-phosphate hydrolysis. If the rate of hydrolysis exceeds that of phosphorylation, a net release of glucose ensues in the liver cell and this sugar passes to the blood. In contrast, when the rate of phosphoryl-ation exceeds that of glucose 6-phosphate hydrolysis, a net uptake of glucose from the blood by the hepatocyte occurs. At some critical 'null point' glucose concen-tration, approximating the ambient blood glucose concentration, the two opposing reaction rates are equal and no *net* transfer of glucose occurs be-tween the liver cell and the blood.

Earlier experiments, analyses and discussions of these tuning mechanisms were reviewed in *TIBS*[2] and elsewhere[3]. Results of this analysis are summarized in Fig. 2, which shows why the classical idea that glucose 6-phosphate is syn-

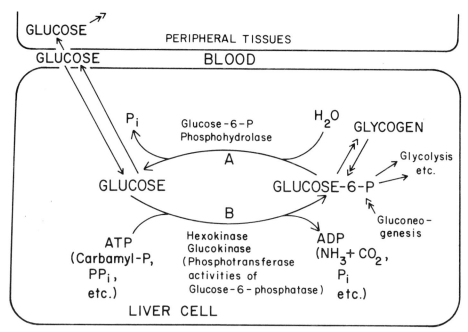

Fig. 1. Interrelationships among liver, blood, and peripheral tissues with respect to glucose flow and utilization. Net rate and direction of flux of glucose between blood and the homeostatic organ, liver, are determined by the relative rates of glucose phosphorylation (B) and glucose 6-phosphate hydrolysis (A), as generally postulated by Hastings and co-workers[1]. Inclusion of synthetic activity of glucose-6-phosphatase is suggested by the present author. From Nordlie[2]; reproduced by permission of Academic Press.

thesized by glucokinase* and hydrolysed by glucose-6-phosphatase had to be modified. If the traditional idea was correct, then at some concentration of glucose approximating the physiological concentration, the kinase and phosphatase activities should be equal and intersect on the graph; they do not. Unconstrained glucose-6-phosphatase activity of normal, fed rat liver exceeded that of glucokinase at all concentrations of glucose considered (Fig. 2a). A cross-over equivalence point in activities of the enzymes of glucose utilization and production could be obtained when glucose-6-phosphatase was adjusted for latency and inhibitions by known metabolite-inhibitors; however, this cross-over was obtained with approximately 10 mM glucose (Fig. 2b). A comparable analysis, with the use of

glucokinase and adjusted glucose-6-phosphatase activities of diabetic rat liver and normal, fed chicken liver resulted in no cross-over equivalence points with glucose-6-phosphatase and glucokinase at glucose concentrations ranging to 60 mM (Fig. 2c and d).

It follows then, that these results can be explained in one of three ways: (1) The further repression of glucose-6-phosphatase or activation of glucokinase. (2) The concentrations of glucokinase *in vivo* are higher than those observed in conventional *in vitro* techniques. (3) Glucokinase activity is not the only mechanism for glucose phosphorylation. Possibility (1), that glucose-6-phosphatase may be regulated by covalent modifications involving protein phosphorylation/ dephosphorylation was examined and proved to be incorrect[4]. Glucokinase is an allosteric enzyme, but only negative inhibition is known, and in any case,

*Hexokinase does not play a significant role in the liver.

given the low concentrations of glucokinase in diabetic rat liver or normal
chicken liver, the enzyme activity would
have to increase many-fold to produce a
satisfactory cross-over point of equivalence commensurate with observed concentrations of blood glucose (see Fig. 2c
and d). This low concentration of glucokinase also makes the second possibility
unlikely.

More recent studies have, therefore,
been devoted to the possible participation of an auxiliary enzyme in hepatic
glucose phosphorylation.

Liver perfusion studies

The first of these studies was an
attempt to correlate observed rates of
net glucose uptake by isolated perfused
livers of rats which had been fed or
fasted for 48 h with relevant enzyme
activities measured in the same livers[5].
At most concentrations of glucose
tested, rates of net glucose uptake significantly exceeded rates that would be
expected from observed glucokinase
activities (the net change in glucose
uptake is the rate of glucose phosphorylation minus the rate of activity of
glucose-6-phosphatase). The disparity
between glucokinase activity and net
glucose uptake became progressively
greater as the glucose concentration
increased, consistent with the involvement of a second glucose phosphorylating
enzyme with high K_m for glucose.

The tuning–retuning hypothesis

These and other experiments suggested that the synthetic activities of
glucose-6-phosphatase are the adjunct
to glucokinase activity in hepatic
glucose phosphorylation[3]. Figure 3
depicts concisely the biosynthetic and
hydrolytic functions of glucose-6-
phosphatase, which have been described
more fully elsewhere[2,3,6,7]. Carbamyl-
phosphate and PP_i are the most effective
phosphoryl donors in the phosphotransferase reaction typified by the equation:

$$PP_i + \text{D-glucose} \rightarrow \text{D-glucose 6-phosphate} + P_i$$

The involvement of two enzymes
rather than one in phosphorylating
glucose led to the development of the
tuning–retuning hypothesis for glucose
homeostasis[2,3]. Glucokinase is positively
induced by insulin and has a K_m for
glucose of 5–10 mM. In contrast, the
phosphotransferase activity of glucose-
6-phosphatase increases in the absence
of insulin and has a much higher K_m for
glucose (40–125 mM). When the proportion of phosphotransferase activity
increases relative to that of glucokinase
the reaction velocity curve (see Fig. 2)
'flattens' indicating that for any given
concentration of glucose, the rate of
phosphorylation is reduced. This,
together with an increase in the
phosphohydrolase activity of glucose-6-
phosphatase causes the equivalence null
point glucose concentration to shift to
the right (see Fig. 2c and d compared
with b). Applying this system to diabetes
mellitus, in all but the severest cases of
insulin deficiency a hyperglycemic
steady-state is reached which favours
(via mass action) the uptake of glucose
by peripheral tissues, whereas insulin
would be necessary for significant
glucose uptake at the normal steady-
state glucose concentration. The blood
glucose concentration of birds is usually
several times that of mammals, presumably to provide the extra energy needed
for flight. This is concomitant with
concentrations of hepatic glucose phosphorylating enzymes approximating
those in the diabetic rat. Thus, Nature
appears to have provided a most
interesting, subtle and effective means
of 'tuning' the homeostatic machinery to
the steady-state glucose concentration
most advantageous to the individual
organism, and for 'retuning' this blood-
glucose plateau concentration in a
perturbed situation (such as diabetes).

**Glucose phosphorylation in diabetic
livers**

If the concepts outlined above have
substance, glucose phosphorylation must

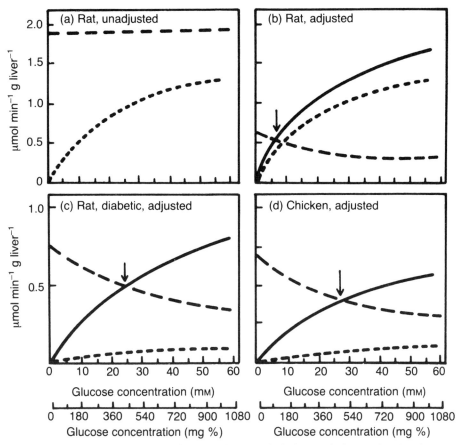

Fig. 2. *Rates of hepatic enzymes of glucose 6-phosphate hydrolysis and glucose phosphorylation at presumed physiological phosphoryl substrate levels and varied concentrations of glucose. Dashed lines depict glucose 6-phosphate phosphohydrolase and dotted lines glucokinase. Solid lines indicate rates of glucose phosphorylation necessary if cross-over points are to correspond with observed physiological values. (a) and (b) include data for normal rats, (c) for diabetic rats, and (d) for normal chickens. In (a), glucokinase and unadjusted glucose-6-phosphatase rates are portrayed. In (b), (c), and (d) glucose 6-phosphate phosphohydrolase rates have been adjusted for apparent inhibition by indicated glucose levels and competitive inhibitions by physiological levels of various metabolites. Arrows indicate 'cross-over' equivalence points where rates of glucose 6-phosphate hydrolysis and of glucose phosphorylation are equal. To the left of this arrow, the hydrolysis rate is greater than the phosphorylation rate, and glucose flows from the liver to blood; to the right, the phosphorylation rate is greater than hydrolysis, and a net uptake of blood glucose by the liver ensues. Redrawn from Nordlie[3]; reproduced by permission of Academic Press.*

be demonstrable in livers of diabetic rats, where glucokinase is virtually absent. Nordlie *et al.*[8] recently demonstrated this phenomenon with isolated perfused livers of alloxan-diabetic rats (see Fig. 4). Utilization of D-[U-^{14}C] glucose was seen at all concentrations of glucose studied (9.5–71 mM). Demonstration of net uptake of unlabeled

glucose by perfused livers of diabetic rats is generally complicated by vigorous gluconeogenesis from endogenous substrates. Net glucose *production* was thus observed with perfusate glucose concentrations of < 22 mM. However, when this gluconeogenesis was inhibited by 3-mercaptopicolinate (a competitive inhibitor of the key gluconeogenic enzyme phosphoenolpyruvate carboxykinase) net uptake of glucose was seen with perfused diabetic livers at all concentrations > 4 mm. This decrease in null-point glucose concentration brought about by 3-mercaptopicolinate correlated directly with reduced steady-state concentrations of hepatic glucose 6-phosphate. This latter observation is directly consistent with the 'tuning–retuning' concept.

Hepatic glucose/glucose 6-phosphate: the main regulatory mechanism

A number of recent studies have supported the significance of controlled flux between hepatic glucose and glucose 6-phosphate (see Fig. 1). For example, Lawson and Veech[9] concluded from 'far from equilibrium' considerations that hepatic glucose, glucose 6-phosphate, PP_i, and P_i are involved in a metabolic control point. El-Refai and Bergman[10] have concluded, on the basis of their computer-simulation metabolic studies, that the interaction of hepatic glucose and glucose 6-phosphate primarily affects the glucose concentration-dependent flux from glucose to glycogen. Nordlie et al.[11] have experimentally confirmed the latter hypothesis by demonstrating a glucose concentration-dependent increase in hepatic glucose 6-phosphate in isolated perfused rat livers (Table I). This substantiation of a metabolic 'push' by glucose at the glucose/glucose 6-phosphate couple as the prime mode of action is in direct contradiction to the concepts of Hue and Hers[12], who advocate a glucose-induced metabolic 'pull' by hepatic glycogen synthase.

Further mechanistic insight of this glucose-dependent metabolic push via glucose/glucose 6-phosphate was provided by recent work of Nordlie and Sukalski[13]. They showed that all non-competitive inhibition by glucose, partial latency, and competitive inhibitions by physiological levels of P_i, HCO^-_3, and Cl^- served to constrain hydrolysis of glucose 6-phosphate, by as much as

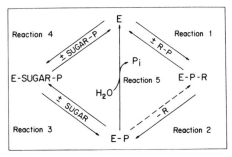

Fig. 3. Kinetic mechanism of multifunctional glucose-6-phosphatase phosphotransferase. E represents enzyme and R-P is the generalized phosphoryl substrate (e.g. carbamyl-P or PP_i). Reactions 4 + 3 + 5 describe glucose 6-phosphate hydrolysis; reactions 1 + 2 + 5 depict hydrolysis of R-P; and reactions 1 + 2 + 3 + 4 represent R-P:glucose phosphotransferase. E-P is protein-bound N-3 phosphoryl histidine. Competition between water and glucose for this phosphoryl group is apparent (i.e. competition between hydrolytic and synthetic reactions) as is the initial competition between the substrates glucose 6-phosphate and R-P for enzyme. Modified from Nordlie[3]; reproduced by permission of Academic Press.

75%. Nonetheless, these phenomena in themselves were insufficient to balance highly active glucose-6-phosphate phosphohydrolase against comparatively low levels of hepatic glucokinase. The need for an hepatic concentration-dependent glucose phosphorylative function beyond glucokinase, as hypothesized earlier (see above), was thus quantitatively established in livers of fed rats and rats starved for 48 h[13].

Phosphotransferase activities of glucose-6-phosphatase as an hepatic glucose phosphorylative system

The involvement of phosphotransferase activity of glucose-6-phosphatase in hepatic glucose phosphorylation under certain conditions is supported by our recent work with perfused livers and intact and permeable isolated hepatocytes. Alvares and Nordlie[5] demonstrated that ornithine, which may drain endogenous carbamyl-P via ornithine transcarbamylase, effectively diminished net glucose uptake in isolated perfused

Table I. Glucose 6-phosphate concentrations in livers of fasted rats perfused with various glucose loads. (Steady-state hepatic glucose 6-phosphate concentrations before perfusion and after perfusion with the indicated loads of glucose are presented.)

Perfusate glucose concentration[a] (mM)	No. of livers	Hepatic glucose 6-phosphate concentration[a] (μmol/g liver)
Initial	19	0.051 ± 0.005
5.4 ± 0.8	3	0.061 ± 0.013
11.9 ± 0.2	9	0.063 ± 0.009
16.1 ± 0.3	9	0.142 ± 0.025[b]
31.1 ± 0.5	9	0.153 ± 0.021[b]
44.7 ± 0.7	7	0.104 ± 0.025[b]
67.1 ± 2.5	5	0.103 ± 0.015[b]

[a]Mean values ± SE.
[b]Differences between indicated and initial values are statistically highly significant ($p < 0.05$).
(From Nordlie et al.[11]; reproduced by permission of American Society of Biological Chemists.

rat livers. 3-O-Methyl-D-glucose has been employed as a discriminating probe in liver perfusion studies by Nordlie et al.[5]. This sugar, which is an effective substrate for the phosphotransferase activity of glucose-6-phosphatase but is totally inactive with glucokinase, inhibited glucose uptake when perfused with glucose[5] and was itself phosphorylated when perfused alone[14] (i.e. it is an inhibitor of the phosphotransferase activity on glucose).

N-Acetylglucosamine, an effective competitive inhibitor of glucose phosphorylation by glucokinase, has also been used as a probe in the study of glucose utilization by isolated perfused rat livers. Sukalski and Nordlie[15] demonstrated an extensive inhibition by this compound of glucose uptake by livers from fed rats, as would be anticipated. However, in perfused livers from 48 h starved rats, in which glucokinase activity was markedly diminished and activities of glucose-6-phosphatase were elevated, little or no inhibition of glucose utilization by this compound was seen. Phosphotransferase activities of glucose-6-phosphatase were insensitive to inhibition by N-acetylglucosamine and thus constitute a credible system for N-acetylglucosamine-insensitive hepatic

glucose phosphorylation in livers from fasted rats[15].

Results of studies by Singh and Nordlie[16] of the effects of progressive starvation on glucose phosphorylation by isolated, intact rat hepatocytes involving endogenous phosphoryl donor(s) constitute some of the most convincing evidence yet accrued of a high-K_m enzyme acting in supplement to glucokinase. In these studies, we measured concurrently the rates of glucose phosphorylation and concentrations of glucokinase in hepatocytes from rats starved for 0, 24, 48 and 72 h, and showed by extrapolation that a significant proportion of total hepatic glucose phosphorylation remained even when no glucokinase was present. Concomitantly, the experimental K_m value for glucose increased from 33.4 ± 2.3 mM in fed rats to 47.5 ± 0.9 mM in 72 h starved rats. Similarly high K_m values were calculated by us either by Lineweaver–Burk analysis of the data of Katz et al.[17] or by totally independent experimentation and kinetic analysis[13]. K_m values of this magnitude greatly exceed the value of 5 to 10 mM usually attributed to glucokinase, but agree reasonably with values for phosphotransferase activity of glucose-6-phosphatase[3].

Major contra-indications in the past to physiological functions for phosphotransferase activities of glucose-6-phosphatase related to the high degree of latency and low pH optimum of the PP_i-glucose phosphotransferase[3]. These characteristics were seen with the enzyme of isolated membrane fragments – microsomes. Jorgenson and Nordlie[18] studied the enzyme in the endoplasmic reticulum, *in situ*, with isolated hepatocytes which were rendered permeable to phosphate substrates by treatment with filipin. These studies showed that the physical state of the cellular membranous element influences profoundly the catalytic behavior of glucose-6-phosphatase contained therein. With these cellular preparations in which the endoplasmic reticulum remained intact, significant phosphotransferase activity was seen at pH 7.4 with PP_i as well as with carbamyl-P. The degree of latency of activities also was much lower than with microsomes: 18, 27, 56 and 54% with PP_i-glucose phosphotransferase, glucose-6-phosphate phosphohydrolase, carbamyl-P:glucose phosphotransferase, and mannose-6-phosphate phosphohydrolase, respectively. All of these observations are consistent with metabolic roles for phosphotransferase as well as phosphohydrolase activities of multifunctional glucose-6-phosphatase.

Availability of cellular PP_i and carbamyl-P

The question of availability within the hepatocyte of putative phosphoryl substrates at concentrations sufficient for activity has been a continuing impediment to the acceptance of phosphotransferase function of glucose-6-phosphatase as an hepatic glucose-phosphorylating system. Some recent studies suggest that this may not be a major problem, however. Veech and colleagues[19] demonstrated that a rat hepatic PP_i level of 5 mM (which

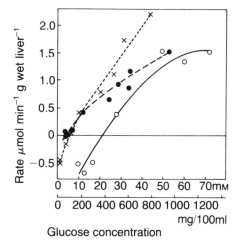

Fig. 4. *Effects of varied glucose concentration on net uptake rates in perfused livers from fed control (X) and glucagon-treated alloxan-diabetic rat livers perfused in the absence (O) and presence (●) of 4 mM mercaptopicolinate. Cross-over points from net glucose production to net glucose utilization were observed at 6, 22, and 4 mM glucose with livers from control, diabetic, and mercaptopicolinate-supplemented diabetic preparations, respectively. From Nordlie et al.*[8]; reproduced by permission of Elsevier Publishing Co.

approximates the K_m for PP_i in the phosphotransferase reaction) may be reached following intraperitoneal administration of fatty acids. This PP_i is formed concomitantly with fatty acyl-CoA synthesis. The free fatty acid concentration in serum is markedly increased in fasting or diabetic conditions – situations in which we previously have suggested that phosphotransferase activity of glucose-6-phosphatase may be especially involved in hepatic glucose phosphorylation[3]. In the past, the synthesis of 3′,5′-cyclic AMP via adenylate cyclase as a significant source of PP_i was ignored due to the low concentrations of cellular cAMP. However, recent work by Goldberg and associates[20] indicates a tremendous rate of turnover of cAMP in cells, involving the entire cellular adenylate pool within minutes. PP_i thus generated with the synthesis of each cAMP molecule, may prove ultimately to be a principal source of phosphoryl substrate for phosphotransferase activity of glucose-6-phosphatase.

The involvement of carbamyl-P as a phosphoryl substrate with glucose-6-phosphatase-phosphotransferase has been questioned because most of the hepatic carbamyl-P synthetase is located intramitochondrially. However, Cohen et al.[21] have shown that carbamyl-P generated in liver mitochondria can be available for extramitochondrial reactions. An increase in carbamyl-P synthetase I seen in fasting or diabetes (see Ref. 5) can thus make increased amounts of carbamyl-P available for cytosolic glucose phosphorylation under these circumstances, consistent with our tuning/retuning hypothesis. Lueck and Nordlie previously demonstrated the utilization of carbamyl-P formed via mitochondrial carbamyl-P synthetase for microsomal glucose phosphorylation, in vitro[3]. The feasibility of this pathway under physiological conditions within the cell is considerably strengthened by the recent demonstration by Katz et al.[22] of a physical continuum between the membrane of the mitochondrion and the smooth endoplasmic reticulum of the liver.

Discriminant regulation of the various activities of glucose-6-phosphatase

For the hydrolytic and synthetic activities of glucose-6-phosphatase to function efficiently, they should each be under discriminant, selective control. Ideally, factors that would favor transferase would have no effect on, or even reduce, glucose-6-phosphate phosphohydrolase, and vice versa. Copper ions (Cu^{2+}) have been shown by Johnson and Nordlie[23] to be one such factor. We demonstrated, in vitro, that micromolar concentrations of Cu^{2+} activate the synthetic function and inhibit the glucose-6-phosphate phosphohydrolase activity of the enzyme. These effects are brought about through the lowering of the affinity

of the enzyme for the product of the former reaction (i.e. glucose 6-phosphate) and for the substrate of the latter reaction (also glucose 6-phosphate). As discussed in Ref. 23, these observations are consistent with hyperglycemia observed accompanying Cu^{2+} deficiency.

Other specific inhibitions and activations have also been demonstrated recently. Vanadate was shown by Singh et al.[24] to inhibit competitively both transferase and hydrolase activities of disrupted and intact microsomes and permeable hepatocytes. The inhibition of transferase ($K_i = 1.3$ μM) was several times more pronounced than of glucose 6-phosphate phosphohydrolase ($K_i = 5.6$ μM). The polyamines spermine, spermidine, putrescine, and polylysine were shown by Nordlie et al.[25] to activate glucose-6-phosphate phosphohydrolase more extensively than transferase. These effects of polyamines contrast diametrically with general detergent effects which are much more pronounced with the transferase than with glucose-6-phosphate phosphohydrolase, and are thus supportive of the control of activities of the enzyme through discriminant modulations at the membrane-conformational level[7,25].

Inherent in the multicomponent glucose-6-phosphatase system recently proposed by Arion and colleagues[26] is the capacity for highly selective, substrate-specific control. They have proposed that the glucose-6-phosphatase-phosphotransferase system includes a catalytic unit of broad specificity located on the luminal side of the endoplasmic reticulum membrane. Working in conjunction with this catalytic unit are several 'translocases' which are responsible for transport of specific substrates from the cellular cytosol to the catalytic unit. Two putative translocases have been identified, one for glucose 6-phosphate ('T_1') and a second for carbamyl-P and PP_i ('T_2'). It follows that metabolites, covalent modifications, membrane-associated perturbations, drugs, and the like may selectively modify T_1, T_2, the catalytic unit, or combinations thereof. To date, a selective inhibition of T_1 has been seen with two compounds – phlorizin[27] and 4,4'-diisothiocanostilbene-2,2'-disulfonic-acid[28]. No inhibitor specific for T_2 has yet been described. A defect in T_1 was identified by Lange et al.[29] in Type Ib glycogenosis, while Nordlie et al.[30] demonstrated that T_2 was non-functional, at least in the out $\rightarrow$ in direction, in Type Ic glycogenesis. These observations correlated with alterations in blood glucose levels predicted to accompany aberrant glucose-6-phosphatase function as depicted in Fig. 1 (see Refs 29 and 30). The increase in T_1 capability seen in response to glucocorticoids, fasting, or diabetes involves an in situ activation of existing translocase molecules rather than enhanced protein biosynthesis[3,28]. The potential for control of blood glucose levels through selective inhibitions or activations of components of the glucose-6-phosphatase–phosphotransferase system through mechanisms just discussed is now very apparent. Selective modulations of this sort can be exploited in the design of chemotherapeutic agents to raise or lower blood glucose levels as desired, based on concepts depicted in Fig. 1. Modulations favoring transferase activity would serve to lower blood glucose while those perturbations favoring the hydrolysis of glucose 6-phosphate over transferase would act to raise ambient blood glucose concentrations. With the emergence of these new concepts of glucose-6-phosphatase mechanism and composition, it appears that this intriguing area of investigation is just beginning to open up.

Acknowledgements

The author is grateful to Katherine Sukalski and Cathrine Snyder for their able editorial assistance. Studies from the author's laboratory were supported by Research Grant AM07141 from the National Institutes of Health, US Public Health Service.

References

1 Cahill, G. F., Ashmore, J., Renold, A. E. and Hastings, A. B. (1959) Am. J. Med. 26, 264–282
2 Nordlie, R. C. (1976) Trends Biochem. Sci. 1, 199–202
3 Nordlie, R. C. (1974) in Current Topics in Cellular Regulation (Horecker, B. L. and Stadtman, E. R., eds), Vol. 8, pp. 33–117, Academic Press
4 Singh, J., Martin, R. E. and Nordlie, R. C. (1983) Can. J. Biochem. Cell Biol. 61, 1085–1089
5 Alvares, F. L. and Nordlie, R. C. (1977) J. Biol. Chem. 252, 8404–8414
6 Nordlie, R. C. (1981) in Regulation of Carbohydrate Formation and Utilization in Mammals (Veneziale, C. M., ed.), pp. 291–314, University Park Press, New York
7 Nordlie, R. C. and Sukalski, K. A. (1985) in The Enzymes of Biological Membranes (Martonosi, A., ed.), 2nd edn, Vol. 2, pp. 349–398, Plenum Press
8 Nordlie, R. C., Alvares, F. L. and Sukalski, K. A. (1982) Biochim. Biophys. Acta 719, 244–250
9 Lawson J. W. R. and Veech, R. L. (1979) J. Biol. Chem. 254, 6528–6537
10 El-Refair, M. and Bergman, R. N. (1976) Am. J. Physiol. 231, 1608–1619
11 Nordlie, R. C., Sukalski, K. A. and Alvares, F. L. (1980) J. Biol. Chem. 255, 1834–1838 ·
12 Hue, L. and Hers, H.-G. (1974) Biochem. Biophys. Res. Commun. 58, 540–548
13 Nordlie, R. C. and Sukalski, K. A. (1982) in Developments in Biochemistry – The Biochemistry of Metabolic Processes (Stratman, F. W., Lennon, D. L. F. and Zahlten, R. N., eds), pp. 125–138, Elsevier Biomedical, New York
14 Nordlie, R. C., Sukalski, K. A., Singh, J. and Alvares, F. L. (1982) Abstr. 12th Int. Congr. Biochem., p. 121
15 Sukalski, K. A. and Nordlie, R. C. (1983) Fed. Proc. 42, 2165
16 Singh, J. and Nordlie, R. C. (1982) FEBS Lett. 250, 325–328
17 Katz, J., Golden, S. and Wals, P. A. (1979) Biochem. J. 180, 389–402
18 Jorgenson. R. A. and Nordlie, R. C. (1980) J. Biol. Chem. 255, 5907–5915
19 Veech, R. L., Cook, G. A. and King, M. T.

(1980) *FEBS Lett.* 117, K65–K72

20 Walseth, T. F., Gander, J. E., Eide, S. J., Krick, T. P. and Goldberg, N. D. (1983) *J. Biol. Chem.* 258, 1544–1558

21 Cohen, N. S., Cheung, C. W. and Raijman, L. (1980) *J. Biol. Chem.* 255, 10248–10255

22 Katz, J., Wals, P. A., Golden, S. and Raijman, L. (1983) *Biochem. J.* 214, 795–813

23 Johnson, W. T. and Nordlie, R. C. (1977) *Biochemistry* 16, 2458–2466

24 Singh, J., Nordlie, R. C. and Jorgenson, R. A. (1981) *Biochim. Biophys. Acta* 678, 477–482

25 Nordlie, R. C., Johnson, W. T., Cornatzer, W. E., Jr and Twedell, G. W. (1979) *Biochim. Biophys. Acta* 585, 12–23

26 Arion, W. J., Wallin, B. K., Lange, A. J. and Ballas, L. M. (1975) *Mol. Cell. Biochem.* 6, 75–83

27 Arion, W. J., Lange, A. J. and Walls, H. G. (1980) *J. Biol. Chem.* 255, 10387–10395

28 Zaccoli, M. A., Hoopes, R. R. and Karnovsky, M. L. (1982) *J. Biol. Chem.* 257, 11296–11300

29 Lange, A. J., Arion, W. J. and Beaudet, A. L. (1980) *J. Biol. Chem.* 255, 8381–8384

30 Nordlie, R. C., Sukalski, K. A., Muñoz, J. M. and Baldwin, J. J. (1983) *J. Biol. Chem.* 258, 9739–9744

R. C. Nordlie is at the Department of Biochemistry and Molecular Biology University of North Dakota School of Medicine, Grand Forks, North Dakota 58202, USA.

Multiple roles of ATP in the regulation of sugar transport in muscle and adipose tissue

Michael K. Gould

ATP can function as a feedback inhibitor of sugar transport in skeletal muscle. This regulates the availability of the sugar according to the metabolic needs of the cell. In muscle and adipose tissue, ATP has a permissive effect on the stimulation of sugar transport by insulin, which has been explained as the provision of energy for the process of translocation of glucose carriers to and from the plasma membrane. Inhibitory effects of exogenous ATP on insulin binding and action and the recent demonstration that the insulin receptor is a tyrosine-specific protein kinase, indicate that there may be several disparate mechanisms whereby ATP may influence sugar transport.

Transport of glucose across the cell membrane is the initial rate-limiting step in its utilization by skeletal muscle and adipose tissue. This process is subject to regulation by external factors (e.g. insulin) and internally by the metabolic status of the cell itself. This review will consider the way in which energy metabolism can influence sugar transport, both directly and indirectly by modifying the action of insulin.

ATP as a feedback inhibitor of sugar transport

Randle and Smith[1] observed that sugar transport in muscle was stimulated when oxidative energy metabolism was interrupted by anoxia or uncouplers of oxidative phosphorylation. This, and the insulin-like effect of work, suggested that ATP could act as a feedback inhibitor to regulate the entry of glucose. This theory is very attractive from a teleological point of view. However, although it can readily be shown that the stimulation of sugar transport by anoxia and uncouplers is accompanied by a fall in the level of ATP, it has been difficult to establish a cause–effect relationship between these two observations. In skel-

etal muscle it has not been possible to demonstrate a temporal relationship between the depletion of ATP levels by anoxia and the stimulation of sugar transport, consistent with the feedback regulation of transport by ATP[2]. Furthermore, under certain conditions it can be shown that changes in sugar transport are not accompanied by changes in ATP. Thus, if rat soleus muscle is incubated at 27°C instead of the more usual 37°C, anoxia stimulates sugar transport without altering the ATP level[2].

On first appraisal these observations appear to refute the proposed regulatory role of ATP on sugar transport. However, if one considers the source rather than the total concentrations of the ATP in the muscle under the various experimental conditions described above, then it is possible to reconcile these results with a feedback system with a specific requirement for mitochondrial as distinct from glycolytic ATP[2]. This is still not an adequate explanation. As shown in Fig. 1, the mitochondria in skeletal muscle tend to be localized within the interior of the cell, arranged between the myofibrils closely associated with glycogen granules. In view of the barrier to diffusion imposed by the myofibrils, it is difficult to see how the ATP generated by these mitochondria could be more readily available for the regulation of sugar transport than that produced *in the same region* by glycolysis. Figure 2 shows that in addition to these interfibrillar mitochondria some of the mitochondria are localized on the periphery of the fibre, often in dense aggregations. According to Korbl *et al.*[2], by virtue of their localization, the ATP produced by these subsarcolemmal mitochondria could be specifically involved in such a feedback system.

These considerations do not apply to adipose tissue in which ATP-depletion does not stimulate sugar transport[3].

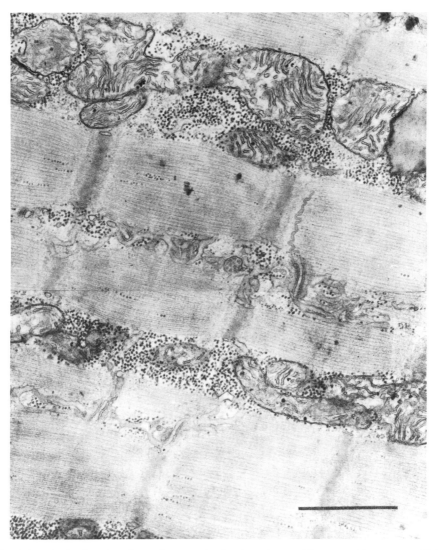

Fig. 1. Longitudinal section of rat soleus muscle, showing mitochondria arranged between myofibrils in association with glycogen granules. In Figs 1 and 2 bar = 1 μm. Electron micrographs by Mr B. Veitch.

Effects of exogenous ATP on sugar transport

One approach to the role of ATP in the regulation of sugar transport has been to study the effect of exogenously added ATP. In view of the popular opinion that ATP cannot cross cell membranes, one might question the significance of experiments involving the addition of ATP to intact tissues. This certainly was our attitude when Irshad Chaudry and I considered this type of experimentation in 1970. We were surprised when we were unable to find any direct evidence in the literature showing that ATP could not cross the cell membrane, and subsequently we were able to show that externally-added ATP did in fact enter soleus muscle[4]. This raises the possibility that the effects of exogenous

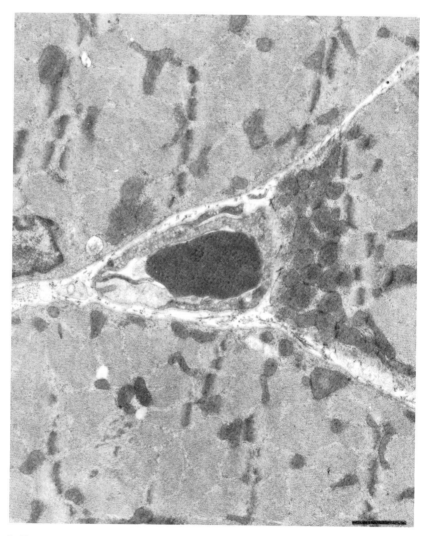

Fig. 2. Transverse section of rat soleus muscle, showing three muscle cells surrounding a blood capillary. Interfibrillar mitochondria can be seen inside the cells. The cell on the right has an aggregation of subsarcolemmal mitochondria on the periphery, next to the capillary. These mitochondria would be at an advantage in obtaining oxygen under conditions which limit the oxygen supply to the muscle.

ATP result from its action in intracellular metabolism. Chaudry found that externally-added ATP inhibited the uptake of glucose by soleus muscle under anaerobic but not aerobic conditions[5].

Chang and Cuatrecasas[6] observed that very low concentrations of ATP (50 μM), which had no effect under basal conditions (no insulin), inhibited the stimulatory effect of insulin on glucose utilization and sugar transport by adipocytes. This effect did not involve the binding of insulin to its receptor. Higher concentrations of ATP (above 0.8 mM) inhibited both basal and insulin-stimulated glucose utilization; however, this was considered to represent a different effect of the nucleotide. Other workers have been unable to detect this inhibitory effect of ATP. Loten et al.[7] confirmed that ATP did inhibit insulin-stimulated glucose utilization and sugar transport in the adipocyte, but found that this required higher concentrations of ATP (1 mM) than those used in the experiments of Chang and Cuatrecasas[6].

The mechanism by which ATP may inhibit sugar transport is not clear. Similarly, since insulin activates sugar transport without depressing muscle ATP, the relationship between the effect of insulin and the proposed ATP-feedback system is also unknown. Chang et al.[8] found that the inhibitory effect of exogenous ATP on sugar transport by the adipocyte was associated with the phosphorylation of two membrane proteins by a cyclic AMP-dependent protein kinase located in the membrane itself. This recalls Randle's original suggestion that the action of ATP on sugar transport could involve the phosphorylation of the transport carrier, or some closely associated membrane protein.

In contrast to the inhibitory effects of ATP discussed thus far, Newsholme and Randle[9] observed that externally added ATP actually stimulated sugar transport in the intact diaphragm.

Permissive effects of ATP on insulin-stimulated sugar transport

In 1952, Walaas and Walaas showed that insulin stimulated anaerobic glucose uptake by rat hemidiaphragm but this effect was short-lived. They related the loss of insulin-responsiveness to the depletion of ATP and explained this in terms of the then current 'hexokinase theory' of insulin action (see Ref. 3).

Later experiments by Kono and Colowick (reviewed in Ref. 3) showed that the action of insulin on the uptake of non-metabolizable sugars by diaphragm was inhibited by uncouplers of oxidative phosphorylation. Our interest in this effect was kindled by experiments which showed that insulin stimulated the uptake of xylose in soleus muscles treated with 2,4-dinitrophenol when this was measured in freshly isolated muscle, but not after pre-incubation in the presence of the uncoupler[2]. This suggested that there could be some ATP-dependent step involved in the action of insulin on sugar transport. Subsequent studies in this laboratory lent further support to this theory[10]. The stimulatory effect of insulin on xylose uptake was progressively lost when rat soleus muscles were preincubated under anaerobic conditions for longer than 30 min; after 90 min these muscles were completely insensitive to insulin. This effect was associated with the loss of muscle ATP. When the breakdown of ATP was retarded, either by lowering the pre-incubation temperature or by pre-incubation with glucose, the effect of insulin in anaerobic muscle was correspondingly prolonged.

ATP appears to have a similar effect in the adipocyte, where uncouplers and respiratory inhibitors also inhibit insulin-stimulated sugar transport[3]. In adipocytes, reducing the ATP level by 50–70% lowers the rate of activation and reduces insulin sensitivity, but does not affect the maximum response of the sugar transport system. Conversely, depletion of ATP abolishes insulin stimulation completely[11].

In soleus muscle, ATP-depletion also inhibits ^{125}I-insulin binding (Ref. 12, see also below). From experiments using insulin alone, it is not possible to say whether the permissive effect of ATP on the activation of sugar transport results entirely from the effect on insulin binding, or whether ATP is also involved in the transmission of the insulin signal. This is not a problem in the adipocyte, where ATP-depletion does not appear to affect insulin binding[11]. Recent work has shown that, in addition to the activity of insulin, the activities of several other insulinomimetic agents are ATP-dependent. This suggests that ATP is involved in some post-receptor event and, furthermore, that this function of ATP may be fundamental to the process of activation, regardless of the triggering agent.

Studies by Chaudry et al.[13], concerned with the insulin resistance induced by hemorrhagic shock, also indicate that permissive effects of ATP are associated with the action of insulin at a post-receptoral level. They found that supramaximal concentrations of insulin (in excess of 0.1 U/ml) were required to stimulate glucose uptake by soleus muscles from rats after hemorrhagic shock. This was associated with low levels of ATP in these muscles and could be overcome by the administration of ATP either in vivo or in vitro. There are many differences between this effect and the permissive effect of ATP observed after prolonged anoxia or exposure to uncouplers. Thus (1) shock muscles are demonstrably aerobic, (2) sugar transport in ATP-depleted muscle does not respond to supramaximal concentrations of insulin, and (3) exogenous ATP is considerably less effective in ATP-depleted muscle than in shock muscle. Most importantly, the insulin resistance in hemorrhagic shock is not associated with any decrease in the binding of ^{125}I-insulin by the muscle.

In adipocytes, deactivation of sugar transport following insulin stimulation also requires ATP[3]. Depletion of cellular ATP after insulin treatment locks sugar transport into an activated state, which can only be reversed by restoring energy metabolism. From these observations Kono concluded that ATP is required as an energy source for the process of reversible translocation of glucose carriers between the plasma membrane and intracellular storage sites[3,14]. In soleus muscle, ATP-depletion following insulin stimulation does not preserve the activated state of sugar transport, but promotes rapid deactivation[15]. At present it is not clear whether this is because the muscle system is fundamentally different from that in adipose tissue, or whether it is because ATP-depletion induces the dissociation of bound insulin from muscle, but not from adipocytes.

There are several other ways in which ATP could be involved in the transmission of the insulin signal from the receptor to the transport system. It is generally considered that the intracellular action of insulin promotes the dephosphorylation of certain key metabolic enzymes such as glycogen synthase and pyruvate dehydrogenase. However, insulin also stimulates phosphorylation of certain proteins (ATP-citrate lyase, acetyl-CoA carboxylase and the ribosomal subunit S6), apparently without affecting their metabolic activity[16]. Thus, ATP may be required for the phosphorylation of an essential component of the system. It has been shown that insulin promotes the phosphorylation of an endogenous protein (mol. wt 15 000) in sarcolemma[17] and of a specific protein (120 000–140 000) in adipocytes[18]. Whether or not these are concerned with the regulation of sugar transport has yet to be established.

Interest in the potential role of phosphorylation reactions in the action of insulin has been stimulated by recent reports that insulin activates a protein kinase present in the β-subunit of the insulin receptor[19]. This catalyses the tyrosine-specific auto-phosphorylation of the 95 000 subunit and phosphorylation of exogenous substrates. Other agents which mimic insulin action (e.g. lectins, anti-insulin receptor antibody and trypsin) also stimulate receptor protein kinase activity. This could imply that receptor phosphorylation is an early event in insulin action. Noting that tyrosine-specific protein kinase activity is also exhibited by the epidermal growth-factor receptor and by the transforming proteins of RNA tumour viruses, Houslay and Heyworth[20] suggested that the insulin receptor kinase could be concerned with the long-term growth promoting actions of insulin, rather than with its more rapid metabolic effects.

Permissive effect of ATP on insulin binding

Yu and Gould[12] found that the binding of ^{125}I-insulin by soleus muscle was depressed when ATP was depleted either by prolonged incubation under anaerobic conditions, or more rapidly in the presence of the uncoupler, 2,4-dinitrophenol. Subsequently, we have consistently observed that agents which lower ATP concentration inhibit ^{125}I-insulin-binding in soleus muscle[21]. There was no effect on the binding of ^{125}I-insulin when muscle protein synthesis was inhibited by prolonged incubation with cycloheximide[22]. This suggests that the effects of prolonged anoxia discussed above were not simply caused by the lack of ATP for the synthesis of the receptor, but by some more direct effect of ATP. We have proposed that the 'activity' of the insulin receptor may be regulated by a phosphorylation/dephosphorylation mechanism involving either the receptor itself or some closely related membrane protein. According to this hypothesis, the receptor could bind insulin only when it was in the phosphorylated state.

In the adipocyte, insulin binding is also diminished by ATP-depletion; however, it has generally been considered that this effect is concerned with the ATP-dependent internalization of bound hormone, rather than the initial binding step[3,11]. However, using conditions which excluded internalization, Steinfelder and Joost[23] have shown that ATP-depletion does affect adipocyte insulin binding. Draznin et al.[24] found that ATP-depletion (with 2,4-dinitrophenol) reduced ^{125}I-insulin-binding by hepatocytes. In these studies, ATP-dependent internalization of the bound hormone was also reported. We have observed that ATP-depletion (by 2,4-dinitrophenol) does not affect ^{125}I-insulin binding by hepatocytes, when binding is determined at 10°C, at which temperature internalization is essentially eliminated (S. Kelemen, unpublished results).

Because insulin binding by whole-cell preparations is generally measured under conditions where internalization is a factor, it is essential to distinguish between effects of ATP on internalization and on binding itself. Accordingly, using two different binding assays which minimized internalization of bound ^{125}I-insulin, we have confirmed that insulin binding is depressed in ATP-depleted soleus muscle[21]. In marked contrast to the effects described above, depletion of cellular ATP actually increased ^{125}I-insulin binding by cultured IM-9 cells[25]. The same laboratory has reported that exogenously added ATP inhibited insulin binding by rat liver and human placental membranes[26]; insulin binding by a purified human placental insulin receptor was even more sensitive to inhibition by ATP. This effect of ATP did not appear to be mediated by a phosphorylation reaction.

In view of the multiplicity of reactions involving ATP, it is not altogether surprising that a number of these may be involved in the process by which muscle-sugar transport is regulated. The studies reviewed here indicate that ATP can both inhibit sugar transport and permissively promote the stimulatory effect of insulin. In demonstrating the overall scope of these roles, this review also shows how incomplete our knowledge is in this area.

Acknowledgements

It is a pleasure to acknowledge the collaborative efforts of Dr Irshad Chaudry, Dr John Forsayeth, Mrs Solveiga Hall, Mr Robert Kaldawi, Mrs Sylvie Kelemen, Dr Gary Korbl, Dr Izabela Kozka, Miss Yoke Hoon Lim, Miss Barbara Scher, Dr Ian Sloan and Dr Kin Yu in the studies reported from this laboratory.

References

1 Randle, P. J. and Smith, G. H. (1958) *Biochem. J.* 70, 501–508

2 Korbl, G. P., Sloan, I. G. and Gould, M. K. (1977) *Biochim. Biophys. Acta* 465, 93–109

3 Kono, T. (1983) *Recent. Progr. Horm. Res.* 39, 519–557

4 Chaudry, I. H. and Gould, M. K. (1970) *Biochim. Biophys. Acta* 196, 320–326

5 Chaudry, I. H. and Gould, M. K. (1970) *Biochim. Biophys. Acta* 196, 327–335

6 Chang, K.-J. and Cuatrecasas, P. (1974) *J. Biol. Chem.* 249, 3170–3180

7 Loten, E. G., Regen, D. M. and Park, C. R. (1976) *J. Cell Physiol.* 89, 651–660

8 Chang, K.-J., Marcus, N. A. and Cuatrecasas, P. (1974) *J. Biol. Chem.* 249, 6854–6865

9 Newsholme, E. A. and Randle, P. J. (1961) *Biochem. J.* 80, 655–662

10 Yu, K. T. and Gould, M. K. (1978) *Amer. J. Physiol.* 234, E407–416

11 Haring, H. U., Rinninger, F. and Kemmler, W. (1981) *FEBS Lett.* 132, 235–238

12 Yu, K. T. and Gould, M. K. (1978) *Amer. J. Physiol.* 235, E606–613

13 Chaudry, I. H., Sayeed, M. M. and Baue, A. E. (1976) *Can. J. Physiol. Pharmacol.* 54, 736–741

14 Simpson, I. A. and Cushman, S. W. in *Molecular Basis for Insulin Action* (1985) (Czech, M. P., ed.), Plenum Publishing Co.

15 Kaldawi, R. E., Yu, K. T. and Gould, M. K. (1983) *Arch. Biochem. Biophys.* 226, 612–617

16 Avruch, J., Alexander, M. C., Palmer, J. L., Pierce, M. W., Nemenoff, R. A., Blackshear, P. J., Tipper, J. P. and Witters, L. A. (1982) *Fed. Proc.* 41, 2629–2633

17 Walaas, O., Walaas, E., Lystad, E., Alertsen, A. R., Horn, R. S. and Fossum, S. (1977) *FEBS Lett.* 80, 417–422

18 Avruch, J., Leone, G. R. and Martin, D. B. (1976) *J. Biol. Chem.* 251, 1511–1515

19 Kasuga, M., Fujita-Yamaguchi, Y., Blithe, D. L., White, M. F. and Kahn, C. R. (1983) *J. Biol. Chem.* 258, 10973–10980

20 Houslay, M. D. and Heyworth, C. M. (1983) *Trends Biochem. Sci.* 8, 449–452

21 Lim, Y. H. and Gould, M. K. (1983) *Biochem. Int.* 6, 163–169

22 Yu, K. T. and Gould, M. K. (1979) *Biochem. Biophys. Res. Commun.* 87, 9–16

23 Steinfelder, H. J. and Joost, H. G. (1983) *Biochem. J.* 214, 203–207

24 Draznin, B., Solomons, C. C., Toothaker, D. R. and Sussman, K. E. (1981) *Endocrinology* 108, 8–17

25 Vigneri, R., Maddux, B. and Goldfine, I. D. (1984) *J. Cell Biochem.* 24, 177–186

26 Trischitta, V., Vigneri, R., Roth, R. A. and Goldfine, I. D. (1984) *Metabolism* 33, 557

Michael K. Gould is at Monash University, Melbourne, Australia, 3168.

Energy metabolism in muscle and its regulation during individual contraction–relaxation cycles

David F. Wilson, Katsuyuki Nishiki and Maria Erecińska

Muscles can attain efficiencies in excess of 40% in utilizing energy to do work, a tribute in part to their extraordinarily effective metabolic regulation. Only a small fraction of the tissue content of ATP and creatine phosphate (CrP) is hydrolysed during a single contraction–relaxation cycle and metabolic responses to changes in work load are the cumulative effect of several cycles.

The conversion of metabolic energy to mechanical work by muscle is one of the most fascinating expressions of the role of energy metabolism in living organisms. During each contraction–relaxation cycle (beat) of the heart or twitch of skeletal muscle, ATP – the primary source of energy in the process – is hydrolysed to ADP and inorganic phosphate and then resynthesized to ensure a constant level of mechanical performance. A close coordination must, therefore, exist *in vivo* between the contractile apparatus and the energy-synthesizing machinery which allows muscles to function continuously and effectively over a wide range of working conditions.

A. V. Hill in his book 'Trails and Trials in Physiology'[1] summarized the development of ideas and experimental endeavours in the field of muscle energetics up to the mid-1960s. Several reviews have appeared since which either emphasize various aspects of the problem[2-3] or focus on certain type of muscle[4]. Much less attention has been paid to the regulation of energy metabolism during individual contractions largely because of paucity of accurate experimental information.

During recent years, however, procedures have been developed for the measurements of energy parameters in intact cells and tissues. These include on the one hand, improvements of conventional biochemical methods and on the other applications of sophisticated biophysical techniques such as nuclear magnetic resonance. In addition, progress has been made in understanding the mechanisms which may be involved in regulation of energy metabolism[5-7]. These advances have allowed us to approach the problem of changes in energy metabolism on a beat to beat (or single twitch) basis. The discussion which follows places special emphasis on heart muscle because the beating perfused heart provides a convenient model for evaluating the energy requirement for a single contraction–relaxation cycle.

The content of 'high-energy' phosphate compounds and their rate of synthesis in a beating perfused rat heart

We have used in the analysis, experimental results from our own work in which the relevant parameters were measured with conventional biochemical techniques (Table I). There are two reasons for doing so; firstly, our data are in excellent agreement with those of other authors[8,9]. Secondly, even with the advent of ^{31}P NMR, the conventional techniques provide the only methods by which quantitative values of *all* relevant parameters can be obtained. (^{31}P NMR does not measure concentration of creatine and that of ADP is below the level for detection. Moreover quantitation of NMR results, although possible in principle, still presents a problem. Most investigators express their data in relative terms, e.g. ATP/P_i or CrP/P_i, and then 'calculate' concentrations using [ATP] or [CrP] measured by standard biochemical assays.)

A beating rat heart perfused with glucose hydrolyses ATP (5.2×10^{-6} mol/g wet wt) to ADP (1×10^{-6} mol/g wet wt) and inorganic phosphate (3×10^{-6} mol/g wet wt) in order to provide the energy for muscular work. The ATP which is hydrolysed during the contraction–relaxation cycle is subsequently resynthesized by cellular energy-yielding reactions. In a heart perfused with 5.5 mM glucose as the only oxidizable substrate, essentially all synthesis of ATP comes from glucose metabolism either by complete oxidation to CO_2 and water

$$\text{Glucose} + 6O_2 + 36\,\text{ADP} + 36\,P_i \rightarrow$$
$$6CO_2 + 6CH_2O + 36\,\text{ATP} \qquad (1)$$

or by glycolysis alone

$$\text{Glucose} + 2\text{ADP} + 2P_i \rightarrow$$
$$2\,\text{lactate} + 2\text{ATP} \qquad (2)$$

With a sufficient supply of oxygen the latter reaction (anaerobic glycolysis) provides only a minor fraction of the cellular ATP requirement ($\leq 5\%$)[10]. (*In vivo* the predominant energy source for the heart is fatty acids[11] which are oxidized via the tricarboxylic acid cycle and oxidative phosphorylation to CO_2 and water to yield approximately the same amount of ATP per molecule of O_2 as in the oxidation of glucose.) The rate of ATP synthesis in the perfused beating heart can be calculated from the rates of oxygen consumption and lactate production (Table I). It is assumed in these calculations that 6 mol of ATP are produced per mol of oxygen utilized and that 1 mol of ATP is formed per mol of lactate produced. Table I shows that oxygen consumption is 9.0×10^{-6} mol/min/g wet wt while lactate production is 1.8×10^{-6} mol/min/g wet wt. This gives an ATP production rate of 5.58×10^{-5} mol/min/g wet wt.

Comparison of energy requirement during the contraction–relaxation cycle in different muscles

The perfused hearts (Table I) were electronically paced at 4 Hz; this means that they utilized 2.33×10^{-7} moles of ATP per beat per g wet weight.

The energy requirements for an isometric contraction–relaxation cycle have been reported for frog sartorius[12,13] and cat papillary muscle[14]. In the former, ATP hydrolysis was expressed as the decrease in creatine phosphate, whereas in the latter the estimates were made from changes in the rate of oxygen consumption. These values are summarized in Table II along with the measurements for different perfused heart preparations. When the amount of ATP utilized per beat (heart) or per twitch (sartorius and papillary) is calculated, the values are the same within experimental error and range from 1.0×10^{-7} mol. ATP/beat (or twitch)/g wet wt to 2.93×10^{-7} mol ATP/beat or twitch/g wet wt with a mean of $2.07 \pm 0.70 \times 10^{-7}$ mol ATP/beat or twitch/g wet wt. This value is, however, dependent on the work condition[8,15] and refers only to the average work-load.

Enthalpy and free energy changes associated with a single contraction–relaxation cycle in a beating perfused rat heart

Production of heat (ΔH) in the beating perfused heart arises exclusively from net metabolism of glucose to either CO_2 and H_2O (reaction 3: $\Delta H = 2.8 \times 10^3$ kJ/mol) or to lactate + H^+ (reaction 4: $\Delta H = 1.49 \times 10^2$ kJ/mol glucose)

Table I.

A. Metabolite concentrations in an isolated perfused rat heart[a]

Adenosine triphosphate	5.21×10^{-6} mol/g wet wt
Adenosine diphosphate	1.00×10^{-6} mol/g wet wt
Orthophosphate	3.07×10^{-6} mol/g wet wt
Creatine phosphate	6.22×10^{-6} mol/g wet wt
Creatine	4.12×10^{-6} mol/g wet wt
Oxygen consumption	$9.0 \ \times 10^{-6}$ mol/min/g wet wt
Lactate production	1.83×10^{-6} mol/min/g wet wt

B. Thermodynamic constants for glucose combustion and glycolysis *in vivo*

Reaction	ΔH	ΔG
Glucose $+ 6O_2 \rightarrow 6H_2O + 6CO_2$	-2813 kJ/mol (Ref. 16)	-2878 kJ/mol (Ref. 17)
?Glucose $\rightarrow 2$ lactate $+ 2H^+$	-149 kJ/mol (Ref. 16)[b]	-208 kJ/mol (Ref. 17)

[a] The heart was perfused essentially by the method of Langendorff[18] at 37°C with 80 cm H_2O aortic pressure and paced at 4 Hz. Data taken from Ref. 7.

[b] Data taken from Ref. 16 but corrected for the heat of neutralization of the protons released under physiological conditions[19].

$$Glucose + 6O_2 \rightarrow 6CO_2 + 6H_2O \quad (3)$$
$$Glucose \rightarrow 2 \text{ lactate} + 2H^+ \quad (4)$$

The total energetics of the heart muscle may therefore be calculated from the rates of oxygen consumption and lactate production (Table I). Such calculation shows that metabolic enthalpy change (ΔH) occurs at a rate of 4.35 J/min/g wet wt or 18.7 mJ/beat/g wet wt.

The perfused heart preparation analysed here represents a steady-state system. This means that metabolites which are hydrolysed to provide energy for contraction or relaxation are resynthesized to their original levels during the same single beat. Therefore the calculated heat production (18.7 mJ/beat/g wet wt) incorporates the 'recovery heat', i.e. the energy 'cost' for metabolic regeneration of various reactants (including ATP and creatine phosphate). In contrast, most direct measurements of heat production were made for experimental conditions in which ATP and creatine phosphate were not resynthesized and consequently yielded lower values by about 35–50% (see (Ref. 3) and references therein). (In systems which perform net work, the measured heat production is lower than the calculated maximal metabolic enthalpy change by the amount of work done. The data of Table I are, however, for a Langendorff preparation of perfused rat heart[7] in which the net work performed is zero.)

The ΔH value per beat/g wet weight estimated above for the rat heart is considerably higher than the 5.3–10.6 mJ of heat produced/beat/g wet wt obtained by Coulson[19] with steady-state isovolumic rabbit hearts. The reported oxygen consumption rates were also correspondingly lower which indicates a lower metabolic requirement per beat in his system. This may have resulted in part from the lower temperature of measurements (25°C v. 35°C in our experiments) and in part from mechanical differences in the heart muscle preparation (isovolumic contractions[19] v. contractions at a constant aortic pressure[7]).

The ability of the heart to do work is determined by the associated free energy changes (ΔG). The ΔG values for reactions 3 and 4 are approximately -2.88×10^3 and -2.08×10^2 kJ/mol glucose respectively at 25°C. Since the rate of ATP synthesis is known (Table I), it can be calculated that the rate of metabolic free energy production is 4.51 J/min/g wet wt (or 18.8 mJ/beat/g wet wt). If we now use the value of 53.5 kJ/mol[7] for the free energy of ATP synthesis under the same conditions, we can estimate that the metabolic efficiency for production of intracellular ATP is approximately 66%; that is, two-thirds of the total available free energy from combustion of glucose is conserved by synthesizing ATP from ADP and P_i. (It should be mentioned that the value for the free energy of ATP synthesis in muscle tissue is still under debate. The free Mg^{2+} concentration is not accurately known nor is the amount of cytosolic ADP bound. Recent measurements by NMR[20,21] have suggested that the actual ΔG value may be more negative than that used above by about -5.7 kJ/mol. This would increase the calculated efficiency for production of intracellular ATP to 73% but would not significantly alter the other calculations or conclusions in this paper.)

The efficiency of muscles in utilizing metabolic energy to work

An evaluation of the efficiency of different muscles in utilizing metabolic energy to work (and defined as the ratio of the work accomplished to the total metabolic free energy change utilized) has been attempted by a number of investigators (see Refs 1, 3 and 4 for review). Among the highest overall efficiencies for individual muscles are those reported for isolated frog sartorius[22] and tortoise[3] muscles of about 35–40%. Burton[23] has estimated that human heart *in vivo* functions with an overall efficiency of 10% and that this can rise to 20–30% in vigorous exercise. It may be calculated that a 68 kg man carrying a 25 kg load up a vertical ladder at a speed of 11.9 m/min accomplishes work at a rate of 10.5 kJ/min using 106 kJ of metabolic energy per minute. This corresponds to an overall efficiency of 10% based on moving both his body weight and the load up the ladder. Since it has been estimated above that about 66% of the free energy change generated during oxidation of glucose is conserved as ATP, this man's efficiency of utilization of ATP to do work is approximately 17%. It would appear to be generally true that individual muscles are capable of working at overall efficiencies of at least 40% but this value declines with increasing complexity of the motion and number of muscles involved, as well as the increased cost of maintenance metabolism when whole tissues and animals are considered.

Regulation of muscle energy metabolism during the contraction–relaxation cycle

Regulation of energy metabolism in a beating heart poses the question as to what extent the metabolic rate changes during each contraction–relaxation cycle. The available data allow direct evaluation of changes in the energetic parameters and therefore possible metabolic rate changes. As indicated in Table I each beat utilizes approximately 4.5% of the total ATP content of the heart. If we assume that ATP hydrolysis occurs essentially instantaneously at a single point in the contraction–relaxation cycle and that the measured values of ATP, ADP and P_i give good approximations of their cytosolic concentrations then hydrolysis of this much ATP increases ADP by 24% and P_i by 7.7%. Consequently the cytosolic $[ATP]/[ADP][P_i]$, would be expected to decrease by approximately 29%. However the heart (as well as skeletal muscle) contains a system which 'buffers' changes in ATP and ADP. This consists of creatine phosphate (CrP) and creatine (Cr) and the enzyme, creatine phosphokinase which catalyses the near equilibrium reaction:

$$ADP + CrP \rightleftharpoons ATP + Cr$$

Because of the near equilibrium relation

between the adenine nucleotides and the creatine compounds[24,25], creatine phosphate serves to increase the available 'pool' of ATP whereas creatine fulfills the same function for ADP. One can calculate therefore that the amount of ATP which is utilized for each heart beat (2.33×10^{-7} mol/g wet wt) causes only a 2.1% decrease in the (ATP + CrP) pool and gives rise to a 4.6% increase in the (ADP + Cr) pool. Since the change in [P_i] is the same as that calculated above (7.7%) the real decline in [ATP]/[ADP][P_i] during each contraction–relaxation cycle of the beating perfused heart is only 13%. This change in [ATP]/[ADP][P_i] refers to the ratio of free cytosolic [ATP] and free cytosolic [ADP] because as long as the creatine compounds are free in the cytosol, at a large concentration (in relation to the adenine nucleotides) and linked to their respective adenine nucleotides through a near equilibrium relation the decrease in [ATP]$_f$/[ADP]$_f$ must be equal to that in [CrP]/[Cr]. This also means that the change in the [ATP]$_f$/[ADP]$_f$[P_i] calculated above (13%) is independent of the actual concentration of free ADP because the alterations in [ATP]$_f$/[ADP]$_f$[P_i] are dominated by changes in [CrP]/[Cr] owing to the much larger concentrations of the latter compounds. It follows that the 'buffering power' of the creatine phosphate/creatine pool depends on its size, i.e. the larger the concentrations of CrP plus Cr with respect to that of ATP and ADP, the smaller the changes in [ATP]/[ADP] and therefore in [ATP]/[ADP][P_i]. If, for example, the concentrations of CrP and Cr were each three times higher in the heart, the decrease in [ATP]/[ADP][P_i] during each beat would be of only 8%. It should finally be emphasized that the assumptions that ATP hydrolysis occurs at a single point in time during the contraction–relaxation cycle, gives the maximum possible decline in [ATP]$_f$/[ADP]$_f$[P_i]. The corresponding physiological change should be less than the estimated 13%.

One very important point which becomes obvious is that [P_i] is of major importance in the regulation of metabolism in muscle. Many muscles contain high concentrations of creatine phosphate and creatine (or other high energy phosphates in non-mammalian systems) and in resting muscle [P_i] is much lower than [creatine][20,25]. Under such conditions increase in [P_i] produced by hydrolysis of creatine phosphate following muscular contraction is the major contributing factor to a work-induced change in [ATP]/[ADP][P_i]. In rat thigh muscle for example[25], the tissue contents of creatine phosphate, ATP, ADP and creatine are 23, 6.2, 0.7 and 8.8×10^{-6} mol/g wet wt, respectively. The cytosolic [P_i], in contrast, is unlikely to exceed 1.6×10^{-6} mol/g wet wt[20,25]. Thus hydrolysis of 1.3×10^{-6} mol/g wet wt of total high energy phosphate (ATP + CrP) would give rise to a change in [ATP]$_f$/[ADP]$_f$ of 17% while [P_i] would increase by as much as 81%!

It follows from the foregoing discussion that changes in the [ATP]/[ADP][P_i] which occur during a single contraction–relaxation cycle of the heart muscle do not exceed 13%. Similar, if not smaller changes, occur during a single twitch of skeletal muscle since ATP utilization is of the same magnitude as in the heart (Table II) whereas the concentrations of the creatine compounds are usually larger[20,25]. The question then arises is whether such small perturbations give rise to 'visible' changes in cellular metabolism.

It has been demonstrated that the respiratory rate of mitochondria is quantitatively dependent both *in vitro*[5,7] and *in vivo*[6,7] on the extramitochondrial (cytosolic) [ATP]/[ADP][P_i]. The experimental data have been fitted to a model (described in detail elsewhere[5,7]) which allows us to calculate that for a change of 13% in the [ATP]/[ADP][P_i] at a constant intramitochondrial [NAD$^+$]/[NADH] the

Table II. Energy cost of a single contraction–relaxation cycle

Material	Condition	Compound measured	Chemical change		Ref.
			Amount/SCRC (μmol/g wet wt)	ATP/SCRC[a]	
Sartorius muscle (R. pipiens)	Isometric	CrP	−0.286	0.286	13
Sartorius muscle (R. temporaria)	Isometric	CrP	−0.293	0.293	12
Papillary muscle (cat)	Isometric	O_2	−0.0147–0.0188	0.088–0.113	14
Whole heart (rat)	Langendorff heart preparation (AP = 80 cm H_2O)	O_2	−0.0255	0.153	8,9
	Working heart prep. (LAP = 10 cm H_2O)	O_2	−0.034	0.204	8
	Working heart prep. (LAP = 10 cm H_2O)	O_2	−0.030	0.180	8
	Langendorff heart preparation (AP = 80 cm H_2O)	O_2	−0.038	0.235	7
		Lactate	+0.0076		

[a]The original values described in the indicated references were recalculated to get a per beat (or twitch) value. Except for Ref. 7, the glycolytic ATP production was ignored in accounting the free energy change. Abbreviations used: SCRC, single contraction–relaxation cycle; CrP, creatine phosphate; AP, static aortic pressure, LAP, left atrial pressure.

expected increase in respiratory activity would also be 13%. If the [NAD$^+$]/[NADH] remains constant, this increase in respiration must result from the increase in the reduced steady state level of cytochrome aa_3 and cytochrome c. In agreement with this suggestion Ramirez[26] has observed changes in the order of 2–6% in the state of reduction of the cytochromes during a single beat of amphibian heart which returned to the original level after the cycle was completed. In order to attain a *new* steady-state level of reduction of the respiratory chain components, 4–6 twitches (10–20 s) were required and with cessation of stimulation, 10–20 s were necessary to return to the former steady-state. Similarly, oxygen consumption by embryonic heart[27] followed a time course requiring 10–20 s to acquire a new steady-state and so did the changes in pyridine nucleotide fluorescence[28] associated with twitches of rabbit papillary muscle (the reported rapid fluorescence artifacts should be neglected in order to evaluate the results). It seems therefore that changes in energy metabolism in the heart during single contraction–relaxation cycle are small and that regulation of metabolic responses to alterations in work loads occur through steady-state mechanisms which are expressed as the cumulative effect of several beats. This conclusion is also in agreement with the results of Chance and Connelly[29] who noted that three times as many twitches were needed in skeletal muscle (as compared to amphibian heart muscle) to reach half the maximum oxidation–reduction change in the respiratory pigments and that the cytochrome changes persisted several minutes after a short tetanus. The difference in the behavior of heart and skeletal muscle arises from a much higher content of the creatine phosphate/creatine pool in the latter which very effectively buffer changes in the [ATP]/[ADP][P$_i$].

The role of creatine phosphokinase reaction in muscle energetics

The role of creatine and creatine phosphate in muscle tissue is not fully understood. It has generally been considered to form a 'buffer' for cellular ATP supply which smoothes the metabolic response to work transients and provides a reservoir of ATP for brief periods of anoxia. However, these effects are probably not the primary function of the creatine phosphokinase reaction. Muscle tissue must have the capability to synthesize ATP very rapidly and efficiently in the mitochondria and export it to the muscle fibers (site of its utilization) where it is hydrolysed to ADP and phosphate. Finally ADP must return to the mitochondria for ATP resynthesis. The necessity for maintaining high (>10) values of [ATP]$_f$/[ADP]$_f$ ratio in the muscle tissue results in very low concentrations of free ADP (less than 0.3×10^{-3} M with some estimates as low as 3×10^{-6} M[21]). This is too low for ADP to meet the required large diffusional fluxes. Creatine, on the other hand, is a small molecule with a high diffusion rate and is present at free concentrations of 10–1000 times higher than that of ADP. Thus the presence of creatine phosphokinase throughout the cytoplasm enhances the rate of diffusion of the dephosphorylated forms of the 'high energy' phosphate compounds (ADP plus creatine) by approximately 20- to 100-fold in heart muscle and 100- to 1000-fold in skeletal muscle as compared to ADP alone. This ensures sufficiently rapid rates of ATP synthesis to sustain continuous muscular activity.

Acknowledgement

This work was supported by USPHS GM 12202 and 21524. Maria Erecińska is an Established Investigator of the American Heart Association.

References

1 Hill, A. V. (1965) in *Trails and Trials in Physiology*, Arnold, London

2 Abbott, B. C. and Howarth, J. V. (1973) *Physiol. Rev.* 53, 120–158

3 Woledge, R. C. (1971) *Prog. Biophys. Mol. Biol.* 22, 39–74

4 Gibbs, C. L. (1978) *Physiol. Rev.* 58, 174–254

5 Holian, A., Owen, C. S. and Wilson, D. F. (1977) *Arch. Biochem. Biophys.* 181, 164–171

6 Erecińska, M., Stubbs, M., Miyata, Y., Ditre, C. M. and Wilson, D. F. (1977) *Biochim. Biophys. Acta* 462, 20–35

7 Nishiki, K., Erecińska, M. and Wilson, D. F. (1978) *Am. J. Physiol.* 234, C73–C81; C82–C89

8 Neely, J. R., Liebermeister, H., Battersby, E. J. and Morgan, H. E. (1967) *Am. J. Physiol.* 212, 804–814

9 Hassinen, I. E. and Hiltunen, K. (1975) *Biochim. Biophys. Acta* 408, 319–330

10 Nishiki, K., Erecińska, M. and Wilson, D. F. (1979) *Am. J. Physiol.* 237, C221–C230

11 Bing, R. J. (1965) *Physiol. Rev.* 45, 171–213

12 Carlson, F. D., Hardy, D. J. and Wilkie, D. F. (1967) *J. Physiol.* 189, 209–235

13 Carlson, F. D. and Siger, A. (1960) *J. Gen. Physiol.* 44, 33–60

14 Coleman, H. N., Sonnenblick, E. H. and Braunwald, E. (1971) *Am. J. Physiol.* 221, 778–783

15 Evans, C. L. and Hill, A. V. (1914) *J. Physiol. (London)* 49, 1–16

16 Fruton, J. S. and Simmonds, S. (1958) in *General Biochemistry*, John Wiley & Sons, New York, N.Y.

17 Burton, K. and Krebs, H. A. (1953) *Biochem. J.* 54, 94–107

18 Langendorff, O. (1895) *Pfluegers Arch.* 61, 29–332

19 Coulson, R. L. (1976) *J. Physiol. (London)* 260, 45–53

20 Ackerman, J. J. H., Grove, T. H., Wong, G. G., Gadian, D. G. and Radda, G. K. (1980) *Nature (London)* 283, 167–170

21 Gupta, R. K. and Moore, R. D. (1980) *J. Biol. Chem.* 255, 3987–3993

22 Brandt, P. W. and Orentlicher, M. (1972) *Biophys. J.* 12, 512–527

23 Burton, A. C. (1965) in *Physiology and Biophysics of the Circulation*, Chicago: Yearbook, 109

24 McGilvery, R. W. and Murray, T. W. (1974) *J. Biol. Chem.* 249, 5845–5850

25 Beis, I. E. and Newsholme, E. C. (1975) *Biochem. J.* 152, 23–32

26 Ramirez, J. (1959) *J. Physiol. (London)* 147, 14–32

27 Eisenberg, S. and Ramirez, J. (1963) *J. Physiol.* 169, 799–815

28 Chapman, J. B. (1972) *J. Gen. Physiol.* 59, 135–154

29 Chance, B. and Connelly, C. M. (1957) *Nature (London)* 179, 1235–1237

D. F. Wilson, K. Nishiki and M. Erecińska are at the Department of Biochemistry and Biophysics and Department of Pharmacology, University of Pennsylvania School of Medicine, Philadelphia, Pennsylvania 19104, USA.

Addendum

It is instructive to compare the energy cost of a single contraction–relaxation cycle in working muscle to that in a non-working preparation. When isolated rat cardiac cells are stimulated electrically they beat without work and consume 0.2×10^{-7} mol ATP/beat/g wet wt in the absence of isopreterenol and 0.32×10^{-7} mol ATP/beat/g in its presence (calculated from Table 3 in Ref. 30). The corresponding value for perfused rat heart obtained by extrapolation to zero pressure was 0.23×10^{-7} mol ATP/beat/g wet wt[8] which is not far removed from 0.35×10^{-7} mol ATP/beat/g in dog heart preparation shunted to prevent pressure

development[31]. Comparison of these values with those in Table II shows that in cardiac muscle under a moderate work load, 80–90% of ATP generated is used to develop tension (pressure). Under higher work loads the energy cost per beat can attain values as high as 8×10^{-7} mol ATP/g wet wt (calculated from Ref. 32). This means that in intensely working heart, 'basal' metabolism (i.e. that not involving pressure development) consumes a negligible portion of the overall ATP utilized.

Attempts have been made recently to measure directly changes in high energy phosphate compounds during the cardiac contraction–relaxation cycle[33,34]. The measurements were carried out in isolated rat hearts perfused with saline containing high glucose as the respiratory fuel and operating at high work loads. Two methods were used: standard chemical assays of freeze-clamped tissue[34], and ^{31}P NMR[33]. It was found that the levels of CrP, ATP and Pi oscillated during the cardiac cycle; highest levels of the high energy phosphate compounds were present at minimum aortic pressure and lowest at maximum pressure. The decreases in ATP and CrP (maximum to minimum) were of approximately the same magnitude and their sum amounted to about 15% of the total tissue content of the high energy phosphate compounds as measured by NMR[33] and 7.8–14% (Tables 4 and 2 of Ref. 34, respectively) as determined by chemical analysis. The changes of 14–15% correspond to approximately 20×10^{-7} mol ATP utilized/beat/g wet wt, i.e. more than twice the amount of ATP used per beat than the value calculated from the steady state rate of O_2 utilization for very similar experimental conditions (8×10^{-7} mol ATP; Ref. 32). Moreover, the oscillations appeared to be substrate specific since they were not observed when pyruvate was used instead of glucose[34]. It is difficult to explain the nature of these oscillations on several grounds: (1) oscillations in the high-energy phosphate compounds cannot exceed significantly the consumption of ATP (oxygen) per beat; (2) true metabolic oscillations in ATP and CrP should not have an all or nothing substrate-dependence; and (3) near equilibrium of the CPK (creatine phosphokinase) reaction and the steady-state levels of adenylates and creatine compounds should have yielded larger alterations in the levels of CrP than in ATP, not the nearly equal changes reported in the studies above. These considerations suggest that the oscillations which were observed do not reflect the behavior of hearts under physiological conditions

but may have been due, in part, to pressure-induced tissue hypoxia which can arise in preparations perfused with saline (which has low-oxygen carrying capacity) and operating at a high work load. During systole, muscular contraction decreases vascular volume and increases vascular resistance which allows respiration to deplete the perfusion medium, and the tissue, of oxygen thus leading to a transient tissue hypoxia and lowering of the high-energy phosphate compounds. This situation is reversed during diastole when fresh, oxygen-containing medium reperfuses the heart. Hence the oscillations reported should largely disappear when whole blood is used for perfusion or lower pressures are developed in the hearts.

The view that the role of creatine phosphate, creatine and creatine phosphokinase is to buffer the cellular ATP supply *and* to facilitate transport of ATP and ADP (see last section of the review) has received wide and independent support[35–37]. Meyer et al.[37] summarized the results of recent investigations and presented elegant calculations of the effect of CPK on the diffusional fluxes of ATP and ADP in muscle. They demonstrated that both functions depend quantitatively on the equilibrium constant for the enzyme, on the total concentrations of adenylates and creatine and on the [ATP]/[ADP] ratio. The binding of CPK isoenzymes near sites of ATP production or utilization serves to raise the local enzyme activity where the net flux is greatest, thus ensuring overall near equilibrium. It has been concluded that no physical or functional compartmentation or diffusion barrier to adenylates (see for example Refs. 38 and 39) need be postulated to explain the currently available results.

References

30 Haworth, R. A., Hunter, D. R., Berkoff, H. A. and Moss, R. L. (1983) *Circ. Res.* 52, 342–351
31 Gibbs, C. L., Papadoyannis, D. E., Drake,

A. J. and Noble, M. I. M. (1980) *Circ. Res.* 47, 408–417

32 Neely, J. R., Rovetto, M. J., Whitmer, J. T. and Morgan, H. E. (1973) *Am. J. Physiol.* 225, 651–658

33 Fossel, E. T., Morgan, H. E. and Ingwall, J. S. (1980) *Proc. Natl Acad. Sci. USA*, 77, 3654–3658

34 Wikman-Coffelt, J., Sievers, R., Coffelt, R. J. and Parmley, W. M. (1983) *Amer. J. Physiol.* 245, H354–H362

35 Bessman, S. P. and Geiger, P. J. (1981) *Science* 211, 448–452

36 Seraydarian, M. W. (1982) *Trends Biochem. Sci.* 7, 393–395

37 Meyer, R. A., Sweeney, H. L. and Kushmerick, M. J. (1984) *Am. J. Physiol.*, 246, C365–C377

38 Bessman, S. P., Yang, W. C. T., Geiger, P. J. and Erickson-Viitanen, S. (1980) *Biochem. Biophys. Res. Commun.* 96, 1414–1420

39 Saks, V. A., Kupriyanov, V. V., Preobrazhenskii, A. N. and Jacobus, W. E. (1982) *J. Mol. Cell. Cardiol.* 14, 1–12

What governs ethanol metabolism? Biochemists have an alcohol problem

A. G. Dawson

The question of which factors are most influential in determining the rate of ethanol metabolism in the liver, and hence the speed at which ethanol is eliminated from the body, is of considerable importance. Not only does it exercise the minds of quite a few biochemists – a fact which alone may be thought sufficient evidence of that importance – but it also has social and clinical implications in relation to possible therapeutic measures that might be taken to alleviate severe intoxication by ethanol.

It has been pointed out[1] that one such measure would be to accelerate the elimination of ethanol by administering a suitable agent. As yet, however, only large intravenous doses of fructose have been proved effective in this respect in man[2,3]. This kind of therapy is inconvenient and can have undesirable side effects, although it is no doubt more acceptable than the only other procedures so far observed to be effective in experimental animals, i.e. excessive stress[4], castration[5-7] or treatment with oestradiol[7]. Given this resistance of ethanol metabolism to easy manipulation, it seems that we need to know more about the way it is regulated if better means of accelerating ethanol elimination are to be devised.

Metabolic pathways involved

The process of ethanol metabolism is, by comparison with many other catabolic sequences, very simple. It is practically confined to the liver and involves only the oxidation of ethanol to acetaldehyde which, in turn, is oxidized to acetate. This last product is released from the liver and becomes available for other tissues to use as an energy source.

Earlier controversy over the relative importance of various enzymatic mechanisms able to oxidize ethanol to acetaldehyde has largely faded. It is now widely accepted that, under all but the most exceptional circumstances, alcohol dehydrogenase, a cytosolic NAD-dependent enzyme, is predominantly responsible for the transformation. Oxidation of acetaldehyde to acetate is catalysed by another NAD-dependent enzyme, aldehyde dehydrogenase. At least two types of this enzyme exist, residing in various parts of the liver cell; however, it is fairly certain that, in rats at least, nearly all acetaldehyde oxidation takes place in the mitochondria under the influence of the high-affinity isoenzyme[8].

Despite the apparently uncomplicated nature of this principal pathway of ethanol metabolism, there is strong disagreement over what governs the rate of metabolic flux through the pathway. This is mainly because the pathway is integrated with other metabolic processes and could, therefore, be controlled to a greater or lesser extent by factors that regulate these other processes. For example, ethanol oxidation can be sustained only if cytosolic NADH is reoxidized at a sufficient rate to maintain the supply of NAD to alcohol dehydrogenase. As illustrated in Fig. 1, this normally requires the mediation of hydrogen shuttles capable of moving reducing equivalents from cytosol to mitochondria[9] and can also be influenced by factors involved in the regulation of mitochondrial respiration. Indeed, it is on this question of the adequacy of the NAD supply that the current argument over the control of ethanol metabolism hinges.

NAD level or enzyme level?

Two contrasting concepts of how the rate of ethanol metabolism is governed have developed over the past decade. In simple terms, one states that the liver contains ample alcohol dehydrogenase, but that its activity is limited by the rate at which NAD is regenerated. The opposing view is that the amount of alcohol dehydrogenase *per se* is the crucial factor and that its activity is not normally restricted by the availability of NAD. Both hypotheses are supported by substantial arguments but both have weaknesses.

There seems little doubt that the rate of reoxidation of NADH can severely restrict ethanol metabolism in freshly isolated hepatocytes[10-12], but such cell preparations are known often to be depleted of substrates involved in hydrogen shuttles[11,13]. When these substrates are supplied, or when the oxidation of cytosolic NADH is more directly stimulated by adding pyruvate, the rate of ethanol metabolism rises, but only to the level normally seen *in vivo*[11,14]. Attempts to promote ethanol metabolism *in vivo* by stimulating NADH oxidation have yielded conflicting results[15,16], though some believe that the positive effect of fructose is brought about in this way[17]. Israel and his colleagues, however, contend that the acceleration of ethanol metabolism that accompanies the induction of a 'hypermetabolic state' can be attributed to an

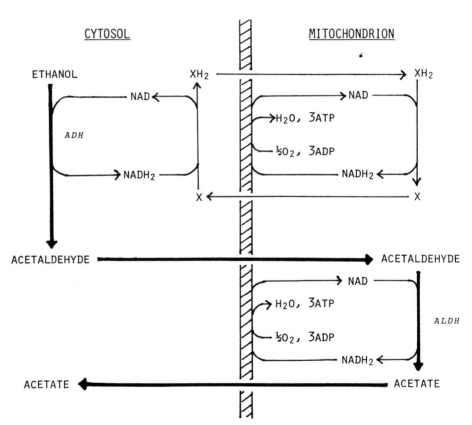

Fig. 1. The principal pathway of ethanol metabolism in the liver cell. *ADH = alcohol dehydrogenase, ALDH = aldehyde dehydrogenase, X = oxidized intermediate of hydrogen shuttle, XH_2 = reduced intermediate of hydrogen shuttle. It is important to note that most hydrogen shuttles are more complex than is indicated here.* For more details see Ref. 9.

increase in the rate of intramitochondrial NADH oxidation, prompted by a raised ADP/ATP ratio[18].

Other evidence purported to favour the concept of limitation by the coenzyme level was recently reported by Kashiwagi *et al.*[19]. Using the perfused rat liver they examined ethanol metabolism and the associated changes in NADH concentration in different regions of the liver lobule. The rationale for this approach was that earlier histochemical studies had indicated that alcohol dehydrogenase activity is higher in the periportal region of the lobule than in the pericentral region[20], whereas NAD and NADH were thought to be evenly distributed. It was reasoned, therefore, that the relative rates of ethanol metabolism in the two regions should show whether enzyme activity or NAD supply was the principal rate-determining factor. The experiments were performed by perfusing media containing various concentrations of ethanol through the liver, in either the anterograde (portal vein → vena cava) or retrograde (vena cava → portal vein) direction and monitoring changes in NADH fluorescence by means of a micro-light guide placed over pericentral or periportal areas. Because the tip of the guide was only 170 μm across (one-third of the average diameter of a liver lobule) there seemed little chance that recordings of fluorescence changes in one region would be unduly influenced by changes in the other. The data obtained led these workers to conclude that pericentral and periportal regions oxidized ethanol at similar rates, consistent with the distribution of NAD but not with that of alcohol dehydrogenase.

However, this work while technically sophisticated, is of questionable value on at least three counts. First, rates of ethanol oxidation were not measured directly but were calculated from the observed increases in NADH fluorescence. This not only begs the question but, because it links higher rates of ethanol metabolism with higher levels of NADH,. and hence with lower levels of NAD, argues against the authors' general conclusions. Second, the statement that similar maximal fluorescence changes occurred in the two regions was not borne out by the data which showed a 25% greater increase in the periportal region than in the pericentral region, consistent with the assumed distribution of alcohol dehydrogenase. The last count, one which confuses the whole issue, is that alcohol dehydrogenase might not be distributed as assumed by Kashiwagi *et al.*[19]. Using immunohistochemical techniques Buehler *et al.*[21] found that pericentral, rather than periportal, regions of human liver contained the most alcohol dehydrogenase, a finding which agrees with that made by Morrison and Brock[22] on both human and rat liver.

Among those who dispute the idea that the rate of ethanol oxidation is determined by the rate at which NAD is regenerated and who, instead, consider the level of alcohol dehydrogenase to be the crucial factor, Kathryn Crow and her colleagues have been prominent. Braggins and Crow[16] described experiments in which they administered ethanol to live rats through the exteriorized opening of a cannula dwelling in the hepatic vein and then followed the rate at which the ethanol disappeared from the blood. They were unable to detect any stimulation of ethanol metabolism by pyruvate and in fact found that the rate at which ethanol was eliminated correlated positively with the lactate/pyruvate ratio. This implied that the highest rates of ethanol metabolism occurred in association with the lowest NAD levels.

Braggins and Crow[16] also measured the hepatic alcohol dehydrogenase activity of each of the rats used in the experiments on ethanol elimination. They calculated that the average activity was just sufficient to account for the average rate of ethanol clearance *in vivo*. This finding, if taken at face value, appears to support the same group's earlier contention (based largely on an analysis of the kinetics of alcohol dehydrogenase) that the amount of enzyme, and not the availability of NAD, governs the rate at which ethanol is metabolized *in vivo*[23]. However, two points might be noted: first, it might not be judicious to draw too firm conclusions concerning the activity of an enzyme in its cellular environment from measurements made under contrived assay conditions and, second, analysis of the data from individual rats used in these experiments revealed no correlation between liver alcohol dehydrogenase activity and the rate of ethanol clearance. This lack of correlation must devalue the hypothesis that the alcohol dehydrogenase level alone is important.

Hormonal effects

Other evidence relevant to the question of whether the alcohol dehydrogenase level governs the rate of ethanol metabolism comes from studies on the effect of hormones. Experiments with certain strains of rat have shown that, in males, castration or treatment with oestradiol raises both the rate of ethanol metabolism and the specific activity of liver alcohol dehydrogenase[5-7]. Testosterone has the opposite effect in females[7]. These data suggest a positive link between the alcohol dehydrogenase level and ethanol elimination but it must be remembered that hormonal effects on enzyme levels are rarely very specific. The activities of enzymes involved in other possible regulatory mechanisms were not looked at in any of these studies. In addition, it has been observed that thyroidectomy leads to an increase in hepatic alcohol dehydrogenase without any corresponding increase in the rate of ethanol metabolism[24], while rats acclimatized to cold conditions are reported to metabolize ethanol more quickly, despite suffering a small fall in liver alcohol dehydrogenase activity[25]. Observations such as these throw considerable doubt on the idea that the level of alcohol dehydrogenase is the sole governor of ethanol metabolism.

What other factors could be involved?

As neither of the two main hypotheses provides a totally satisfactory explanation of how ethanol metabolism is controlled it is worthwhile considering what other factors might be involved. Perhaps the most likely candidate for a regulatory role is acetaldehyde, which has long been known to act as an inhibitor of liver alcohol dehydrogenase[26], although at concentrations higher than those at one time considered to obtain *in vivo*. However, some recent work suggests that the role of acetaldehyde, and especially the relationship between alcohol dehydrogenase and aldehyde dehydrogenase activities, merits further attention[27,28]. Direct regulation by acetaldehyde at least explains why the concentration of this potentially cytotoxic intermediate does not rise to intolerably high levels. This point is not always addressed by other hypotheses, despite the knowledge that aldehyde dehydrogenase activity in the liver is probably no higher than alcohol dehydrogenase activity and would therefore have to operate with maximum efficiency to prevent such an occurrence.

Much remains to be learned in this area and, in relation to the overall control of ethanol metabolism *in vivo*, it is just one more element to be considered in what remains a very open question.

References

1 Linnoila, M. and Mattila, M. J. (1981) *Pharmac. Ther.* 15, 99–109
2 Brown, S. S., Forrest, J. A. H. and Roscoe, P. (1972) *Lancet* ii, 898–900
3 Sprandel, U., Troger, H.-D., Liebhardt, E. W. and Zollner, N. (1980) *Nutr. Metab.* 24, 324–330
4 Mezey, E., Potter, J. J. and Kvetnansky, R. (1979) *Biochem. Pharmac.* 28, 657–663
5 Mezey, E., Potter, J. J., Harmon, S. M. and Tsitouras, P. D. (1980) *Biochem. Pharmac.* 29, 3175–3180
6 Cicero, T. J., Bernard, J. D. and Newman, K. (1980) *J. Pharmac. Exp. Ther.* 215, 317–324
7 Rachamin, G., Macdonald, J. A., Wahid, S., Clapp, J. J., Khanna, J. M. and Israel, Y. (1980) *Biochem. J.* 186, 483–490
8 Eriksson, C. J. P., Marselos, M. and Koivula, T. (1975) *Biochem. J.* 152, 709–712
9 Dawson, A. G. (1979) *Trends Biochem. Sci.* 4, 171–175
10 Meijer, A. J., Van Woerkom, G. M., Williamson,

J. R. and Tager, J. M. (1975) *Biochem. J.* 150, 205–209

11 Crow, K. E., Cornell, N. W. and Veech, R. L. (1978) *Biochem. J.* 172, 29–36

12 Rognstad, R. (1981) *Biochim. Biophys. Acta* 676, 270–273

13 Krebs, H. A., Cornell, N. W., Lund, P. and Hems, R. (1974) in *Regulation of Hepatic Metabolism* (Lundquist, F. and Tygstrup, N., eds), pp. 726–750, Academic Press, New York

14 Berry, M. N., Fanning, D. C., Grivell, A. R. and Wallace, P. G. (1980) *Biochem. Pharmac.* 29, 2161–2168

15 Wendell, G. D. and Thurman, R. G. (1979) *Biochem. Pharmac.* 28, 273–279

16 Braggins, T. J. and Crow, K. E. (1981) *Eur. J. Biochem.* 119, 633–640

17 Scholz, R. (1977) in *Alcohol and Aldehyde Metabolizing Systems* (Thurman, R. G., Williamson, J. R., Drott, H. R. and Chance, B., eds), Vol. 3, pp. 271–284, Academic Press, New York

18 Israel, Y., Videla, L., Fernandez-Videla, V. and Bernstein, J. (1975) *J. Pharmac. Exp. Ther.* 192, 565–574

19 Kashiwagi, T., Ji, S., Lemasters, J. J. and Thurman, R. G. (1982) *Molec. Pharmac.* 21, 438–443

20 Greenberger, N. J., Cohen, R. B. and Isselbacher,

K. J. (1965) *Lab. Invest.* 14, 264–271

21 Buehler, R., Hess, H. and Von Wartburg, J.-P. (1982) *Am. J. Path.* 108, 89–99

22 Morrison, G. R. and Brock, F. E. (1967) *J. Lab. Clin. Med.* 70, 116–120

23 Cornell, N. W., Crow, K. E., Leadbetter, M. G. and Veech, R. L. (1979) in *Alcohol and Nutrition* (Li, T.-K., Schenker, S. and Lumeng, L., eds), pp. 315–330, US Government Printing Office, Washington, DC

24 Mezey, E. and Potter, J. J. (1981) *Gastroenterology* 80, 566–574

25 Videla, L., Flattery, K. V., Sellars, E. A. and Israel, Y. (1975) *J. Pharmac. Exp. Ther.* 192, 575–582

26 Wratten, C. C. and Cleland, W. W. (1963) *Biochemistry* 2, 935–941

27 Dawson, A. G. (1981) *Biochem. Pharmac.* 30, 2349–2352

28 Dawson, A. G. (1983) *Biochem. Pharmac.* 32, 2157–2165

A. G. Dawson is at the Department of Biochemistry, School of Biological and Biomedical Sciences, The New South Wales Institute of Technology, Australia.

Addendum

The balance of opinion on this question now appears to be shifting towards the view that the level of hepatic alcohol dehydrogenase is the dominant governing factor. In recent articles both Cornell[29] and Crabb et al.[30] suggest that once the activity of alcohol dehydrogenase has been determined *in vitro*, and assuming that the intrahepatic concentrations of substrates and products *in vivo* are known, the rate of ethanol metabolism can be predicted simply by fitting these data and the appropriate kinetic constants to be steady-state rate equation for the alcohol dehydrogenase-catalysed reaction. According to Cornell[29], this approach indicates that, *in vivo*, alcohol dehydrogenase is not greatly restricted either by lack of substrates or accumulation of products, and the enzyme level is therefore the most important determinant of flux through

the ethanol metabolic pathway. Crabb et al.[30] reach a similar conclusion.

This appears, on the surface, a remarkably simple and, indeed, self-evident solution to the biochemists' alcohol problem but it should be treated with some reservation. At the very least it must be asked how closely alcohol dehydrogenase activity determined *in vitro* represents the true *in vivo* activity, whether or not the measured kinetic constants are valid for the enzyme *in situ*, and how accurate are the values for the concentrations of reactants, especially NADH and acetaldehyde, at the enzymic site. Middleton and Kacser[31], in a paper dealing with alcohol dehydrogenase activity and metabolic flux in *Drosophila melanogaster*, caution against a too literal translation of *in vitro* measurements to the *in vivo* state, and it is worth noting that Cornell[29] and Crabb et al.[30] offer substantially different values for some kinetic constants even though both claim to have used 'physiological' conditions for their determination. If, in fact, the two different sets of kinetic constants are used in conjunction with one or other set of velocity and concentration terms the predicted rates vary considerably and the apparent value of the approach suffers accordingly. As to the concentrations of reactants, there is always some degree of unreliability in values for NADH based upon hepatic lactate/pyruvate ratios and there is evidence to suggest that the concentration of acetaldehyde within the liver cells might be considerably higher than either Cornell[29] or Crabb et al.[30] allow. Uncertainties such as these highlight the difficulties inherent in this kind of direct approach to the question of how ethanol metabolism is controlled.

In an alternative approach, Sturtevant and Garber[32] attempted to shed light on the problem by looking at the circadian rhythm of alcohol dehydrogenase in the rat. Peak activity was at the mid-point of the dark phase of a 12 h light/12 h dark cycle and was twice the activity measured at the mid-point of the light phase. The higher enzyme activity in the dark period was accompanied by a substantially higher rate of clearance of ethanol from the blood, suggesting a direct link between alcohol dehydrogenase activity and metabolic flux. Unfortunately, the activities of other enzymes that might directly or indirectly influence the rate of ethanol metabolism via the alcohol dehydrogenase pathway were not measured, and so the specificity of the association between the circadian rhythms of ethanol clearance and alcohol dehydrogenase activity remains in doubt.

Hence, while recent articles may lean towards alcohol dehydrogenase as the single most important governor of the rate of ethanol metabolism, there is plenty of scope for more definitive evidence to be adduced.

References

28 Dawson, A. G. (1983) *Biochem. Pharmac.* 32, 2157–2165

29 Cornell, N. W. (1983) *Pharmac. Biochem. Behav.* 18 (Suppl. 1), 215–221

30 Crabb, D. W., Bosron, W. F. and Li, T-K. (1983) *Arch. Biochem. Biophys.* 224, 299–309

31 Middleton, R. J. and Kacser, H. (1983) *Genetics* 105, 633–650

32 Sturtevant, R. P. and Garber, S. L. (1984) *Proc. Soc. Exp. Biol. Med.* 175, 299–303

Biochemists' alcohol problem: a case of addiction to the wrong concepts?

H. Kacser

In his concise and informative review on the problems of ethanol metabolism, Dr Dawson (see p. 87 of this book) exposed opposing hypotheses of 'what governs the rate of metabolic flux through the pathway'. He presented the conflicting evidence from a variety of authors and approaches which attempted to answer the question 'whether enzyme activity or NAD supply was the principal rate-determining factor'.

By coincidence, in another recent TIBS article, Dr Porteous (see p. 29 of this book) discussed a fundamentally different approach to such problems, in the development of which I have played some part. May I therefore be permitted to make a few general remarks although I must stress that my experience in the field of ethanol metabolism is minimal.*

It would be absurd to suggest that either alcohol dehydrogenase activity or NAD 'supply' played *no* part in the metabolic flux and the various authors do not say this. What they do, however, appear to believe is that *one* of these factors must be 'the most influential'.

It is at this point that I must give my opinion that the questions which are being asked and the concepts which they reveal are based on a profound misapprehension of the kinetic nature and organization of metabolic systems. Let me pursue the 'walk-through-the-system' which Dr Dawson began in his diagram. The NAD

'supply' to the cytosol is clearly dependent on metabolic events within the mitochondrion, hydrogen shuttles, ADP/ATP- ratios (which in turn depend on other well-known ATP generating pathways). Acetaldehyde, which may act as an effector as well as a product is further transformed to acetate (dependent on NAD, ATP, etc.). All the associated enzymes and transport systems, apart from interacting with a variety of effectors, are subject to genetic control. The signals, which affect their synthesis and hence 'control' their concentration, are themselves generated within the system. Acetate enters further pathways going to acetyl CoA etc. etc. (Please consult a reliable textbook or wall chart for the continuation of your 'walk'. At the end the diligent reader will find himself having traversed the whole of the biochemical world.) It is therefore clear that any particular flux (or other variable) is coupled, in some way, to every element in the system and hence, in principle, is affected by all of them. The question which 'factors' 'govern' or 'control' the flux must therefore be answered by: All factors. A systemic property, such as flux, is just that – the whole system is involved in determining its magnitude. Left at that, this would be a depressingly empty conclusion.

We can, however, *start* from this and ask further questions: Are all factors equally involved? If not, is factor A more 'important' than factor B? What is the definition of 'importance' and what criteria should we apply? In attempting to answer such questions a quantitative theory of control has been developed. This

---

* Middleton, R. J. and Kacser, H. (1983). Enzyme variation, metabolic flux and fitness: Alcohol Dehydrogenase in *D. Melanogaster. Genetics* 105, 633–650

is not the place to expound this in any detail (which can be found in the publications cited in Dr Porteous' letter). The central concept derives from the measurement of the response of a chosen variable to a small (in principle, infinitesimal) change in a chosen factor. This is expressed as a dimensionless number, a coefficient, whose magnitude represents precisely the effectiveness of a factor and the share among all the factors investigated in controlling the variable. There is no place in the theory for such *a priori* notions as 'rate-determining factor', 'sufficient supply' or 'excess enzyme' nor does it tolerate the confusion of treating enzyme concentrations and effector concentrations as equivalent. The systems analysis enables us to devise experiments (different from the traditional ones) which yield the quantitative parameters of 'control'. The experimental evidence available indicates that the major share of the control is usually distributed among many enzymes and translocators.

The insight gained from such an analysis then convinces us that the question: 'Is it the enzyme level or the NAD level which governs ethanol metabolism?' is unanswerable. What is answerable is a series of questions concerned with the distribution of control and with the quantitative evaluation of the various interactions using a methodology demanded by the theory. If this is done we shall end up with a precise array of numbers, the control coefficients, describing the absolute and relative role which each element plays.

The biochemists' alcohol problem which Dr Dawson diagnosed is a reflection of a more general malaise. The lack of progress in certain areas of biochemistry (and genetics) has, in my opinion, been due to the addiction of its practitioners to false concepts and, like all addicts, they are not very effective workers. The pushers in this trade are, of course, the writers-of-books and the givers-of-lectures. They corrupt the young who are then hooked. All is not bleak, however. There *is* a cure. In the last few years a number of strong minded people have undergone the cold turkey treatment. This consists of reading the relevant papers until one has understood them. Once free of the addiction, unlike an ex-alcoholic, one is cured for life.

H. Kacser is at the Department of Genetics, University of Edinburgh, West Mains Road, Edinburgh EH9 3JN, UK.

Futile cycling in glucose metabolism

Joseph Katz and Robert Rognstad

When interconversion of two compounds occurs by irreversible reactions, and the enzymes catalysing these reactions are both active, there is 'futile cycling', with dissipation of energy without a corresponding change in metabolites. There is now evidence for such cycling in glucose metabolism. How do we measure such cycling? Are futile cycles utile, and if so, what is their function?

According to body needs animal cells have the capacity to synthesize and catabolize a large variety of cell constituents. For example, triglycerides are synthesized and deposited in fat tissue of the fed animal, and on fasting are hydrolysed to glycerol and fatty acid which are exported via the blood stream. Thus there must be effective controls of the opposite pathways. Unexpectedly, experiments with radioisotopes *in vitro* indicated that in adipose tissue simultaneously with active lipogenesis there was also extensive lipolysis, so that fatty acids were continuously recycled.

Activation of fatty acids to acyl-CoA esters requires energy, ultimately derived from ATP, so that recycling dissipates energy without any metabolic gain, and hence the designation 'futile cycling'. We have estimated that in epididymal fat pad tissue of fed rats, the rate of lipolysis is about one-half that of esterification, and that about 10% of the ATP production is used up in this cycling[1]. There is a host of reactions that potentially could constitute futile cycles, but there is experimental evidence for very few of them. So far the only system studied in animal tissue has been carbohydrate metabolism in liver.

There are three irreversible steps in the interconversion of glucose and pyruvate, between (a) glucose and glucose 6-P, (b) fructose 6-P and fructose 1,6-P_2, and (c) between pyruvate and P-enolpyruvate. Cycling has been established to occur at all three steps *in vitro*. Here we will limit ourselves to the first two cycles. We will discuss briefly the methods to detect and quantitate these cycles and their presumed physiological role. A detailed exposition is available[2].

The irreversible reactions between glucose and glucose 6-P, and fructose 6-P and fructose 1,6-P_2 are catalysed in the direction of glycolysis by two kinases [glucokinase and phosphofructokinase (PFK)], and in the direction of gluconeogenesis by the phosphatases [glucose-6-phosphatase (G6Pase) and fructose-1,6-diphosphatase (FDPase)], as shown below.

$$\text{glucokinase}$$
$$\text{ATP + glucose} \longrightarrow \text{glucose 6-P + ADP} \quad (1a)$$

$$\text{G6Pase}$$
$$\text{glucose 6-P} \longrightarrow \text{glucose} + P_i \quad (1b)$$

$$\text{Sum: ATP} \longrightarrow \text{ADP} + P_i$$

$$\text{PFK}$$
$$\text{ATP + fructose 6-P} \longrightarrow \text{fructose 1,6-}P_2 + \text{ADP} \quad (2a)$$

$$\text{FDPase}$$
$$\text{fructose 1,6-}P_2 \longrightarrow \text{fructose 6-P} + P_i \quad (2b)$$

$$\text{Sum: ATP} \longrightarrow \text{ADP} + P_i$$

If the two opposite reactions proceed simultaneously the result is ATP breakdown not accompanied by a net change in substrates or products. Assays *in vitro* show that two kinases and two phosphatases are active in liver tissue; however, the enzymes could be largely or even completely inhibited. There is no way to detect cycling, except by using isotopes.

The glucose–glucose 6-P cycle

Simultaneous operation of hexo- (and gluco-) kinase and G6Pase in liver was first observed in the mid-fifties by the investigators in Baird-Hastings Laboratory at Harvard. In their pioneering studies with ^{14}C-labeled glucose, summarized by Cahill[3], they observed with rat-liver slices incorporation of ^{14}C into CO_2, glycogen and lactate, in the absence of any net glucose uptake or even during glucose production. They concluded that glucose was phosphorylated to glucose 6-P, which in part was metabolized, and in part hydrolysed back to glucose and pointed out that the incorporation of ^{14}C from glucose in liver does not provide a measure of net glucose utilization. This work, however,

had little impact and recycling was largely neglected for about 25 years. It was 'rediscovered' in our laboratory when the metabolism of [14]C- and ^{3}H-labeled glucose were compared using isolated rat hepatocytes. It was found that the yield of water from [2-^{3}H]glucose greatly exceeded the incorporation of ^{14}C into products (mainly lactate and CO_2)[4]. Isotope uptake occurred also when there was net glucose production, either from glycogen or from added precursors.

The formation of water from [2-^{3}H]-glucose serves to measure the rate of glucose phosphorylation. The method is based on the exchange of tritium from position 2 of glucose 6-P with the protons of water. The hexose 6-P isomerization represents a transfer of hydrogen between C-2 of an aldose to C-1 of a ketose. In each transfer about one-half the hydrogen is exchanged with protons of the medium and one-half retained in the ester[5]. When [2-^{3}H] glucose is phosphorylated the tritium is retained, but will be partially lost in the isomerization. If the isomerization is very rapid, as an upper theoretical limit,

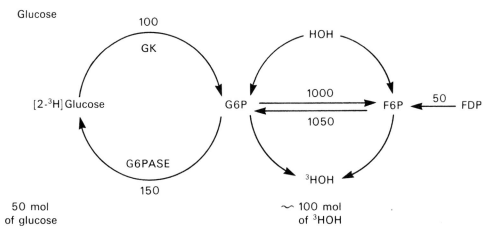

Fig. 1. The detritiation of [2-³H]glucose. There is inflow of 50 mol from fructose 1,6-P₂ (FDP) and net synthesis of 50 mol of glucose. However, glucokinase (GK) is active and per unit time 100 mol of glucose are phosphorylated and 150 dephosphorylated with a net formation of 50 μmol of glucose. The rate of phosphohexose isomerase is 1000 mol, so that the glucose 6-P loses its tritium before reconversion into glucose, with a yield of 100 mol of ³HOH although there was no net uptake of glucose.

glucose 6-P will contain no tritium and the glucose once phosphorylated will lose its entire tritium (see Fig. 1).

With [2-^{3}H, U-^{14}C]glucose as substrate the specific activity of [^{14}C]glucose 6-P will be that in the medium, but if detritiation is complete the ^{3}H:^{14}C ratio will be close to 0, and under those conditions the yield of labeled water will provide a simple means to determine the rate of glucose phosphorylation (see Fig. 1). In reality, however, the isomerization of the hexose phosphate is not rapid enough to bring about complete detritiation and the ^{3}H:^{14}C ratios in glucose 6-P (as compared to glucose) range from 0.25 to 0.5[6]. Thus to calculate the rate of phosphorylation from the labeled water yield it is necessary to correct for incomplete detritiation. Two procedures for this have been proposed. One of these requires the isolation and determination of the relative specific activity of glucose 6-P derived from [2-^{3}H] glucose, an exacting and tedious procedure. An easier method[7] is to measure the incorporation of [2-^{3}H]-galactose into glucose and water. The ratio ^{3}H in water + ^{3}H in glucose : ^{3}H in water provides a correction factor for incomplete detritiation of [2-^{3}H]glucose. The two methods were compared and gave identical results[8].

Cycling between the fructose phosphates

One criterion for this cycling is based on the detritiation from positions 3 or 5 of glucose, and is similar in principle to that described for [2-^{3}H]glucose. [3-^{3}H, 5-^{3}H]-fructose 1,6-P$_2$ is formed glycolytically from tritiated glucose and cleaved by aldolase to dihydroxyacetone-P and glyceraldehyde 3-P, containing tritium on C-1 and C-2 respectively. This tritium is exchanged with protons of the medium in the triose-P isomerase reactions[5]. If the aldolase and triose-P isomerase reactions are close to equilibrium, most of the tritium in fructose 1,6-P$_2$ will be replaced by hydrogen, and

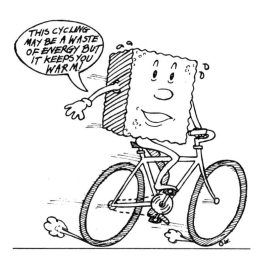

if PFK and FDPase are both active there will be dilution of the specific activity of the hexose 6-phosphates. If the labeled glucose is labeled with ^{14}C and tritium, the ^{3}H:^{14}C ratio in fructose 1,6-P$_2$ and the hexose phosphates will be less than that of substrate glucose. This approach was first applied by M. Clark et al.[9] in bumblebee flight muscle (see below).

In perfused liver[10] and rat hepatocytes[6] there was detritiation of [3-^{3}H]- and [5-^{3}H]glucose during glucose formation from lactate indicating the operation of PFK during gluconeogenesis. However, more label in water was formed from positions 5 than from 3. Detritiation of [3-^{3}H]- and [5-^{3}H]glucose may also occur via the pentose cycle or by exchange reactions[11] casting doubts on the validity of the methods based on tritiated glucoses. Also there is no simple procedure to correct for incomplete detritiation.

An alternate criterion for the simultaneous activity of PFK and FDPase is provided by randomization of ^{14}C in hexose phosphates[12]. [1-^{14}C]Galactose will form hexose phosphates and glucose without randomization when there is no recycling, but if PFK and FDPase are both active ^{14}C will be introduced into position 6. The extent of randomization will depend also on the

Table I. Glucose phosphorylation and G6Pase activity in rat hepatocytes

Diet	Lactate	Δ Glucose	Glucose phosphorylation	G6Pase
Fed	−	−24	106	82
	+	+22	102	124
Fasted	−	+6	32	38
	+	+34	26	60
Diabetic, fed	−	+4	7.8	12
	+	+46	4.0	50

Cells were incubated with [2-³H]glucose, 15 mM, with or without 10 mM lactate. (After Ref. 4, corrected for incomplete detritiation.) All quantities are expressed as μmol h^{-1} (g wet wt)$^{-1}$

activities of aldolase and hexose-6-P isomerase, complicating quantitative estimates of recycling.

Futile cycling *in vitro* and *in vivo*

Glucose phosphorylation and G6Pase rates are shown for hepatocytes obtained from meal fed, fasted and streptozotocin diabetic rats (Table I). The phosphorylation of glucose is greater in the fed than in the fasted animal, and is much reduced in the diabetic. This is as expected from the response of glucokinase to diet and diabetes[13]. The rate of glucose phosphorylation was found to depend primarily on the concentration of medium glucose as expected with a high K_m (10–20 mM) enzyme such as glucokinase. The phosphorylation was not affected by glucagon[6,8] which stimulates glucose synthesis. Under most conditions the detritiation is 60–70% of the theoretical maximum[9]. However, in the presence of fructose, detritiation is greatly depressed (to 20–30% of maximum), because of extensive inhibition of hexose-6-P isomerase by fructose 1-P[14] and the correction ranges from 350 to 500%.

It should be stressed that the method described here measures glucose 6-P formation by any and all enzymes by whatever mechanism. The phosphorylation rate parallels the activity of glucokinase. It is low in the diabetic where G6Pase is very high and glucokinase depressed. This makes phosphorylation

of glucose via G6Pase, as suggested by Nordlie[15], rather unlikely.

In Table II, rates of action of PFK and FDPase in hepatocytes of fasted rats, calculated from the randomization of ¹⁴C from [1-¹⁴C]glucose, are presented. Glucose contained from 2 to 5% of its activity in carbon 6. The rate of action of PFK, calculated from this randomization, ranged from 12 to 30% of that of FDPase[12]. Glucagon but not epinephrine markedly depressed randomization, increased glucose production from dihydroxyacetone by 15–25%, and greatly depressed PFK activity to as low as 2% of the rate of FDPase. The increase in glucose production by glucagon can only partially be accounted for by a depression of PFK activity.

The calculations are based on several yet unproven assumptions but most likely indicate the order of magnitude and direction of the effects. In hepatocytes of fed animals randomization is much higher and recycling is likely to be more extensive. However, calculations of the rates for the fed state are much more complex, and the methods which were used for the fasted state are not adequate for the fed.

Results in perfused liver resemble those in hepatocytes. The rate of detritiation of [2-³H]- [5-³H]- and [3-³H]glucose are much higher than those of [1,6-³H] glucose and of ¹⁴C uptake[16]. *In vivo* the turnover of [2-³H]glucose is much higher than that of other tritiated glucoses and of $^{14}C^{16}$. However, as distinct from *in vitro* there appears to be little difference between the turnover of 3-, 5- or [6-^{3}H]glucose[16]. Some 10–15% of the total turnover of [2-^{3}H]glucose could be due to futile cycling between glucose and glucose 6-P. On the other hand it appears that there is as yet no evidence for appreciable cycling between fructose 6-P and fructose 1,6-P$_2$ *in vivo*.

Physiological role of futile cycling

There has been a great deal of speculation on the utility of 'futile' cycles. The functions most commonly suggested are in heat generation and metabolic control. Newsholme[17–19] has advanced the role of cycling in numerous processes in health and disease. The most likely functions are in thermogenesis and in metabolic control.

Thermogenesis

Since the energy dissipated in cycling appears as heat it was reasonable to attribute to it a role in body temperature regulation. Good evidence for such a role has been provided in bumblebees. For flight the temperature the flight muscle has to attain is about 30°C. In cold weather bumblebees forage for nectar, whereas honeybees are not able to fly and remain in the hive. Newsholme et al.[20] measured the activity of PFK and FDPase in flight muscle of a number of species of the genera *Apis* (honeybees) and *Bombus* (bumblebees). Both genera have high levels of PFK. There was virtually no activity of FDPase in honeybees, but in bumblebees the level of FDPase was about the same as that of PFK. Newsholme suggested that in bumblebees a futile cycle between fructose 6-P and fructose 1,6-P$_2$ provides heat, to permit flying in cold weather. Clark et al.[9] indeed showed that futile cycling occurs in bumblebee muscle at low temperature (5°C) but not at 30°C. However, Newsholme pointed out[19] that at most, cycling between the fructose phosphates could provide 10–15% of the heat requirement for flight.

Since muscle lacks pyruvate carboxylase and PEP carboxykinase, mammalian muscle was thought to lack the capacity of glycogen synthesis from pyruvate. The function of FDPase in white muscle fibers was puzzling. It was proposed to play a role in thermogenesis. Calculations, however, reveal that the contribution of this cycle to heat production in mammals would be very small. Most recently, the glycogen synthesis from lactate was convincingly demonstrated by Hermansen and Vaage in human muscle[21]. Thus while the mechanism of phosphoenolpyruvate synthesis in muscle is still obscure, it is most likely that FDPase is still involved in glycogen synthesis. The fact that FDPase is restricted to white muscle fibers, whose major fuel

Table II. PFK and FDPase activities in hepatocytes of fasted rats

Expt. No.	Additions	Formation of: glucose (μmol min^{-1} g^{-1})	lactate	C6:C1 ratio in glucose	FDPase (μmol min^{-1} g^{-1})	PFK	PFK/ FDPase
1	None	86	47	0.024	99	13	0.13
	0.1 μM Glucagon	113	16	0.004	115	2	0.018
	1 μM Epinephrine	90	45	0.023	102	12	0.12
2	None	87	43	0.045	121	34	0.28
	0.01 μM Glucagon	100	24	0.011	107	6.8	0.064
	10 mM Ethanol	86	14	0.017	94	8.0	0.085

Cells were incubated for 30 min with 10 mM dihydroxyacetone and trace amounts of [1-^{14}C]galactose. (After Ref. 12.)

is glycogen, and is absent in red fibers and cardiac muscle, whose fuel is mainly fat, supports this conclusion.

Metabolic control

PFK and FDPase are allosteric enzymes, affected by several ligands, the most important of which is probably AMP. It inhibits FDPase, but counteracts the inhibition of PFK by ATP. Attempts to correlate carbohydrate metabolism in liver with ligand concentration have, however, been unsuccessful. Newsholme[17-19] proposed that cycling would amplify the response to ligands, and he has provided an extensive theoretical analysis of such an effect. The concept can be best explained by an example. Suppose that the rate of PFK is 100 and of FDPase is 90, with a net glycolytic flux of 10 (arbitrary units). Suppose a small increase in ADP concentration stimulates PFK by 5%, and depresses the rate of FDPase by an equal amount. Then the rate of glycolysis would be 108−85 or 20 units. This illustrates that when recycling is much higher than the flux, small changes in ligand levels, not readily detectable by analysis, would markedly affect rates of flux, and could readily reverse its direction. For efficient modulation the two rates must be of similar magnitude and the rate of cycling must be much higher than the net flux, an energetically rather wasteful mode of regulation. Actually, as described above, the rate of PFK in hepatocytes is 10–30% that of FDPase and PFK is virtually inactive in the presence of glucagon. Thus cycling provides only a small gain in sensitivity of control under these conditions.

Glucokinase and glucose-6-Pase are high K_m enzymes (10 and 2–4 mM respectively). The concentration of glucose is of the order of the K_m for glucokinase and that of glucose 6-P one order of magnitude less than the K_m values. Neither of these enzymes is under significant allosteric control. Thus the rates of these enzymes in any one dietary state would be largely determined by the concentration of their substrates. A regulatory role in maintaining the level of blood glucose has been attributed to the glucokinase–G6Pase catalysed cycling, with rates of flux and its direction determined mainly by changes in the concentration of glucose 6-P in the liver cell[22]. Glucose 6-P is a major metabolic crossroad, with inputs and outputs to and from 3-carbon precursors, glycogen, glucose and the pentose-cycle system. The interplay of all enzymes including glucokinase and G6Pase will determine the magnitude and direction of the various metabolic flows. It is difficult, however, in such a system to distinguish cause from effect and to assign a definite regulatory 'function' to cycling.

In our opinion it is still not clear whether the phenomenon of cycling has evolved as a regulatory mechanism. Cycling might simply be due to the 'imperfection' of regulatory mechanisms. To use an analogy, it could be akin to a leaky water supply system. Unfortunately, experimental data are so limited, that generalizations are risky.

Summing up

For many years the idea was prevalent that metabolic control operates in a manner analogous to an electric flip-flop switch, simultaneously turning on one reaction and shutting off the other. At another extreme several physiological functions have been attributed to cycling, and it has been suggested that it plays a role in a number of pathological conditions and in aging. The results described here show the first idea to be not generally tenable.

There is still very little evidence to support speculations about the function of cycling. The elucidation of its function requires reliable quantitative measurements. This is a difficult task and has been achieved only for few systems, all *in vitro*. So far the studies have been restricted to very few laboratories. The authors hope that this problem will in the near future attract more extensive experimental studies, and that novel improved methods will be developed to measure cycling *in vitro* and *in vivo*.

References

1 Rognstad, R. and Katz, J. (1966) *Proc. Natl Acad. Sci. USA* 55, 1148–1156

2 Katz, J. and Rognstad, R. (1976) in *Current Topics in Cell. Regulation*, Vol. 10, 237–289

3 Cahill, C. F., Ashmore, J., Renold, A. E. and Hastings, A. B. (1959) *Am. J. Med.* 26, 264–282

4 Clark, D. G., Rognstad, R. and Katz, J. (1973) *Biochem. Biophys. Res. Commun.* 54, 1141–1148

5 Rose, I. D. and Rose, Z. B. (1969) *Comp. Biochem. Physiol.* 17, 93–161

6 Katz, J., Wals, P. A., Golden, S. and Rognstad, R. (1975) *Eur. J. Biochem.* 60, 91–101

7 Rognstad, R. (1976) *Int. J. Biochem.* 7, 221–228

8 Katz, J., Wals, P. A. and Rognstad, R. (1978) *J. Biol. Chem.* 253, 4530–4536

9 Clark, M. G., Bloxham, D. P., Holland, P. C. and Lardy, H. A. (1973) *Biochem. J.* 134, 589–597

10 Clark, D. G., Lee, D., Rognstad, R. and Katz, J. (1975) *Biochem. Biophys. Res. Commun.* 67, 212–219

11 Hue, L. and Hers, H. G. (1974) *Biochem. Biophys. Res. Common.* 58, 532–539

12 Rognstad, R. and Katz, J. (1976) *Arch. Biochem. Biophys.* 177, 337–345

13 Weinhouse, S. (1976) in *Current Topics in Cell. Regulation*, Vol. 11.

14 Zalitis, J. and Oliver, I. T. (1967) *Biochem. J.* 102, 735–759

15 Nordlie, R. I. (1976, 1974) in *Current Topics in Cell. Regulation* Vol. 8, 33–117

16 Katz, J., Golden, S., Dunn, A. and Chenoweth, M. (1976) *Hoppe-Seyler's Z. Physiol. Chem.* 357, 1387–1394

17 Newsholme, F. A. and Gevers, W. (1967) *Vitam. Horm.* 25, 1–87

18 Newsholme, F. A. and Crabtree, B. (1976) *Biochem. Soc. Symp.* 41, 61–109

19 Newsholme, F. A. and Start, C. (1973) *Regulation in Metabolism*, Wiley and Sons

20 Newsholme, F. A., Crabtree, B., Higgins, S. J., Thornton, S. D. and Start, C. (1972) *Biochem. J.* 128, 89–97

21 Hermansen, L. and Vaage, O. (1977) *Am. J. Physiol.* 233, E422–E429

22 Hue, L. and Hers, H. G. (1974) *Biochem. Biophys. Res. Commun.* 58, 540–548

J. Katz and R. Rognstad are at Cedars-Sinai Medical Center, Los Angeles, CA 90048. USA.

Substrate cycles: their role in improving sensitivity in metabolic control

E. A. Newsholme, R. A. J. Challiss and B. Crabtree

Substrate cycles can be shown, theoretically, to be one of a series of mechanisms for improving sensitivity of enzymes, enzyme-systems or transport processes to changes in the concentrations of effectors. The rates of four cycles, the triacylglycerol/fatty acid, glucose/glucose 6-phosphate, fructose 6-phosphate/fructose bisphosphate and glycogen/glucose 1-phosphate cycles, are all increased either by the stress hormones or by changes in physiological conditions. These findings provide experimental support for the view that cycles improve sensitivity in metabolic regulation.

In many biochemical or physiological processes a weak stimulus produces a large or massive response (e.g. activation of the blood clotting process, activation of glycolytic flux in muscle, increase in the flux through the Krebs cycle in avian pectoral or insect flight muscle in the transition from rest to flight, the maintenance of a *precise* concentration of an ion or a specific protein in the cell). This ability can be represented diagrammatically as follows:

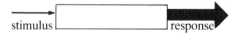

It invites an answer to the question, how does the 'black box' in the diagram convert the weak stimulus into the large response? Unfortunately, it is all too easy to state 'the process is switched on by the increase in concentration of Ca^{2+} ions or cyclic AMP or . . . . . .', or to suggest that it is achieved by a cascade mechanism without defining what is meant by any of these terms. A simple analysis of the physical chemistry of interactions between concentration of a regulator and enzyme activity demonstrates the magnitude of the problem contained within such statements.

Sensitivity in metabolic regulation can be defined as the quantitative relationship between the relative change in enzyme activity and the relative change in concentration of the regulator.† For example, if an enzyme activity increases 100-fold, to produce the necessary change in metabolic flux, how large an increase in concentration of regulator is required? The greater the response of enzyme activity to a given increase in regulator concentration, the greater is the sensitivity[1].

In order to understand how sensitivity can be improved, it is necessary to appreciate the basic mechanism of the regulation of enzyme activity. It is probable that all regulators modify the activity of an enzyme by binding in a reversible manner to a protein; such binding, which is described as equilibrium binding, will control the activity of the enzyme as follows:

$$E + X \rightleftharpoons E^*X$$

†If the concentration of a regulator (x) changes by Δx, the relative change is $\Delta x/x$; similarly, if the flux (J) changes by ΔJ, the relative change is $\Delta J/J$. The sensitivity of J to the change in x is given by the ratio $(\Delta J/J)/(\Delta x/x)$.

where E is the inactive form of the enzyme and E* is the active form. The asterisk indicates that the binding of X has changed the conformation of the catalytic site, so that the enzyme is now in the active form. The normal response of enzyme activity to the binding of the regulator is hyperbolic, and this response is relatively 'inefficient' for metabolic regulation; for example, on the most linear portion of the response, a two-fold change in regulator concentration will change the enzyme activity by no more than two-fold (i.e. the maximum sensitivity is unity). (The same argument applies to the interaction of a hormone or a neurotransmitter with a specific receptor.) Application of this important point to the above statement concerning 'switches' illustrates the problems. To decrease the activity of E to zero, or almost to zero, the concentration of X must decrease to zero, or almost zero, whereas to elicit a maximal response (i.e. a 'switch') the concentration of X would need to increase to infinity. Such changes are impossible. Even the sarcoplasmic reticulum, which is very extensively distributed throughout a muscle fibre, only produces about a 100-fold change in Ca^{2+} concentration, from 10^{-8} M (not zero) to 10^{-6} M (Ref. 2).

Consequently, mechanisms must exist to raise the sensitivity above that of simple equilibrium binding[3,4]. One simple means is via a high catalytic activity of the enzyme so that it catalyses a near-equilibrium reaction – such reactions are sensitive to changes in concentrations of substrates or products, and especially co-substrate and co-product but not to allosteric effectors. More complex mechanisms are, however, required at non-equilibrium reactions.

Mechanisms for improving sensitivity at non-equilibrium reactions

There are several different mechanisms for improving sensitivity; these include multiplicity of regulators, co-operativity, interconversion cycles and substrate cycles. If an enzyme can respond to several different effector molecules, concentration changes in all these effectors could result in a large change in activity; a good example is muscle 6-phosphofructokinase[5].

The response of the activity of some enzymes to substrate or regulator concentration is sigmoid or cooperative. Hence, for part of the concentration range of the regulator, the sensitivity will be greater than that provided by the hyperbolic response (i.e. greater than unity). A limitation of this mechanism is that the extent of the improvement in sensitivity is fixed depending on the degree of sigmoidicity[6].

An increasing number of enzymes are considered to be regulated by interconversion cycles. The enzymes exist in two forms, conventionally designated a and b, one being a covalent modification of the other, and only one form (a) has significant catalytic activity, so that the flux can be regulated by altering the amount of enzyme in this form. The covalent modification may involve phosphorylation, adenylation, methylation, acetylation or ADP-ribosylation. The interconversions between the forms are catalysed by enzymes, one for each direction, the activity of which can be modified by regulators. Theoretical analysis of this mechanism demonstrates that a large increase in sensitivity is possible[7], but direct experimental evidence that the system improves sensitivity is still lacking.

An enzyme that catalyses a reaction in the forward direction of a pathway (i.e. A → B) may be 'opposed' by an enzyme that catalyses a reaction in the reverse direction as follows:

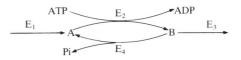

If the two enzymes are simultaneously active a substrate cycle results. Since both forward and reverse reactions are non-equilibrium, each turn of the cycle must involve the conversion of chemical energy into heat (i.e. hydrolysis of ATP) so that such cycles are sometimes termed 'futile'. The theoretical role of such cycles in improving sensitivity[3,4] is described briefly below.

Substrate cycles and sensitivity

In some metabolic pathways, it may be necessary during 'resting' conditions to decrease the flux through a reaction to almost zero. Even with a sigmoid response this would require that the concentration of an activator be lowered to almost zero or that of an inhibitor increased to almost infinity. Such enormous changes in concentration probably never occur in living organisms; they may cause osmotic or ionic problems and unwanted side reactions (even small increases in the concentration of blood glucose can result, over a period of time in marked damage to basement membranes, probably due to the interaction of the glucose molecule with protein molecules[4,8]). However, the net flux through a reaction can be decreased to very low values (approaching zero) via a substrate cycle. Thus, in the above scheme, as the product of the forward enzyme (i.e. B) is produced, most of it could be converted back into substrate A by the reverse enzyme (E_4). Hence, the net flux (i.e. A to B) is *very* low despite a finite activity of the forward enzyme and a moderate concentration of an activator of E_2. Now, if the concentration of this activator is increased, by only a small amount above that at which the activities of the two enzymes are almost identical (and the flux is almost zero), the activity of E_2 will increase so that the net flux through the reaction will increase from almost zero to a moderate rate‡. Such a cycle therefore provides a large improvement in sensi-

tivity; indeed, it can be seen as a means of producing a threshold response (or a 'switch' or 'gate' mechanism) using a simple metabolic system[9]. It must, however, be emphasized that, similarly to the other mechanisms described above, the improvement in sensitivity applies only to the rate of conversion of A to B and *not* to the pathway as a whole. Other cycles or other means of improving sensitivity must occur at other non-equilibrium reactions of the pathway.

Evidence for the role of substrate cycles in metabolic regulation

So far, the discussion on the role of substrate cycles has been theoretical. The question can be raised, do cycles exist and, if so, do they play any role in metabolic regulation? There is no doubt that substrate cycles exist; that is, that the activities of forward and reverse reactions occur simultaneously: these include glucose/glucose 6-phosphate[11,12], fructose 6-phosphate/fructose bisphosphate[13,14], phosphoenolypyruvate/pyruvate[15], adenosine/AMP[16], glycogen/glucose 1-phosphate[17], triglyceride/fatty acid[18], glutamate/glutamine[19]. Furthermore the turnover of protein, effected by the processes of protein synthesis and protein degradation, can be considered to be an amino acid/protein cycle and, similarly, the turnover of cell Na^+, effected by the Na^+-ATPase and the Na^+-leak process, can be considered to be a Na^+-translocation cycle[3]; (these cycles may be involved, not so much in the control of flux, but in the control of the *precise* concentration of a given pro-

‡This means for improving sensitivity has been criticized on the grounds that an increase in activity of E_2 will lead to an increase in the concentration of B which will only stimulate a greater rate of cycling via an increase in the activity of E_4 (Ref. 10). This can be avoided by several means including the following: substrate saturation of E_4; activation of E_3 so that there is little or no increase in the concentration of B; inhibition of E_4 by the same effector that stimulates E_2.

tein or that of intracellular Na^+)§. However, the demonstration that cycling occurs does not prove that they play a role in metabolic regulation; indeed it has been proposed that cycles represent imperfections in evolution of metabolic control[21].

An important prediction of the hypothesis that cycles are involved in metabolic regulation is that the cycling rate will vary from one condition to another, and that some hormones, especially the stress hormones, will specifically increase the rate of cycling. In other words, variations in the cycling rate are expected since the requirement for sensitivity will vary from one condition to another. Such variations have now been demonstrated for a number of cycles, and it is predicted that similar variations in rate will be eventually observed for most, if not all, substrate cycles.

(1) The precise rate of triacylglycerol/ fatty acid cycle can be measured by comparing the rates of fatty acid and glycerol production by adipose tissue, or by following the rates of incorporation of $[^3H]$ from ^3H_2O into the glycerol and fatty acid moieties of triacylglycerol. The cycling rate was increased markedly by β-adrenergic agents and the effect was abolished by the β-blocker propranolol[18]. Furthermore, the rate of this cycle in white adipose tissue *in vivo* was doubled by feeding and increased five-fold by a β-agonist, and, in brown adipose tissue, it was increased three-fold by a β-agonist and doubled by exposure to the cold (4°C) for 4 h[22].

(2) The precise rate of the glucose/ glucose 6-phosphate cycle can be measured from the changes in the $^3H/^{14}C$ radioactivity ratio in glucose *and* hexose monophosphates after isolation and separation from a tissue that has been utilizing $[2-^3H, 2-^{14}C]$glucose. Such studies demonstrated that the cycling rate was increased 65-fold in the flight muscle of the hawk moth, *Acherontia atropos*, during flight. The rate of cycling at rest was 0.06 and this was increased during flight to 3.9 μmol/min per g; the latter represents 85% of the maximum glucose 6-phosphatase activity determined *in vitro*[12].

(3) The precise rate of the fructose 6-phosphate/fructose bisphosphate cycle can be measured from the changes in the $^3H/^{14}C$ radioactivity ratio in hexose-monophosphates *and* fructose bisphosphate after isolation and separation from a tissue that has been utilizing $[5-^3H, 6-^{14}C]$glucose. The hormone adrenaline, or other β-adrenergic agents, increased the cycling rate up to ten-fold in the isolated epitrochlearis muscle of the rat. This stimulation occurred at physiological concentrations of the hormone and was abolished by the β-blocker propanolol[17].

(4) The rate of the glycogen/glucose 1-phosphate cycle can be measured in an *in vitro* incubated muscle preparation from the difference between the rate of glycogen synthesis and the rate of breakdown. The rate of synthesis has been measured from the incorporation of $[^{14}C]$ from $[^{14}C]$glucose into glycogen. The rate of glycogen degradation has been measured from that of lactate formation: from the difference in lactate concentration when estimated radiochemically (i.e. conversion of $[^{14}C]$-glucose to lactate) and that estimated by

§If the concentration of intracellular Na^+ was dependent only upon the active process of Na^+-extrusion, the rate of the latter would need to be inhibited *totally* when the concentration reached the required intracellular value; this would be impossible to achieve. However, the concentration can be easily but precisely regulated at a given value when the rate of active extrusion equals the rate of leakage into the cell. Similarly, the concentration of a given protein can be more easily maintained by the 'balance' between synthesis and degradation. Since there are probably many proteins whose concentrations must be maintained precisely, it is perhaps not surprising that the protein turnover accounts for at least 20% of the basal metabolic rate[20].

a non-radiochemical assay (i.e. conversion of both glucose and glycogen to lactate). Adrenaline decreased the rate of this cycle in the isolated muscle but it was increased by exposure of the donor animal to the cold (4°C) for 60 h[17].

The changes in the rates of cycling caused by the conditions indicated above, support but do not prove the hypothesis that substrate cycles improve sensitivity in metabolic and endocrine control. It is suggested that one major role of the stress hormones is to increase the rate of substrate cycles that play a role in the mobilization and utilization of fuels. Consequently, if the sensitivity to the stress hormones were decreased or a lower concentration of the hormone were released for a given stimulus, a greater change in the concentration of a regulator (e.g. allosteric effector or other hormone) would be needed to produce a normal increase in flux through reaction or pathway. Since tissues from older animals are less sensitive to the effects of a number of hormones[23] it is tempting to speculate that ageing decreases either the capacity of substrate cycles or the ability of certain tissues to respond to catecholamines. The speculation provides a further means of testing the hypothesis that substrate cycling increases sensitivity in metabolic control.

References

1 Crabtree, B. and Newsholme, E. A. (1978) *Eur. J. Biochem.* 89, 19–22
2 Ashley, C. C. (1983) in *Calcium in Biology* (Spiro, T. G., ed.), John Wiley
3 Newsholme. E. A. and Crabtree, B. (1976) *Biochem. Soc. Symp.* 41, 61–109
4 Newsholme. E. A. and Leech, A. R. (1983) *Biochemistry for the Medical Sciences*, Chapter 7, John Wiley
5 Tejwani, G. A. (1983) *Adv. Enzymol.* 54, 121–194
6 Newsholme, E. A. and Crabtree, B. (1973) *Symp. Soc. Exp. Biol.* 27, 429–460
7 Stadtman, E. R. and Chock, P. B. (1978) *Curr. Top. Cell. Regul.* 13, 53–95
8 Brownlee, M. and Cerami, A. (1981) *Ann. Rev. Biochem.* 50, 385–432
9 Newsholme. E. A. (1978) *Biochem. Soc. Symp.* 43, 183–205
10 Stein, R. B. and Blum, J. J. (1978) *J. Theor. Biol.* 72, 487–522
11 Clark, D. G., Rognstad, R. and Katz. J. (1973) *Biochem. Biophys. Res. Commun.* 54, 1141–1148
12 Surholt, B. and Newsholme. E. A. (1983) *Biochem. J.* 210, 49–54
13 Clark, M. G., Bloxham, D. P., Holland, P. C. and Lardy, H. A. (1973) *Biochem. J.* 134, 589–597
14 Rognstad, R. and Katz. J. (1980) *Arch. Biochem. Biophys.* 203, 642–646
15 Friedman, B., Goodman, E. H., Saunders, H. L., Kostos, V. and Weinhouse, S. (1971) *Arch. Biochem. Biophys.* 143, 566–578
16 Bontemps, F., van den Berghe, G. and Hers, H.-G. (1983) *Proc. Natl Acad. Sci. USA* 80, 2829–2833
17 Challiss, R. A. J., Arch, J. R. S. and Newsholme, E. A. (1984) *Biochem. J.* 221, 153–161
18 Brooks, B., Arch, J. R. S. and Newsholme. E. A. (1982) *FEBS Lett.* 146, 327–330
19 Haussinger, D., Gerok, W. and Seis, H. (1983) *Biochim. Biophys. Acta* 755, 272–278
20 Waterlow, J. C. and Jackson, A. D. (1981) *Brit. Med. Bull.* 37, 5–10
21 Katz, J. and Rognstad, R. (1978) *Trends Biochem. Sci.* 3, 171–174
22 Brooks, B., Arch, J. R. S. and Newsholme, E. A. (1983) *Biosci. Rep.* 3, 263–267
23 Davidson, M. B. (1979) *Metabolism* 28, 688–705

E. A. Newsholme and R. A. J. Challiss are at the Department of Biochemistry, University of Oxford, South Parks Road, Oxford OX1 3QU, UK. B. Crabtree is at the Rowett Research Institute, Bucksburn, Aberdeen, Scotland.

A critical examination of the evidence for the reactions of the pentose pathway in animal tissues

John F. Williams

There are two pentose pathway reaction sequences in tissues. The classical textbook reaction scheme is present in adipose tissue and is now called the F-type pathway. A new pathway has been found in liver, photosynthetic and other tissues and is called the L-type pathway. The evidence for the L-type pathway is reviewed.

Status of and evidence for the pathway

The pentose phosphate pathway of glucose metabolism (Fig. 1) is recognized as an established sequence of intermediary steps for the dissimilation of glucose in many tissues. The pathway has the status of having been accepted in biochemistry for some time and has featured in textbooks of general biochemistry since 1956. It thus has some of the attributes of a canon of biochemical science. The unravelling of the pentose pathway was recently reviewed[1]. The identification of the pathway in tissues conventionally involves one or more of the following observations:

(1) A rate of formation of $^{14}CO_2$ from [1-^{14}C]glucose which is greater than the rate of $^{14}CO_2$ formation from [6-^{14}C]glucose (C-1/C-6 ratio>1).

(2) Conversion by enzymically active tissue extracts of ribose 5-phosphate to hexose 6-phosphate via the intermediates of Fig. 1.

(3) An enzyme composition of the tissue consistent with the catalysed steps of the sequence of Fig. 1.

Given that the above criteria are satisfied, investigators have most often applied [2-^{14}C]glucose to the tissue and quantitatively estimated the percentage contribution of the pathway to total glucose metabolism using the unique degree of ^{14}C isotope distribution into carbon atoms 1 and 3 of glucose 6-phosphate (Fig. 1). It is

invariably the case that a derivative of glucose 6-phosphate (e.g. glucose units of glycogen) is isolated and the ^{14}C isotope distribution measured in the carbon atoms of the degraded hexose[2]. Quantitative methods and estimates of the pentose cycle in tissue have been reviewed[3,4]. In spite of the seeming simplicity of the above procedures, the results of their application in liver tissue are most complicated and defy interpretation using the reaction scheme of Fig. 1[5]. It is thus necessary to be reminded of the weaknesses in the evidence and the limitations of the type of experiment which was used to establish the reaction scheme of Fig. 1. It is also important to note that any change in the ordered reaction sequence of Fig. 1 will invalidate both the degree and distribution of ^{14}C isotope into hexose 6-phosphate and thus nullify the quantitative and predictive value of these methods. It is the aim of this article to review recent evidence which disagrees with the reaction scheme of Fig. 1.

Evidence for the reaction sequence

Before proceeding with the evidence from the recent studies, it is apposite to reiterate briefly the nature and results of the type of experiment which has provided the sole basis for the metabolic pathway outlined in Fig. 1[6,7]. The experiment involved incubating [1-^{14}C]- or [2,3-^{14}C]ribose 5-phosphate with buffer extracts

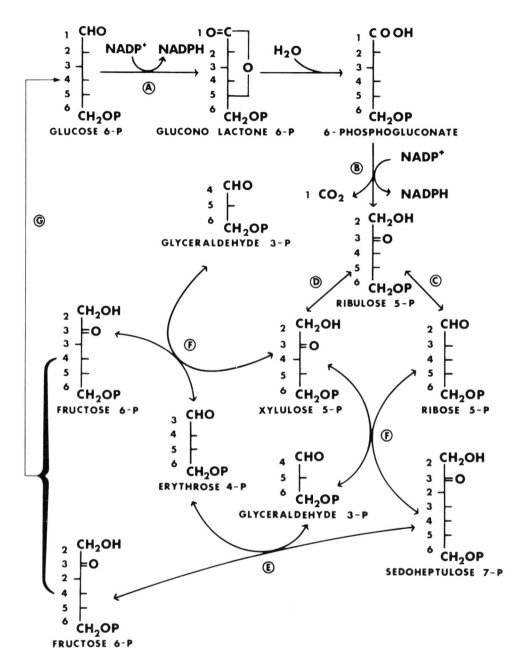

Fig. 1. Reaction sequence of F-type Pentose Pathway. (A) Glucose 6-P dehydrogenase; (B) 6-phosphogluconate dehydrogenase; (C) pentose 5-P isomerase; (D) pentose 5-P-3' epimerase; (E) transaldolase; (F) transketolase; (G) phosphohexose isomerase.

* In Fig. 1 the numbering of the carbon atoms of all the intermediates corresponds to those of the original glucose substrate. In the description of the experiments involving [^{14}C]ribose 5-phosphate (see 'Evidence for the reaction sequence') the redistribution of ^{14}C may be followed in Fig. 1 by substituting [2-^{14}C]glucose 6-P and [3,4-^{14}C]glucose 6-P for [1-^{14}C] and [2,3-^{14}C]ribose 5-P, respectively.

of enzymes from acetone dried powders prepared from rat liver, pea root or pea leaf tissues; [14C]hexose 6-phosphate and triose phosphate were formed. The acetone-dried powder preparations have the advantage over fresh tissue extracts of being free from nucleotides so that the oxidative decarboxylation of glucose 6-phosphate and its recycling is prevented. Such an experiment essentially 'froze' the 14C in the reaction product after only one passage through the sequence of Fig. 1. Formation of hexose 6-phosphate from triose 3-phosphate produced in the pathway was prevented by omitting Mg^{2+} from the reaction mixture, which inhibited the action of hexose bisphosphatase. The incubation with liver enzyme was carried out for 17 h and the reaction product was sampled only at that time. The incubations with pea root and pea leaf enzymes were sampled after 4 and 2 h respectively. Although fructose 1,6-bisphosphatase was specifically inhibited in the liver incubations[6] this enzyme was reported to be most active in both the pea leaf and pea root preparations[7]. With liver the [1-14C]ribose 5-phosphate gave rise to [1,3-14C]hexose 6-phosphate, with 74% of the 14C in C-1 and 24% in C-3 (C-1/C-3 ratio = 3). The [2,3-14C]pentose 5-phosphate yielded glucose 6-phosphate labelled with 14C isotope as follows: 45% in C-4, 28% in C-3 and 7% in C-1. The isotope distributions in hexose 6-phosphate formed by pea root tissue enzyme was essentially the same as that in liver.

These results were tentatively interpreted[6] to occur by reactions (a) to (e):

(a) 2[1-14C]R 5-P $\leftrightharpoons$ 2[1-14C]Xu 5-P

(b) [1-14C]R 5-P + [1-14C]Xu 5-P $\leftrightharpoons$
$\qquad$ [1,3-14C]SH 7-P + GA 3-P

(c) [1,3-14C]SH 7-P + GA 3-P $\leftrightharpoons$
$\qquad$ [1,3-14C]Fru 6-P + Ery 4-P

(d) [1-14C]Xu 5-P + Ery 4P $\leftrightharpoons$
$\qquad$ [1-14C]Fru 6-P + GA 3-P

Sum.

(e) 3[1-14C]R 5-P$\rightarrow$[1,3-14C]Fru 6-P +
$\qquad$ [1-14C]Fru 6-P + GA 3-P

R = ribose, XU = xylulose, Ery = erythrose, Fru = fructose, SH = sedoheptulose, GA = glyceraldehyde.

It is of note that the C-1/C-3 ratio of the hexose 6-phosphate product of reaction (e) is 2/1, whereas the experimental value was 3/1. The experiments involving [2,3-14C]ribose 5-phosphate resulted in a significant labelling of C-1 of hexose 6-P formed by liver and the pea tissue enzymes. Labelling of carbon 1 using this substrate is prohibited by the reaction sequence of Fig. 1.

These anomalies notwithstanding the equations were written as a metabolic pathway[8]. The above experiments and their consequences have been reviewed[9,10].

The development during the years 1958–63 of methods for measuring the pentose cycle revived new interest in the reactions of Fig. 1 and were responsible for much subsequent attention to quantitative carbohydrate metabolism. Liver was a tissue of interest for these studies because it eminently satisfied the three criteria for the presence of the pathway and also because it was one of the two tissues where the reaction sequence of the pathway of Fig. 1 was originally established.

Contradictory evidence

Surprisingly, the short term (5 min) metabolism of [2-14C]glucose by liver *in vivo*[5] and by liver slices[11] indicated that there was less than 3% pentose cycle in spite of liver having a C-1/C-6 ratio varying from 3 to 7 and a rich complement of enzymes which could catalyse the reaction steps of Fig. 1. Following the metabolism of [2-14C]glucose *in vivo* one would predict from the reaction mechanism of Fig. 1 that twice as much 14C isotope should be in carbon 1 as compared to carbon 3. This was not found[5]. Instead there was a heavy 14C labelling in position 6 of the glucose 6-phosphate product. These findings redirected attention to the experimental procedure which initially established the pentose pathway. To this end [1-14C]-ribose 5-phosphate was incubated with rat

Table I. Distribution of ^{14}C in glucose 6-phosphate formed at various times from [1-^{14}C] ribose 5-phosphate as catalysed by the rat liver enzyme preparation

Carbon atom	Sample time						
	1 min	2 min	5 min	30 min	3 h	8 h	17 h
1	1.0	0.5	1.1	2.0	28.2	40.6	57.2
2	45.0	44.0	16.1	12.9	20.9	13.4	10.2
3	1.7	0.1	2.2	1.9	9.8	16.3	25.1
4	10.1	3.1	4.9	6.9	4.5	4.6	2.7
5	0.9	5.9	0.9	0.1	1.9	3.7	1.4
6	41.3	46.4	74.8	76.2	34.7	21.4	3.4
Recovery (%)	98.4	100.3	107.7	97.9	98.9	98.2	98.6

liver enzyme preparation for 1, 2, 5, 30 min and 3, 8 and 17 h[9]. The hexose 6-phosphate product of these reactions was recovered and degraded in order to measure the distribution of ^{14}C in the carbon atoms of each sample (Table I).

The data of Table I show that at 17 h there is some agreement with the 17 h data of the original experiment[6], the C-1/C-3 ratio is 2.3 and thus nearer the theoretical prediction of equation (e) and carbons 4, 5 and 6 are only lightly labelled. There is, however, significant ^{14}C in carbon 2. At all times less than 17 h there was heavy ^{14}C labelling of carbon 6 (76% at 30 min) and carbon 2 remained significantly labelled throughout the timecourse.

The ^{14}C labelling of carbon 6 hexose 6-phosphate was very similar to that found in hexose 6-phosphate formed from [2-^{14}C]glucose metabolism in liver in vivo[5]. It is thus clear that the pentose pathway reactions of Fig. 1 cannot be reconciled with the data of Table I and a new and different sequence of reactions must exist to produce such labelling in liver. Analysis for the intermediates of Fig. 1 in the reaction mixture which was used to generate the data of Table I indicated that up to 20% of the carbon could not be accounted for and no free inorganic phosphate had been formed[9]. Thus it was concluded that the pentose pathway was different in liver from that shown in Fig. 1 and that there were significant quantities of phosphorylated compounds present that were probably connected with the formation of hexose 6-phosphate and their presence was indicated by heavy labelling of carbons 2 and 6 of the final product.

The new L-type pentose pathway

The reaction sequence of Fig. 2 shows a new pathway for the conversion of ribose 5-P to hexose 6-P. The sequence of reactions is consistent with the distribution of ^{14}C noted during the first 8 h incubations shown in Table I. The pathway also contains as intermediates the principal phosphorylated compounds which were discovered during the search for the 20% deficit of substrate carbon noted above[9]. The changing concentrations of these new intermediates during the conversion of ribose 5-P to hexose 6-P are given in Table II.

Fig. 2 shows how carbon 1 of ribose 5-P (C-2 of glucose 6-P) is transferred to position 2 of product glucose 6-P. The heavy labelling of carbon 6 of hexose 6-P (Table I) is not caused by metabolite flux but is entirely due to the actions of ^{14}C exchange reactions catalysed by transketolase[12] and transaldolase[13]. The sequence of these exchange reactions has been described[10, 14].

Distinguishing features of the L-type pathway

Over and above the unique and specific ^{14}C transfers of Fig. 2 and Table I, the

L-type pathway is characterized by the actions of aldolase (reaction H, Fig. 2) and two new enzyme activities, a pentose 5-phosphate 2'-epimerase (reaction E, Fig. 2) and a phosphotransferase, D-*glycero* D-*ido* octulose 1,8-bisphosphate: D-*altro* heptulose 7-phosphotransferase (reaction I, Fig. 2) The *altro* and the *ido* isomers of the octulose phosphates, sedoheptulose 1,7-bisphosphate, *manno*heptulose 7-P and arabinose 5-P were found in pentose pathway reaction mixtures *in vitro* (Table II)[10]. The octulose phosphates and the two heptulose phosphates have recently been found in fresh liver and their concentrations measured[15].

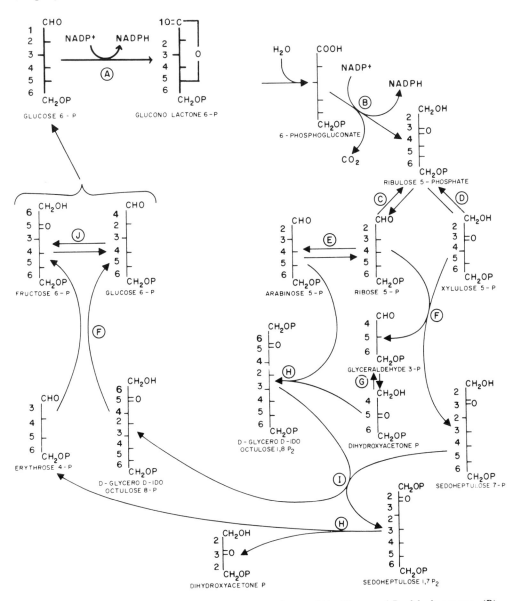

Fig. 2. Reaction sequence of the L-type pentose pathway. (A) Glucose 6-P dehydrogenase; (B) 6-phosphogluconate dehydrogenase; (C) pentose 5-phosphate isomerase; (D) pentose 5-phosphate 3' epimerase; (E) pentose 5-phosphate 2' epimerase; (F) transketolase; (G) triose phosphate isomerase; (H) aldolase; (I) phosphotransferase; (J) phosphohexose isomerase.

Phosphotransferase measurement

Phosphotransferase activity is found in rat liver enzyme preparation, dialysed rat liver cytosol, extracts of *Chlorella pyrenoidosa*, rat heart and rat epididymal fat pad. It is detected by the following reaction sequence and measured using the rate of hexose 6-P formation (reaction sequence f.)

The catalytic activity of the enzyme acting in the reverse direction is measured using the rate of ^{14}C incorporation into the octulose bisphosphate (reaction g)[16].

The addition of liver aldolase antibody to the mixture of reaction (f) when catalysed by rat liver enzyme preparation completely inhibits hexose 6-P formation. The addition of the antibody to the reaction mixture of equation (g) increased the measured value of the phosphotransferase

rate since the aldolase present in the preparation is prevented from breaking down the sedoheptulose-P_2 substrate. The activity of the phosphotransferase enzyme (5.0 $\pm$ 0.35 nmol min^{-1} mg^{-1}) may be among the rate-limiting steps in the formation of hexose 6-P from ribose 5-P by liver (3.5 $\pm$ 0.2 nmol min^{-1} mg^{-1}).

The role of arabinose 5-phosphate

Arabinose 5-P was identified among the pentose phosphates formed by the action of a yeast enzyme preparation on 6-phosphogluconate[17]. ^{14}C labelled arabinose is metabolized by a number of animal species[18] and by man[19]. It is converted to $^{14}CO_2$, and labelled lactate and glycogen by leucocytes[20] and utilized by a variety of rat tissues[10]. Its reactions in the scheme of Fig. 2 are easily shown by incubating [U-

Table II. Composition of reaction mixture and carbon balance at various times for reactions forming hexose 6-phosphate from ribose 5-phosphate catalysed by rat liver enzyme preparation

	Composition				
	Incubation time (h)				
Metabolite	0	0.5	3	12	17
Ribose-5-P	100	55.0	22.9	9.3	7.5
Xylulose-5-P	0	13.6	5.6	0.8	0
Ribulose-5-P	0	0	0	0	0
Arabinose-5-P	0	16.2	5.2	1.2	1.0
D-*altro*-Heptulose-7-P	0	4.0	23.1 ⎫	26.1	18.3
D-*manno*-Heptulose-7-P	0	3.4	10.0 ⎭		
Glyceraldehyde-3-P	0	0.2	0	0	0
Dihydroxyacetone-P	0	1.3	5.3	4.0	3.0
Fructose-1,6-P_2	0	1.7	12.0	8.3	7.4
D-*altro*-Heptulose,1,7-P_2	0	0.2	1.7	2.1	2.3
D-*glycero*-D-*altro*-Octulose-1,8-P_2	0	1.1	2.8	3.5	4.1
D-*glycero*-D-*ido*-Octulose, 1,8-P_2	0	0.1	0.4	0.5	0.5
Erythrose-4-P	0	0	0	0	0
Glucose-1-P	0	0.1	0.3	1.1	1.8
Fructose-6-P	0	0.5	1.8	11.0	16.0
Glucose-6-P	0	1.3	6.0	29.2	36.2
Total	100	98.7	97.1	97.1	98.1
Percentage of original carbon of ribose 5-phosphate not accounted for	0	1.3	2.9	2.9	1.9

(f)   (Phosphotransferase)

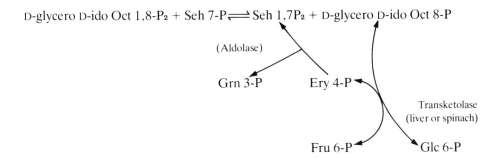

D-glycero D-ido Oct 1,8-P₂ + Seh 7-P ⇌ Seh 1,7P₂ + D-glycero D-ido Oct 8-P

(Aldolase)

Grn 3-P   Ery 4-P

Transketolase
(liver or spinach)

Fru 6-P   Glc 6-P

(g)   [8-¹⁴C]D-glycero D-ido Oct 8-P + Seh 1,7-P₂ ⇌
             Seh 7-P + [8-¹⁴C]D-glycero D-ido Oct 1, 8-P₂

¹⁴C]arabinose 5-P (1 part) and ribose 5-P (5 parts) with rat liver enzyme preparation for 30 min. ¹⁴C labelled glucose 6-P, fructose 6-P, ribose 5-P, xylulose 5-P and ribulose 5-P are the principal ¹⁴C labelled compounds made[16, 10]. The addition of liver aldolase antibody to the above reaction mixture prevents any formation of hexose 6-P. Only the ¹⁴C labelled pentose 5-phosphates and heptulose 7-P are then formed. The above experiment with the aldolase antibody unequivocally demonstrates that the L-type pathway reaction sequence of Fig. 2 is the only pentose pathway in liver, since any activity of the F-type pathway which is independent of aldolase action (Fig. 1) would be revealed by the formation of hexose 6-P.

An as yet unidentified product of arabinose 5-P dissimilation by the rat liver enzyme preparation powerfully inhibits both of the dehydrogenase enzymes of the oxidative segment of the pentose pathway. Arabinose 5-P *per se* does not affect these enzymes[16]. Thus the formation of glucose 6-P from arabinose 5-P after incubation with the preparation is best measured using assays which are based on either glucose 6-phosphatase, or gas–liquid chromatography of the trimethyl silyl derivatives of the dephosphorylated reaction products, or measurement using glucose 6-P dehydrogenase in an extensively diluted mixture of the reaction products. All of the above methods have been employed to demonstrate the conversion of arabinose 5-P to hexose 6-P by the preparation[16, 21].

Arabinose 5-P may also be a regulator of the reactions of the non-oxidative segment of the L-type pentose pathway. It is a competitive inhibitor of ribose 5-P conversion to hexose 6-P (K_i = 40 μM)[16]. This inhibition is unrelated to its inhibition of transaldolase (K_i = 70 μM)[10] since transaldolase has no role in the metabolic flux of Fig. 2. Arabinose 5-P (2.6 mM) has been reported to inhibit yeast transketolase[22]. There is no evidence that it inhibits the enzyme from liver or spinach[23].

Procedures for the recognition and measurement of the L-type pathway

Qualitatively the presence of the L-type pentose pathway in tissues is established by compliance with the following four criteria (1) ribose 5-P conversion to hexose 6-P by an appropriate preparation of tissue enzymes[9]; (2) demonstration that tissue aldolase activity is at least equal to but usually greater than (3–10 times) the activities of transketolase and transaldolase; (3) utilization of [¹⁴C]arabinose 5-P and its conversion to [¹⁴C]hexose 6-P[10]. Because arabinose 5-P has a complex and as yet unresolved inhibitory function in the pentose pathway its average rate of utilization (0.2 nmol min^{-1} mg^{-1}) and conversion to hexose 6-P can be very significantly increased if low concentrations (0.01–0.1 mM) of either glyceraldehyde 3-P, erythrose 4-P or ribose 4-P are included; (4) conversion of D-*glycero* D-*ido* octulose 1,8-P$_2$ (Ref. 24) and sedoheptulose 7-P to hexose 6-P by the tissue enzyme preparation[10].

If the system satisfies these four qualitative criteria it is then worth applying [5-^{14}C]glucose to the tissue for a quantitative measurement of the pathway. The rythmical and ordered sequence of the reaction of Fig. 2 determines that the steady state metabolism of [5-^{14}C]glucose results in the ^{14}C labelling of C-2 of fructose 6-P (Fig. 2). The proportion of this labelling (the C-2/C-5 ratio) is used for the quantitative measurement of the L-type pathway[25, 26]. The quantitative method shows that 22–30% of glucose metabolism in rat liver is by the L-type pathway[26].

The F-type pathway

Extensive investigation of the pentose pathway mechanism[9] in rat epididymal fat pad tissue using ^{14}C-isotope and the above criteria showed that only the F-type pathway (Fig. 1) was present in this tissue[27]. Its contribution to total glucose metabolism is 50–60%. Arabinose 5-P is present and the most active phosphotransferase measurement has been made with fat tissue. However, the level of aldolase in fat pad is only marginally greater than the individual activities of transketolase and transaldolase[28]. It is suggested that aldolase activity is a determining force for the reactions of Fig. 2. The investigations with fat pad show that it is quite feasible to distinguish biochemically the two possible pathways in tissues. Fat pad is the only tissue among 17 different animal and plant preparations examined by us which has the reaction sequence shown in Fig. 1, hence the title F-type pathway for these reactions. We find no evidence for the pathway of Fig. 1 in liver.

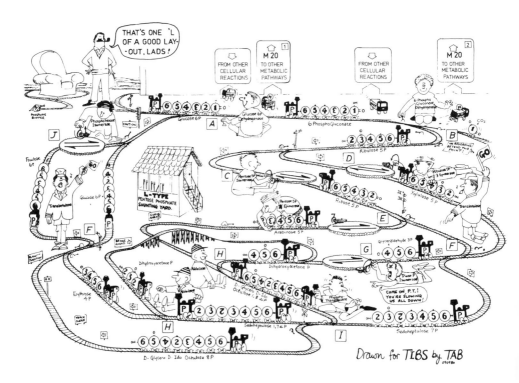

Acknowledgements

This work was supported by Grant No. D276/15829 from the Australian Research Grants Committee. The gift of liver aldolase antibody from Dr B. L. Horecker is gratefully acknowledged.

References

1 Horecker, B. L. (1976) in *Reflections on Biochemistry: in Honour of Severo Ochoa* (Kornberg, A., Horecker, B. L., Cornudella, L. and Oró, J., eds), pp. 65–72, Pergamon Press

2 Katz, J. and Wood, H. G. (1960) *J. Biol. Chem.* 235, 2165–2177

3 Katz, J. (1961) in *Radioactive Isotopes in Physiology, Diagnostics and Therapy* (Schwiegk, H. and Turba, F., eds), pp. 705–751, Springer-Verlag

4 Wood, H. G., Katz, J. and Landau, B. R. (1963) *Biochem. Z.* 338, 809–847

5 Williams, J. F., Reinits, K. G., Schofield, P. J. and Clark, M. G. (1971) *Biochem. J.* 123, 923–943

6 Horecker, B. L., Gibbs, M., Klenow, H. and Smyrniotis, P. Z. (1954) *J. Biol. Chem.* 207, 393–403

7 Gibbs, M. and Horecker, B. L. (1954) *J. Biol. Chem.* 208, 813–820

8 Horecker, B. L. and Mehler, A. H. (1944) *Annu. Rev. Biochem.* 24, 207–274

9 Williams, J. F., Clark, M. G. and Blackmore, P. F. (1978) *Biochem J.* 176, 241–256

10 Williams, J. F., Blackmore, P. F. and Clark, M. G. (1978) *Biochem. J.* 176, 257–282

11 Hostetler, K. Y. and Landau, B. R. (1967) *Biochemistry* 6, 2961–2964

12 Clark, M. G., Williams, J. F. and Blackmore, P. F. (1971) *Biochem. J.* 125, 381–384

13 Ljungdahl, L., Wood, H. G., Racker, E. and Couri, D. (1961) *J. Biol. Chem.* 236, 1622–1625

14 Williams, J. F. and Clark, M. G. (1971) *Search 2.* 80–88

15 Paoletti, F., Williams, J. F. and Horecker, B. L. (1979) *Archiv, Biochem. Biophys.* 198, 620–626

16 Bleakley, P. A., Arora, K. K. and Williams, J. F. (1984) *Biochem. International.* 8, 491–500

17 McNair Scott, D. B. and Cohen, S. S. (1951) *J. Biol. Chem.* 188, 509–530

18 Metzger, R. P., Edwards, K. D., Nixon, C. C. and Mobley, P. W. (1980) *Biochim. Biophys. Acta* 629 482–489

19 Segal, S. and Foley, J. B. (1959) *J. Clin. Invest.* 38, 407–413

20 Stjernholm, R. L. and Noble, E. P. (1963) *Arch. Biochem. Biophys.* 100, 200–204

21 Blackmore, P. F. (1975) Ph.D. Thesis, University of New South Wales, Australia

22 Wood, T. and Gascon, A. (1980) *Archiv. Biochem. Biophys.* 203, 727–733

23 Kapuscinski, M., Franke, F. P., Flannigan, I., MacLeod, J. K. and Williams, J. F. *Carbohydr. Res.* (in press)

24 Paoletti, F., Williams, J. F. and Horecker, B. L. (1979) *Archiv. Biochem. Biophys.* 198, 614–619

25 Longenecker, J. and Williams, J. F. (1980) *Biochem. J.* 188, 847–857

26 Longenecker, J. and Williams, J. F. (1980) *Biochem. J.* 188, 859–865

27 Blackmore, P. F., Williams, J. F., Schofield, P. J. and Power, P. A. (1982) *Int. J. Biochem.* 14, 171–186

28 Novello, F. and McLean, P. (1968) *Biochem. J.* 107, 775–791

J. F. Williams is at the Department of Biochemistry, The Faculties, Australian National University, Canberra, Australia.

The pentose cycle in liver
Joseph Katz

I wish to respond to the article by John Williams (see p. 107 of this book) on the mechanism of the pentose cycle. The pentose cycle (PC) is a reaction sequence in which glucose 6-P is decarboxylated to ribulose 5-P and the pentose phosphate reconverted to hexose 6-phosphate. The net reaction is

$$3 \text{ Hexose 6-P} + 6 \text{ NADPH} \rightarrow 3 \text{ CO}_2 + 2 \text{ Hexose 6-P} + \text{Triose-P} + 6 \text{ NADPH}_2$$

The generally accepted reaction sequence for the re-synthesis of hexose 6-P from ribulose 5-P involves as intermediates xylulose 5-P, ribose 5-P, sedoheptulose 7-P and erythrose 4-P. This scheme, based mainly on studies by Horecker and co-workers, is described in numerous reviews and textbooks. Williams accepts that this scheme operates in adipose tissue, but rejects it as erroneous for liver. He proposes a rather different, more complex reaction sequence which includes the additional intermediates arabinose 5-P, sedoheptulose 1,7-P$_2$, octulose 8-P, octulose 1,8-P$_2$ and dihydroxyacetone P (Ref. 1). His scheme also assumes two non-mixing pools of triose phosphates. Williams designates his scheme the L (liver) pentose cycle, as distinct from the 'classical' F (fat tissue) pentose cycle. According to Williams, the F type of PC is restricted to adipose tissue, and the L type is the only mechanism in liver, photosynthesis, and presumably other tissues. We disagree with his conclusion, and show here that the L scheme is not consistent with Williams' own experimental data and a substantial body of other findings.

The two schemes lead to an altogether different distribution of the carbons in the re-synthesized hexose phosphates, as shown in Fig. 1.

The F cycle is characterized by randomization of the C-2 of glucose into positions 1 and 3 of hexose 6-P, whereas in the L scheme C-2 is not randomized, but C-5 appears in position 2 and C-4 and C-6 in position 1 of hexose 6-P. Incorporation of carbons 5 and 6 into position 2 and 1 respectively, may also occur in liver by re-condensation of the triose phosphates formed by glycolysis, but the incorporation of C-4 into position 1 is altogether unique to the L scheme.

We question the existence of the L

F scheme				
1C		2C	2C	
2C		3C	3C	
3C		2C	3C	
4C		4C	4C	4C
3 5C		5C	5C	5C
6C-OP		6C-OP	6C-OP	6C-OP
Glucose 6-P	CO$_2$	Hexose 6-P		Triose-P

L scheme				
1C		6C	4C	
2C		5C	2C	
3 3C		3C	3C	
4C		4C	4C	2C
5C		5C	5C	3C
6C-OP		6C-OP	6C-OP	2C-OP
Glucose 6-P	CO$_2$	Hexose 6-P		Triose-P

Fig. 1. Two schemes proposed for the pentose cycle.

scheme on the basis of three lines of evidence:

(1) Most of the results published by Williams and co-workers fit poorly with his scheme. For example, in their latest publication Longenecker and Williams[2] incubated rat hypatocytes with [4,5,6-^{14}C] glucose and isolated and degraded glucose 6-P. The ^{14}C pattern was as follows:

Carbon of

glucose 6-P	1	2	3	4	5	6
% of [14]C	2.0	12	2.7	30	24	29

There was indeed incorporation of ^{14}C into position 2 of hexose 6-P, which may have come from C-5. However, according to Williams' scheme, ^{14}C from C-6 and C-4 should appear in C-1, and the ^{14}C yield on C-1 should have been about twice that on C-2, but there was virtually none on C-1. This result alone makes the L scheme untenable in our opinion.

(2) Arabinose 5-P is a key intermediate in the L scheme, serving as precursor for octulose 1,8-P_2. However, in a recent study, Wood and Gascon[3] were not able to confirm Williams' results with this ester. They found arabinose 5-P virtually inert in liver extracts. The discrepancy in the experimental findings remains to be resolved.

(3) Williams and co-workers altogether ignore results with liver *in vivo*[4,5], and studies with hepatocytes[6,7] on the randomization of carbon from position 2 into positions 1 and 3 of glucose, which are consistent with the classical F scheme. Randomization in glucose was increased in hepatocytes from fasted re-fed animals (as expected due to the need for supplying NADPH for fatty acid synthesis) and in the presence of phenazine methosulfate, a known stimulant of NADPH oxidation and of the pentose cycle. In a recent collaborative study with S. M. Cohen and R. G. Shulman of the Merck Institute[8], hepatocytes were incubated with [2-^{13}C] and [2-^{14}C] glycerol and the randomization of carbon in glucose determined by both NMR spectroscopy and by conventional degradation. Both procedures agreed closely. In hepatocytes of starved rats the carbon activities of C-1 and C-3 were, respectively, 11 and 5% that of carbon 2. In the presence of phenazine methosulfate the ^{14}C yields in C-1 and C-3 were increased to 19 and 9% respectively. From this we calculate, according to Rognstad[7], with hepatocytes of fasted rats incubated with 11 mM glycerol, that the rate of glucose 6-P dehydrogenase was 17% of the rate of gluconeogenesis. Upon the addition of phenazine methosulfate the rate of glucose 6-P dehydrogenase was increased to 47% of that of glucose formation. However, there was little randomization and virtually no pentose cycle in perfused liver of starved mice.

Williams claims that the F scheme of the pentose cycle occurs only in adipose tissue and could not be detected in 17 other animal and plant preparations. However, there is convincing evidence for the 'classical' F scheme in lactating mammary glands of ruminants[9] and rats[10]. In other tissues (too extensive for review here), a C_1/C_2 ratio in glucose consistent with the classical scheme has been observed.

To obtain the distribution of ^{14}C, Williams *et al.* have isolated and degraded glucose 6-P. We and nearly everyone else have isolated and degraded glucose or glycogen. Williams has criticized the use of glucose as being 'removed' from glucose 6-P. However, under physiologic conditions liver is predominantly gluconeogenic (at the expense of glycogen or 3 carbon precursors) and glucose formation represents a major flux from glucose 6-P. Also, glucose yields the mean metabolic pattern for the whole experimental period, whereas the ^{14}C pattern in glucose 6-P is that at the moment of termination. Moreover, H. R. Williams and Landau[11] have shown that the ^{14}C distribution in glucose, glycogen and glucose 6-P are quite similar.

Williams and co-workers have discovered novel seven and eight carbon esters in liver and elucidated the mechanism of their biosynthesis. There is in liver and probably other tissues many other yet unknown reactions. When there is no metabolic flux, exchange reactions may be predominant and account for some of the results described by Williams. These exchange reactions are likely to be of minor extent during active metabolism. We conclude that at present there is no adequate evidence for the operation of the L scheme of the pentose cycle during carbodydrate metabolism in liver, and that experimental data support the operation in liver of pentose cycle as in adipose tissue and mammary gland.

References

1 Longenecker, J. P. and Williams, J. F. (1980a) *Biochemistry*, 188, 847–857

2 Longenecker, J. P. and Williams, J. F. (1980b) *Biochemistry*, 188, 859–865

3 Wood, T. and Gascon, A. (1980) *Arch. Biochem. Biophys.* 203, 327–336

4 Sui, P. M. and Wood, H. G. (1959) *J. Biol. Chem.* 234, 2223

5 Hostetler, K. Y. and Landau, B. R. (1967) *Biochemistry*, 6, 1961–1964

6 Rognstad, R. and Katz, J. (1974) *Biochem. Biophys. Res. Comm.* 61, 774–780

7 Rognstad, R. (1976) *Int. J. Biochem.* 7, 222–228

8 Cohen, S. M., Rognstad, R., Shulman, R. G. and Katz, J. (1981) *J. Biol. Chem.* 256, 3428–3432

9 Wood, H. G., Gillespie, R., Joffe, S., Hansen, R. G. and Hardenbrook, H. (1958) *J. Biol. Chem.* 233, 1271

10 Katz, J. and Wals, P. (1972) *Biochemistry*, 128, 879–899

11 Williams, H. R. and Landau, B. R. (1972) *Arch. Biochem. Biophys.* 150, 708–713

J. Katz is at the Cedars-Sinai Medical Center, Los Angeles, CA 90048, USA.

The pentose cycle in animal tissues: evidence for the classical and against the 'L-type' pathway

Bernard R. Landau and Harland G. Wood

There is abundant evidence for the operation in animals of the classical textbook scheme of reactions comprising the pentose cycle, also called the pentose phosphate pathway or pentose pathway. A second pentose pathway has been proposed to operate in many mammalian tissues. We do not find the evidence for this second pathway convincing.

Two different pentose phosphate pathways have been proposed for the metabolism of glucose 6-P. One is the classical pathway (Fig. 1)[1]. The second is a pathway (Fig. 2) proposed by Williams and co-workers[2]. In both pathways, three molecules of glucose 6-P form three molecules of CO_2, two molecules of hexose 6-P, and one molecule of triose-P. However, the redistribution of the carbons of the three molecules of glucose 6-P into the resulting hexose 6-phosphates and triose-P is very different. In the traditional pathway, two molecules of fructose 6-P are formed, one containing carbons 232456 of the glucose 6-P and the other carbons 233456, and one molecule of glyceraldehyde 3-P containing carbons 456 (see Fig. 1, dashed-line enclosures). In the pathway proposed by Williams and co-workers[2] one molecule of glucose 6-P is formed containing carbons 423456 and one molecule of fructose 6-P containing carbons 653456, along with dihydroxy-acetone-P containing carbons 232 (see Fig. 2, dashed-line enclosures).

Williams and his co-workers[3] find distributions of ^{14}C in glucose 1-P, glucose 6-P and glucose 1,6-diP, formed on incubating epididymal fat pads with [2-^{14}C]glucose, in accord with the classical pathway (Fig. 1). They find very different distributions for liver and they propose, for this tissue, the pathway shown in Fig. 2. Williams con-

cludes[2] that the pathway of Fig. 1 occurs only in 'fat tissue' and designates it the 'F-type pathway', while the pathway of Fig. 2 he designates the 'L-type pathway'. He states that the L-type pathway is the pentose pathway present in the fifteen other animal and plant tissues he and his co-workers have examined, but he provides no data or references to support this statement.

First, we will review the information relevant to the quantitative role of the traditional pentose phosphate pathway. Then we will consider the investigations of Williams and co-workers.

[2-^{14}C]Glucose and isotope patterns produced by the traditional pentose phosphate pathway

A distinguishing feature of the traditional pentose phosphate pathway is the labeling pattern of the hexose 6-phosphates that are formed from [2-^{14}C] glucose. Phosphohexose isomerase is active in mammalian tissues and so the pentose phosphate pathway is a cycle as shown in Fig. 1. The ratio of ^{14}C in C-1 to C-2 or in C-3 to C-2 can be used to estimate the amount of glucose metabolized by the cycle and under ideal conditions the ratio of ^{14}C in C-1 to C-3 will be 2, as is apparent from Fig. 1. These conditions are defined in reference 4 and include (1) complete equilibration of glucose 6-P with fructose 6-P, (2) equilibration of fructose 6-P formed in the cycle with fructose 6-P formed in the Embden–Meyerhof pathway and (3) randomization of carbons 1, 2 and 3 of the glucose 6-P and fructose 6-P only as a consequence of metabolism by the cycle functioning in the direction of oxidation.

In practice, glycogen is isolated and the glucose derived from it is degraded. A summary of the extensive series of experiments in which [2-14C]glucose has been administered to rats[5–7] or incubated with or perfused through various tissue preparations[8–14] and glucose from isolated glycogen degraded is shown in Table I. The incorporation of 14C into C-1 is often less than twice that in C-3 and in several cases the activity in C-3 exceeded that in C-1. This is explained by the randomization of carbons that occur in the reversal of the non-oxidative portion of the cycle, i.e.

$$2 \text{ fructose 6-P} + \text{glyceraldehyde 3-P} \rightarrow$$

$$3 \text{ pentose 5-P}$$

by which 14C from [2-14C]glucose can be incorporated into C-3 and not C-1[15]. This reversal allows the synthesis of pentose 5-P without the formation of NADPH. Thus, in

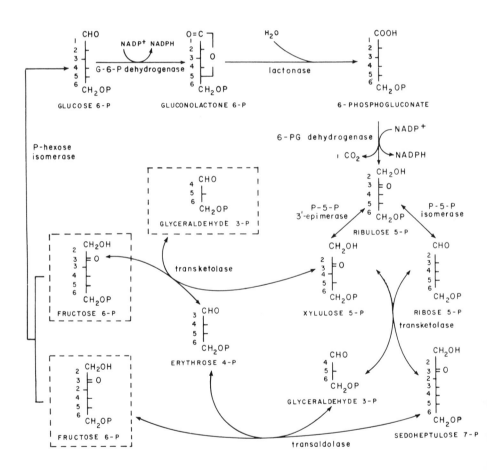

Fig. 1. Reaction sequence of the classical pentose phosphate pathway. Products of the sequence are enclosed by dashed lines and the numbers indicate the carbons of the original glucose 6-P.

rat adipose tissue where NADPH is required for fatty acid synthesis, the oxidative segment of the cycle is active, and C-1/C-3 approaches 2, while in muscle where there is less need for NADPH, C-3 exceeds C-1.

A number of other observations support the scheme of Fig. 1. Glycerol, formed when adipose tissue was incubated with [2-^{14}C]glucose, had almost twice as much ^{14}C in C-1 as in C-3[8]. Since glycerol arises from carbons 1, 2 and 3 of fructose 1,6-bisP, it should reflect (via dihydroxyacetone-P), the distribution of ^{14}C in these carbons of fructose 6-P. Indeed, from the ^{14}C in C-1 and C-3 of glycerol, and that in the glucose from glycogen (reflecting that in glucose 6-P), the extent of equilibration of fructose 6-P with glucose 6-P has been

estimated[8,16]. Horecker and co-workers[1,17] incubated homogenates of liver with specifically ^{14}C-labeled ribose 5-P for 16 to 17 h and found the synthesized glucose 6-P had a distribution of ^{14}C in fair agreement with the cycle as defined in Fig. 1. When the udder of a cow was perfused with [2-^{14}C]glucose[18], the galactose moiety of the lactose had a distribution of ^{14}C in keeping with the classical pentose cycle, i.e. with C-2 in the galactose set to 100, C-1 = 30.6, C-3 = 18.8, C-4 = 0.7, C-5 = 4.9 and C-6 = 0.7.

[2-^{14}C]Glucose and [1-^{14}C]ribose 5-P and the labeling of glucose 6-P

Williams and his co-workers[19] reported that when rabbit livers were perfused for up to 5 min *in situ* with [2-^{14}C]glucose, the

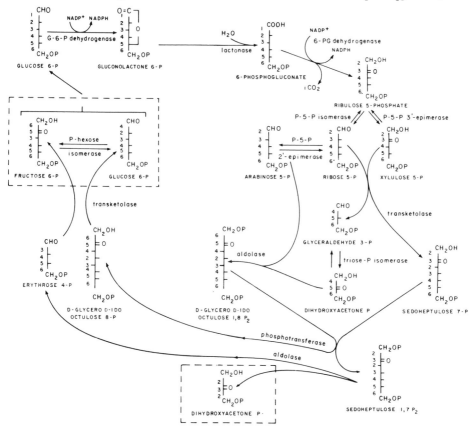

Fig. 2. Reaction sequence of the pentose phosphate pathway proposed by Williams and co-workers. Products of the sequence are enclosed by dashed lines and the numbers indicate the carbons of the original glucose 6-P.

C-6 of glucose 6-P was labeled extensively. During the first 30 min of incubation of [1-^{14}C]ribose 5-P with a rat liver enzyme preparation, 41 to 76% of the ^{14}C in glucose 6-P was in C-6[20]. In addition, at 1.0 and 2.5 min, 45% and 44% of the ^{14}C was in C-2 with lower percentages in C-2 thereafter. Williams concluded[2] that these ^{14}C patterns cannot be reconciled with the sequence of reactions in Fig. 1.

Indeed, the pathway in Fig. 1 is not in accord with the conversions of C-2 of glucose or C-1 of ribose 5-P to C-6 of glucose 6-P, but neither is the pathway in Fig. 2. Williams[2] states that the heavy labeling in C-6 is entirely due to exchange reactions* and is not the result of metabolic flux. However, the exchange reactions have no obvious relation to the pathway in Fig. 2 and provide no support for this pathway. When Longenecker and Williams[22] incubated hepatocytes with [2-^{14}C]glucose they found negligible ^{14}C in C-6 of glucose 6-P.

The incorporation of ^{14}C from [1-^{14}C]ribose 5-P in C-2 of glucose 6-P is in accord with the pathway of Fig. 2. However, Horecker and co-workers[1,23] in incubations similar to those used by Williams,

observed a marked lag phase before the formation of hexose 6-P from ribose 5-P. Horecker[23] states that under the conditions employed by Williams and his co-workers, labeled hexose 6-P in amounts adequate for degradation would not be formed until many minutes after the beginning of incubation. Williams et al.[20] found much less ^{14}C in C-2 and C-6 after several hours than after several minutes of incubation and, indeed, after 17 h the distribution of ^{14}C was in reasonable accord with the scheme in Fig. 1, and the findings of Horecker et al.[1], i.e. in percent of ^{14}C: C-1 = 57.2, C-2 = 10.2, C-3 = 25.1, C-4 = 2.7, C-5 = 1.4 and C-6 = 3.4.

[5-^{14}C]Glucose and isotope patterns produced by the L-type pentose cycle

The scheme of Fig. 2 predicts that C-5 of glucose will be converted to C-2 of fructose 6-P. Longenecker and Williams[22], using [5-^{14}C]glucose, estimated that 22 to 30% of the metabolism of glucose by isolated hepatocytes occurs by the L-type pentose cycle. For this estimation, they[24] derived the expression:

$$PC = r_{H2.5}/(1-r_{H2.5})$$

in which $r_{H2,5}$ is the ratio of ^{14}C in C-2 to that in C-5 of glucose 6-P formed from the labeled sugar and PC is the fraction of the glucose metabolized by the L-type pentose cycle. For this expression to apply[24]: (1) fructose 6-P and glucose 6-P must be maintained in isotopic equilibrium; (2) dihydroxyacetone-P, derived from glyceraldehyde 3-P formed in the transketolase reaction, must react (as shown in Fig. 2) without equilibrating with dihydroxyacetone-P formed in the Embden-Meyerhof pathway; and (3) no reactions may occur which result in a redistribution of carbon other than those produced by the pathway of Fig. 2. With regard to the last requirement, reversal of the Embden–Meyerhof pathway will convert C-5 of glucose to C-2 of fructose 6-P, i.e.:

[5-^{14}C]glucose → [2-^{14}C]triose-P → [2,5-^{14}C]fructose 6-P

---

* Williams and Clark[21] proposed that [1-^{14}C]sedoheptulose 1,7-bisP is formed by the combined action of transketolase-transaldolase catalysed reactions and it gives [6-^{14}C]fructose 6-P from [1-^{14}C]xylulose 5-P arising from [2-^{14}C]glucose and [1-^{14}C]ribose, apparently as follows:

[1-^{14}C]Xu 5-P + Ery 4-P $\overset{TK}{\rightleftharpoons}$ [1-^{14}C]Fru 6-P + GA 3-P

[1-^{14}C]Fru 6-P + Ery 4-P $\overset{TA}{\rightleftharpoons}$ [1-^{14}C]SH 1,7-bisP + GA 3-P

[1-^{14}C]SH 1,7-bisP $\overset{aldolase}{\rightleftharpoons}$ [3-^{14}C]DHA 3-P + Ery 4-P

[3-^{14}C]DHA 3-P $\overset{TI}{\rightleftharpoons}$ [3-^{14}C]GA 3-P

[3-^{14}C]GA 3-P + Fru 6-P $\overset{TA}{\rightleftharpoons}$ [6-^{14}C]Fru 6-P + GA 3-P

Xu = xylulose, Ery = erythrose, Fru = fructose, SH = sedoheptulose, GA = glyceraldehyde, DHA = dihydroxyacetone, TK = transketolase, TA = transaldolase and TI = triose phosphate isomerase. Other than the couplings of these exchange reactions, no explanation has been offered to account for the labeling of C-6 by [2-^{14}C]glucose and [1-^{14}C]ribose.

To find out whether this was occurring, Longenecker and Williams[22] incubated hepatocytes with [4,5,6-^{14}C]glucose, as substrate, as well as with [5-^{14}C]glucose. The distributions of ^{14}C in these substrates and in the glucose 6-P isolated from the reaction mixtures at the completion of the incubation[22] are shown in Table II.

The calculation of 30% pentose cycle from the data with [5-^{14}C]glucose is as follows:

$$r_{H2,5} = (17.7 - 1.3)/70.8 = 0.23; PC = 0.23/(1 - 0.23) = 0.30$$

However, with [4,5,6-^{14}C]glucose, labeling in C-1, C-2, C-3 likewise was almost exclusively in C-2. It should be obvious from Fig. 2 that carbons 1,2 and 3 of glucose 6-P cannot be labeled similarly with both [5-^{14}C]glucose and [4,5,6-^{14}C]glucose. No pathway exists or has been proposed that can account for such a result. [4,5,6-^{14}C]Glucose would form [1,2,3-^{14}C]dihydroxyacetone-P by the Embden–Meyerhof pathway and if hexose 6-P were synthesized from the dihydroxyacetone-P via triose phosphate isomerase, aldolase and fructose diphosphatase, [1,2,3,4,5,6-^{14}C]fructose 6-P would result. Since very little labeling was found in C-1 and C-3 of the glucose 6-P, Longenecker and Williams[22] concluded that this sequence did not occur and that the labeling in C-2 occurred via the L-type pentose cycle. As shown in Fig. 2, ^{14}C from C-6 of the [4,5,6-^{14}C]glucose should then have been incorporated into C-1 of the fructose 6-P and from C-4 into C-1 of the glucose 6-P. C-1 should then have contained twice as much ^{14}C as C-2, i.e. 2(12.1 − 1.6) = 21% (Ref. 25). Williams[26] contends that only 7.4% of ^{14}C would be expected in C-1, but in our opinion his method of making this estimate is not valid.†

We conclude that the calculation of 22 to 30% metabolism by the L-type pentose pathway does not rest on a firm basis. Other studies with labeled glucose, now to be discussed, indicate there is no significant L-type pentose pathway in liver.

The glucose unit of glycogen as an indicator of metabolism

Williams[26] states there is no 'equity or indeed similarity in the distribution of ^{14}C isotope from [2-^{14}C]glucose or [1-^{14}C]-ribose in liver glucose, glycogen units, fructose 6-P or glucose 6-P' and he also states that '^{14}C distribution in the units of glycogen have nothing to do with the metabolic interconversions by reactions of the pentose pathway'. Accordingly, he considers that the results shown in Table I are irrelevant to the pentose cycle and concludes[3] that their 'data provide the first proof of the mechanism of the (classical) pentose pathway in adipose tissue'. We have added the word classical to the quote.

---

†Williams assumed[26] that fructose 6-P labeled from C-6 of the [4,5,6-^{14}C]glucose was not fully equilibrated with glucose 6-P which is labeled directly from C-4 (see Fig. 2). With a 20% pentose cycle, he estimated[26] that there would be a contribution of 5.0% ^{14}C to C-1 of fructose 6-P from C-6 of the [4,5,6-^{14}C]glucose and 5.4% from C-4 to glucose 6-P. He then estimated that only 37% of the fructose 6-P equilibrated with the glucose 6-P, thus giving a total of 7.4% ^{14}C in C-1 [(0.37 × 5.0) + 5.4 = 7.3]. This calculation is in complete contrast to his treatment of the data obtained with the [5-^{14}C]glucose which resulted in his estimate of a 22–30% pentose cycle contribution. For that estimate he assumed there was complete equilibration. However, if the C-2 to C-5 ratio from [4,5,6-^{14}C]glucose is used for the calculation, it gives a 75% cycle [$r_{H2,5} = (12.1 − 1.6)/24.3 = 0.43; PC = 0.43/(1 − 0.43) = 0.75$]. Thus, the use of 20% pentose cycle in reaching the value of 7.4% appears to have no rational basis. Furthermore, if the Williams's correction for non-equilibrium is applied to the results with [5-^{14}C]glucose, PC equals an impossible 170% of glucose utilized [$r_{H2,5} = [(17.7 − 1.3)/(0.37)]/70.8 = 0.63; PC = 0.63/(1 − 0.63) = 1.70$].

Actually, if there was non-equilibration, ^{14}C in C-1 should have been more than twice that in C-2 of glucose 6-P. This is so because then some of the ^{14}C incorporated into C-1 and C-2 of fructose 6-P would not be converted to glucose 6-P, while the incorporation into C-1 of glucose 6-P of ^{14}C from C-4 of the [4,5,6-^{14}C]glucose is not dependent on the conversion of fructose 6-P to glucose 6-P.

There is a vast amount of evidence that glycogen in liver is formed from and contributes to the glucose 6-P pool and that it is a source of glucose produced by liver. We have shown that glucose 6-P formed by liver slices from [2-^{14}C]glucose has essentially the same distribution of ^{14}C as that of the glucose units in glycogen[27]. Further, Rognstad[28] incubated liver cells from starved–re-fed rats with [2-^{14}C]mannose and the glucose formed had a distribution in accord with metabolism via the scheme in Fig. 1, i.e. C-1 = 18, C-2 = 100, C-3 = 12, C-4 = 1.8, C-5 = 10 and C-6 = 2.9. Mannose is metabolized in liver via mannose 6-P to fructose 6-P and, since glucose is formed from glucose 6-P, the glucose almost certainly reflects the ^{14}C pattern that was in fructose 6-P and glucose 6-P.

One of us recently initiated studies (Landau, unpublished results) with [3,4-^{14}C]glucose to obtain further data on whether or not the glucose units of glycogen and the glucose 6-P have similar

Table 1. Distributions of ^{14}C in the glucoses from glycogens formed from [2-^{14}C]glucose in vivo and in vitro[a]

Tissue	Comments	C-1	C-2	C-3	C-4	C-5	C-6	Sources
					in vivo			
Rat, liver	fasted	13.9	100	3.3	2.4	8.4	6.3	Table II, Ref. 5
Rat, liver	regenerating liver	35	100	21	32	28	20	Table II, Ref. 6
Rat, liver	fasted	5.2	100	3.2	0.7	4.7	2.5	Table I, Ref. 7
Rat, muscle	diaphragm	1.9	100	3.0	0.8	1.2	0.9	Table I, Ref. 7
Rat, muscle	skeletal	1.6	100	2.6	0.9	4.0	1.2	Table I, Ref. 7
Rat, muscle	heart	2.1	100	2.9	0.6	2.9	0.4	Table I, Ref. 7
Rat, thyroid		6.1	100	12.4	0.7	4.0	2.4	Table I, Ref. 7
Rat, kidney		7.2	100	8.0	0.8	9.7	2.6	Table I, Ref. 7
Rat, brain		5.4	100	5.5	1.3	5.1	1.9	Table I, Ref. 7
					in vitro			
Rat, adipose		15.2	100	12.8	1.9	13.9	2.9	Table II, Ref. 8
Rat, adipose	insulin	30.7	100	17.9	3.5	14.8	5.3	Table II, Ref. 8
Goosefish, islets	glucose 25/mg/dl	11.1	100	8.3	1.3	15.0	1.7	Table 3, Ref. 9
Goosefish, islets	glucose 100/mg/dl	6.4	100	4.5	1.9	20.2	1.6	Table 3, Ref. 9
Goosefish, islets	glucose 200/mg/dl	4.7	100	4.8	0.8	17.7	0.9	Table 3, Ref. 9
Human, intestine	mucosal strips	10.7	100	8.3	1.7	10.1	2.8	Table 6, Ref. 10
Cow, adrenal		15.7	100	7.9	1.4	11.0	2.1	Table 2, Ref. 11
Cow, adrenal	ACTH	17.0	100	9.3	2.2	9.2	2.2	Table 2, Ref. 11
Cow, thyroid		6.6	100	5.0	0.9	9.6	1.1	Table I, Ref. 12
Cow, thyroid	TSH, 30 min	19.3	100	13.5	2.2	10.3	2.1	Table I, Ref. 12
Cow, thyroid	TSH, 120 min	8.4	100	5.9	2.0	12.1	1.1	Table I, Ref. 12
Monkey, brain	brain stem	10.7	100	3.0	0.6	6.1	2.0	Table 1, Ref. 13
Monkey, brain	cerebellum	12.8	100	5.7	0.7	6.0	0.9	Table 1, Ref. 13
Monkey, brain	hemispheres	10.0	100	4.7	0.7	6.4	1.0	Table 1, Ref. 13
Monkey, brain	hypothalmus	11.6	100	3.8	1.0	7.5[b]	1.3	Table 1, Ref. 13
Mice, muscle	heart-infant	4.6	100	5.7		28.3[b]		Table I, Ref. 14
Mice, muscle	heart-adult	3.4	100	5.2		30.9[b]		Table I, Ref. 14
Mice, muscle	abdominal-infant	0.6	100	1.9		16.7[b]		Table I, Ref. 14
Mice, muscle	abdominal-adult	0.1	100	1.2		19.8[b]		Table I, Ref. 14
Mice, muscle	diaphragm-infant	0.7	100	2.2		19.6[b]		Table I, Ref. 14
Mice, muscle	diaphragm-adult	1.0	100	1.4		10.2[b]		Table I, Ref. 14

[a] Activity in C-2 has been set to 100 and activities in the other carbons are relative to the activity in C-2. Where more than one experiment was done under the same conditions, the average of the activities in each carbon is recorded.

[b] Sum in carbons 4, 5 and 6.

Table II.

C-1	C-2	C-3	C-4	C-5	C-6	
			[5-^{14}C]*Glucose*			
0	1.3	0.9	2.1	94.0	1.7	(substrate)
0.6	17.7	1.9	11.5	70.8	1.4	(glucose 6-P)
			[4,5,6-^{14}C]*Glucose*			
1.2	1.6	1.7	33.0	31.4	31.0	(substrate)
2.0	12.1	2.7	30.0	24.3	28.7	(glucose 6-P)

isotopic patterns and to determine whether or not C-4 of glucose is converted to C-1 of glucose 6-P, as required by the L-type pentose pathway. Livers from fed rats were perfused with [3,4-^{14}C]glucose and after 90 min the glucose in the perfusates, as well as glucose from glucose 6-P and from glycogen in the livers, were isolated, purified and degraded. The distributions are shown in Table III.

The distributions of ^{14}C in the glucose from the glycogen and from the glucose 6-P are very similar. There is no evidence that ^{14}C from C-4 of the [3,4-^{14}C]glucose moves to C-1, as would be expected if there was substantial metabolism of glucose in liver by the L-type pathway. These results indicate a small contribution by the classical pentose cycle by which C-3 of glucose moves to C-2 and C-1 of fructose 6-P and the C-4 remains in C-4 (Fig. 1). Comparison of the ^{14}C in C-1 and C-2 with that in C-5 and C-6 shows that C-1 and C-2 are labeled more than C-5 and C-6 as expected for the cycle. The conclusion from the above experiments is that the ^{14}C pattern of the glucose unit of glycogen does reflect that of glucose 6-P and that the L-type pathway does not occur to a significant extent in liver.

Other considerations

Williams *et al.*[29], using their enzyme preparation from liver, showed the formation of several sugar phosphates from ribose 5-P. These included D-glycero-D-*ido*-octulose 1,8-*bis* P, D-glycero-D-*ido*-octulose 8-P and sedoheptulose 1,7-*bis* P, which are proposed intermediates in the

L-type pathway. Paoletti, Williams and Horecker[30] found the octulose phosphates in fresh liver. Other investigators had previously demonstrated the formation of eight carbon sugars by preparations from yeast, muscle and red blood cells and their presence in fresh erythrocytes (for references see Ref. 23). The existence of these sugar phosphates and the enzymes which form them is not central to the issue of the quantitative role of the L-type pathway. However, there are doubts about the relative importance of these specific compounds. Paoletti, Williams and Horecker[30] found in fresh liver the D-*altro*-octulose mono- and bisphosphates to be in larger concentrations than the *ido* derivatives. In accord with this, much more of the *altro* than *ido* derivatives were formed with the liver enzyme preparation[2][29], even though it is the *ido* derivatives that are the intermediates in the scheme of Fig. 2. Furthermore, Paoletti, Williams and Horecker[31] found that glycero-D-*altro*-octulose-bisP and ribose 5-P were much better substrates for liver aldolase than glycero-D-*ido*-octulose-bisP and arabinose 5-P, the substrates for aldolase in the scheme. T. Wood[32], using a liver enzyme preparation similar to that used by Williams, found no evidence of interconversion between D-arabinose 5-P and other pentose phosphates, nor could he demonstrate its metabolism to triose phosphates or other intermediates of the postulated L-type pathway.

If the pathway proposed by Williams exists in red blood cells, C-6 of glucose would become C-1 of glucose 6-P and therefore [14]CO$_2$ should be formed from [6-^{14}C]glucose. This is not the case[33]. Kuehn and Scholz[34] measured rates of subs-

Table III.

C-1	C-2	C-3	C-4	C-5	C-6	Glucose
1.2	1.3	45.1	51.4	0.4	0.6	added
2.5	2.3	43.4	50.8	0.6	0.4	from perfusate
2.9	4.7	43.4	47.7	0.4	0.9	from glucose 6-P
2.6	4.4	40.7	50.4	1.5	0.4	from glycogen

trate flux through the pentose cycle in perfused rat liver. Their kinetic data are inconsistent with the existence of the L-type pentose cycle in liver. Morgan[35] found that extracts of hamster ovary and lung cells, which were devoid of phosphohexose isomerase, formed fructose 6-P, but not glucose 6-P from ribose 5-P. Since glucose 6-P is a direct product of the L-type pathway, it should have been formed if that pathway were present. Based on these findings, Morgan concluded that only the classical pentose pathway, which does not yield glucose 6-P in the absence of the isomerase, occurs in these cells. Very recently, Rognstad, Wals and Katz[36] have introduced additional evidence for the presence of the classical pathway in liver.

Concluding remarks

Irrespective of which reactions an enzyme catalyses in a subcellular system, or which tissues contain eight-carbon sugar phosphates etc., isotopic tracer studies should yield labeling patterns in intact cells which are consistent with the reactions of the pathway. All patterns obtained to date using intact cell preparations are in keeping with the pentose cycle as depicted in Fig. 1, except for reports of Williams and his co-workers. There are no known pathways, including the pathway in Fig. 2, that can account for their observations.

Acknowledgement

Supported through Grant AM-14507 to Bernard R. Landau from the National Institutes of Health.

References

1 Horecker, B. L., Gibbs, M., Klenow, H. and Smyrniotis, P. Z. (1954) *J. Biol. Chem.* 207, 393–403

2 Williams, J. F. (1980) *Trends Biochem. Sci.* 5, 315–320 (and see p. 107 of this book)

3 Blackmore, P. F., Williams, J. F., Schofield, P. J. and Power, P. A. (1982) *Int. J. Biochem.* 14, 171–186

4 Wood, H. G., Katz, J. and Landau, B. R. (1963) *Biochem. Z.* 338, 809–847

5 Siu, P. M. L. and Wood, H. G. (1959) *J. Biol. Chem.* 234, 2223–2226

6 Horecker, B. L., Damagk, G. and Hiatt, H. H. (1958) *Arch. Biochem. Biophys.* 78, 510–517

7 Hostetler, K. Y. and Landau, B. R. (1967) *Biochemistry* 6, 2961–2964

8 Landau, B. R. and Katz, J. (1964) *J. Biol. Chem.* 239, 697–704

9 Hostetler, K., Cooperstein, S. J., Landau, B. R. and Lazarow, A. (1966) *Am. J. Physiol.* 211, 1057–1062

10 White, L. W. and Landau, B. R. (1965) *J. Clin. Invest.* 44, 1200–1213

11 Weaver, G. and Landau, B. R. (1963) *Endocrinology* 73, 640–646

12 Merlevede, W., Weaver, G. and Landau, B. R. (1963) *J. Clin. Invest.* 42, 1160–1171

13 Hostetler, K. Y., Landau, B. R., White, R. J., Albin, M. S. and Yashon, D. (1970) *J. Neurochem.* 17, 33–39

14 Green, M. R. and Landau, B. R. (1965) *Arch. Biochem. Biophys.* 111, 509–575

15 Katz, J. and Rognstad, R. (1967) *Biochemistry* 6, 2227–2247

16 Landau, B. R. and Bartsch, G. E. (1966) *J. Biol. Chem.* 241, 741–749

17 Gibbs, M. and Horecker, B. L. (1954) *J. Biol. Chem.* 208, 813–820

18 Wood, H. G., Peeters, G. J., Verkke, R., Laurys-sens, M. and Jacobson, B. (1965) *Biochem. J.* 96, 607–615

19 Williams, J. F., Rienits, K. G., Schofield, P. J. and Clark, M. G. (1971) *Biochem. J.* 123, 923–943

20 Williams, J. F., Clark, M. G. and Blackmore, P. F. (1978) *Biochem. J.* 176, 241–256

21 Williams, J. F. and Clark, M. G. (1971) *Search* 2, 80–88

22 Longenecker, J. P. and Williams, J. F. (1980) *Biochem. J.* 188, 859–865

23 Horecker, B. L., Paoletti, F. and Williams, J. F. (1982) *Ann. NY Acad Sci.* 378, 215–224

24 Longenecker, J. P. and Williams, J. F. (1980) *Biochem. J.* 188, 847–857

25 Katz, J. (1981) *Trends Biochem. Sci.* 6, XIV–XV

26 Williams, J. F. (1981) *Trends Biochem. Sci.* 6, XVI–XVII

27 Landau, B. R. (1981) *Trends Biochem. Sci.* 6, XV

28 Rognstad, R. (1976) *J. Biochem.* 7, 221–228

29 Williams, J. R., Blackmore, P. F. and Clark, M. G. (1978) *Biochem. J.* 176, 257–282

30 Paoletti, F., Williams, J. F. and Horecker, B. L. (1979) *Arch. Biochem. Biophys.* 198, 620–626

31 Paoletti, F., Williams, J. F. and Horecker, B. L. (1979) *Arch. Biochem. Biophys.* 198, 614–619

32 Wood, T. (1981) *Trends Biochem. Sci.* 6, XVI

33 Brin, M. and Yonemoto, R. H. (1958) *J. Biol. Chem.* 230, 307–316

34 Kuehn, A. and Scholz, R. (1982) *Eur. J. Biochem.* 124, 611–617

35 Morgan, M. J. (1981) *FEBS Lett.* 130, 124–126

36 Rognstad, R., Wals, P. and Katz. J. (1982) *Biochem. J.* 208, 851–855

Bernard R. Landau and Harland G. Wood are at the Department of Biochemistry, Case Western Reserve University, School of Medicine, Cleveland, Ohio 44106, USA.

The F-pentose cycle doesn't have the answers for liver tissue

John F. Williams, Krishan K. Arora and
John P. Longenecker

For convenience of reference we will use the numbering of Figures and Tables in the paper of Landau and Wood[1] (see p. 119). It is necessary to state that the differences between the proponents of the F-type (Fig. 1) and L-type (Fig. 2) pentose pathways concern results obtained using liver tissues and liver enzyme preparations.

Our Table A details data showing the negligible contribution of the F-type pentose cycle (F-PC) to glucose metabolism in liver. These data illustrate that it is irrational to maintain argument supporting the F-PC reaction sequence in liver when, by a variety of quantitative measurements over nearly thirty years (including the data of Table III)[1], the proponents of the cycle (and other investigators) have shown, using their own impeccable methodology that it has an insignificant role in hepatic glucose metabolism. The failure to ever find the F-PC reaction sequence in liver is the direct consequence of the inappropriate interpretation of the inadequate, inconsistent and erroneous results of the foundational experiments which were used to propose an F-type pentose pathway reaction sequence for liver and plant tissues[2,3]. (See Refs 4 and 5 for reviews of the evidence.) It is most important to note that other workers in very comprehensive investigations have been unable to confirm the results of the foundational experiments, i.e. the reaction sequence of Fig. 1[4,6,7], using liver enzyme preparations, liver slices and intact animals.

It would be quite wrong for scientists to accept without criticism the assortment of ^{14}C distributions in carbons 1 and 3 of the glucose units of glycogen (see Table I) when only eight of the 30 proffered results comply with the predictions of the F-PC, i.e. C-1/C-3 = 2. It is sophistical to anecdotally claim[1] that where C-1/C-3 doesn't

Table A. Quantitative estimates of the F-type pentose cycle in liver

Substrate	Animal	Product isolated for analysis	% F-PC	Ref.
H^{14}CO$_3$	rat (in vivo)	glycogen	<3%	18
[2-^{14}C]glucose	rat (in vivo)	glycogen	2–11% (individual results were 2,5,5,11% respectively)	11
H^{14}CO$_3$	rat (in vivo)	glycogen	too small to calculate	19
[2-^{14}C]glucose [3,4-^{14}C]glucose	rat liver perfused	lactate	<4%	20
[1-^{14}C]ribose	rat liver slices	glucose	zero	6
[1-^{14}C]ribose	mouse (in vivo)	glycogen	zero	7
[2-^{14}C]glucose	rat (in vivo)	glycogen	2.5–2.9	21
[2-^{14}C]glucose	rabbit liver in situ	glucose 6-P fructose 6-P	<4%	22
[2-^{14}C]glucose	rat hepatocytes	glucose 6-P	2.5	12
[1,3-^{14}C]glycerol [2-^{14}C]glycerol [2-^{13}C]glycerol	mouse liver perfused	glucose	negligible	23
[3,4-^{14}C]glucose	rat liver perfused	glucose 6-P glycogen	<2% <2%	1

Table B. Distribution of ^{14}C in glucose 6-phosphate and lactate isolated from normal and regenerating liver cells after metabolism of [2-^{14}C] and [5-^{14}C] glucose (as percentages)

| Intermediate carbon atom of hepatocyte | [2-^{14}C]Glucose | | |
| | Normal liver | | Regenerating liver |
	Glucose 6-P[7]	Lactate[7]	Glucose 6-P[4]
1	2.5 ± 0.8	9.5 ± 0.9	2.7 ± 1.1
2	66.8 ± 5.7	72.1 ± 2.3	66.1 ± 4.2
3	4.2 ± 0.9	18.4 ± 1.6	2.5 ± 0.6
4	1.8 ± 0.4		6.4 ± 2.6
5	21.8 ± 4.0		16.9 ± 1.8
6	2.9 ± 0.9		5.5 ± 2.1
	F-PC = 1.9%		F-PC = 2.13%

| Intermediate carbon atom of hepatocyte | [5-^{14}C]Glucose | | | |
| | Normal liver | | Regenerating liver | |
	Glucose 6-P[4]	Lactate[2]	Glucose 6-P[4]	Lactate[2]
1	0.6 ± 0.2	4.2	0.8 ± 0.3	5.4
2	17.7 ± 2.7	93.1	9.2 ± 1.7	92.7
3	1.9 ± 0.2	2.7	3.1 ± 1.3	1.9
4	11.5 ± 2.7		4.9 ± 2.0	
5	70.8 ± 5.6		81.3 ± 4.1	
6	1.4 ± 0.3		1.6 ± 0.6	
	L-PC = 33.3%		L-PC = 12.76%	

agree with theory (most of the time) then reverse pentose pathway reactions are responsible for the non-compliance and then only support that claim with the data of a theoretical paper.

The glycogen data are of little use because it has been shown[8] using fed and starved rat hepatocytes that ^{14}C labelled glucose (below 12–15 mM) directly exchanges its carbon atoms into glycogen (see Table III for a display of this phenomenon) and only when glucose is well above the physiological portal concentration (20 mM) does net incorporation of glucose into glycogen commence. Maximum incorporation does not occur until glucose concentration is 50–60 mM. The authors' warning is quoted[8] 'Much of the conclusions in the literature based on ^{14}C yields on the role of glucose in hepatic (glycogen) metabolism may require re-examination'. Katz[9] has made an objective and careful appraisal of the considerable inconsistencies in ^{14}C distributions in glu-

cose units of glycogen particularly the differences in F-PC estimations based on C-1/C-2 and C-3/C-2 ratios following [2-^{14}C]glucose metabolism. There was also failure to include the range of liver glycogen data following [2-^{14}C]glucose metabolism by rats[10,11] which highlight the inconsistencies in F-PC estimates using C-1/C-2 and C-3/C-2 ratio data. These data show C-1/C-3 ratios of 4 and 10 and further illustrate results which deny the occurrence of Fig. 1 reactions.

Concerning the L-pentose pathway reactions, we showed[12] in well-founded experiments that glucose with equal C-4, 5 and 6 labelling caused little C-1 and C-3 labelling of hexose 6-phosphate, while [5-^{14}C]glucose gave very high labelling of the C-2 position. The first observation rules out gluconeogenesis from trioses as an explanation of the second and showed labelling patterns which are quite incompatible with the F-PC. Notable C-5 to C-2 transfers were also found with hepatocytes from regenerating liver (Table B) and with Morris hepatoma 5123TC cells where there is extensive utilization and metabolism of the glucose substrate. Unless a compatible explanation for these observations is found the F-type pathway in liver can be regarded as disproved. Katz[13], Rognstad et al.[14] and Landau and Wood[1] have failed to provide such an explanation.

It is known that glucose 6-P and fructose 6-P are not equilibrated by phosphoglucose isomerase although our derived formula to measure the L-PC made this assumption. This was done to simplify the mathematical treatment and to permit feasible experimental application of the formula. We also imposed the strict theoretical caveat that the only triose-P used in the L-pathway reactions contained carbons 4,5 and 6 of glucose. This followed from the results of the study in vitro which established the pathway[4] and was fully justified in that system because there was no glycolytic flux and no mitochondrial reaction. Obviously, in cells this compartmented triose-P assumption is an artificial limitation, but was diagrammatically used (Fig. 2) to illustrate the way that C-5 of glucose labelled position 2 of hexose 6-P.

The composition and distribution of ^{14}C in the carbon atoms of DHAP reflects the ^{14}C distributions in the various triose-P's generated by the metabolism of the specifically-labelled ^{14}C glucose substrates used. We also showed[12,15] that complete equilibration of triose-P's resulted in very high estimates of the L-PC. We elected the most conservative limit in our theoretical treatment, permitting no triose-P equilibration, thus illustrating the introduction of undiluted carbons from C-4 and C-6 of glucose into position 1 of hexose 6-P (Fig. 2). In cells there are numerous processes (e.g. glycerol–glyceride, amino acid metabolism, pyruvate cycling[16]) which act to distribute and influence ^{14}C concentrations in the active metabolic pools of triose-P during one hour of metabolism of our test substrates. The above qualifications account for the statement that the calculated answer for

the L-PC represents a minimum estimate. The †footnote of Ref. 1 only shows that Landau and Wood have arithmetically discovered the difference between the quoted theoretical limits of our model and the reality of the results.

The opponents of the L-PC have based their argument[1,13,14] on the carbon composition of the triose-P's theoretically shown to form the first three carbons of D-g, D-i oct 1,8-P_2 and which ultimately label positions 1 and 2 of hexose 6-phosphate product (Fig. 2). Thus, [4,5,6-^{14}C]glucose as depicted in Fig. 2 should label C-1 of glucose 6-P with at least as much ^{14}C as there is in C-2. This was not found using [4,5,6-^{14}C]glucose[12], [6-^{14}C]glucose[17] or [3,4-^{14}C]glucose[1]. However, [5-^{14}C]glucose labelled C-2[12].

Rather than theorize endlessly, lactate (which may reflect something of the composition of the triose phosphate pool) was isolated from hepatocytes metabolizing [2-^{14}C] and [5-^{14}C]glucose (Table B). The percentage ^{14}C composition of lactate permits the following calculation of the amounts of ^{14}C which may label C-1 of hexose 6-P from carbons 1 and 3 of the triose-P pool by the L-pentose pathway. Using the [5-^{14}C]glucose data of Table B for normal liver, it can be calculated that the contribution of ^{14}C from C-1 of lactate to glucose 6-P is $17.7/93.1 \times 4.2 = 0.8\%$ and from C-3 is $17.7/93.1 \times 2.7 = 0.51\%$, giving a total of 1.31%. Experimentally we found 0.6% in C-1 of glucose 6-P. In regenerating liver the calculated contribution was 0.71% and the experimentally determined value was 0.8%. Thus, the practical contributions of ^{14}C from C-4 and C-6 of glucose substrate, which for these calculations we assume are equivalent to C-1 and C-3 of lactate, do not result in heavy labelling of C-1 of hexose 6-P product by L-PC. Further evidence showing low ^{14}C concentration in C-1 of glucose 6-P is given in Ref. 12 where, using the above calculation and data showing the ^{14}C in lactate and glucose 6-P formed from [2-^{14}C] and [4,5,6-^{14}C]glucose, respectively, a ^{14}C labelling of 4.7% of C-1 is computed. The experimentally determined value was 2%.

The lactate pool is the largest reservoir of trioses in liver and if it is accepted that cellular trioses equilibrate with lactate, then the well-established recycling of lactate through the futile ^{14}C-exchange cycle:

$$Lac \rightarrow Py \rightarrow OAA \rightarrow PEP \rightarrow Py \rightarrow Lac$$

acts to distribute ^{14}C non-equitably in trioses[16]. Evidence for 'lactate pyruvate cycling' is shown by the ^{14}C distribution data in lactate (Table B). Thus, [4,5,6-^{14}C]glucose forms lactate with ^{14}C shifted from C-2 and heavily deposited in C-3 and with a lighter ^{14}C transfer to C-1. Paradoxically, the effect is the opposite when [5-^{14}C] glucose is used as substrate. The effect of the above 'cycle' on the ^{14}C distribution in the DHAP used to form hexose 6-P's by the L-pentose pathway is the production of glucose 6-P with less ^{14}C in position 1 (original C-4 of glucose and C-1 of lactate) than the C-1 (original C-6 of glucose and C-3 of lactate) of fructose 6-P. The slow equilibration of these two hexose 6-phosphates by glucose phosphate isomerase results in significant loss of ^{14}C from the hexose 6-P pool as [14]CO_2 (original C-4 of glucose) from glucose 6-P. The net effect of the above on the ^{14}C labelling of C-1 and C-2 of hexose 6-P using [4,5,6-^{14}C]glucose as substrate is a minimum accumulation of ^{14}C in C-2 from C-5 and an assault on C-1 by the above events. It was for these reasons that we limited the adoption of [4,5,6-^{14}C]glucose to act only as a marker of gluconeogenesis[12,15]. It is obvious that one would not use such a complexly labelled substrate to show L-pentose pathway in hepatocytes by prediction labelling experiments. The above reasoning was briefly and adequately treated in Refs 12 and 15 but has not been understood by the critics[1,13,14] who are more preoccupied with the diagram (Fig. 2) than the narrative and data of Refs 12 and 15.

There is much evidence that results in Ref. 1 have been carefully selected (see, for example, C-1/C-3 ratio data for glycogen in Ref. 11 and compare with Table I). There is also error of fact, e.g. in a footnote (p. 294) they attribute us with the following reaction (which is not a misprint):

$$[1\text{-}^{14}C]\text{Fru 6-P} + \text{Ery 4-P} \overset{TA}{\rightleftharpoons} [1\text{-}^{14}C]\text{SH 1,7-bisP} + \text{GA 3-P}$$

(where Fru = fructose, Ery = erythrose, SH = sedoheptulose, GA = glyceraldehyde and TA = transaldolase)

There is no such reaction in biochemistry and even if there were, TA could not catalyse it. Needless to say, we haven't published meaningless biochemistry. Many other comments are just as unsound, but these matters will be treated in another place.

Acknowledgements

The work reported was supported by Australian Research Grants Scheme Grant No. D28115633R.

References

1 Landau, B. R. and Wood, H. G. (1983) *Trends Biochem. Sci.* 8, 292–296 (see also p. 119 of this book)
2 Horecker, B. L., Gibbs, M., Klenow, H. and Smyrniotis, P. Z. (1954) *J. Biol. Chem.* 207, 393–403
3 Gibbs, M. and Horecker, B. L. (1954) *J. Biol. Chem.* 208, 813–820
4 Williams, J. F., Blackmore, P. F. and Clark, M. G. (1978) *Biochem. J.* 176, 257–282
5 Williams, J. F. (1980) *Trends Biochem. Sci.* 5, 315–320 (see also p. 107 of this book)
6 Katz, J., Abraham, S., Hill, R. and Chaikoff, I. L. (1955) *J. Biol. Chem.* 214, 853–868
7 Hiatt, H. H. (1957) *J. Biol. Chem.* 224, 851–859
8 Katz, J., Golden, S. and Wals, P. A. (1979) *Biochem. J.* 180, 389–402
9 Katz, J. (1961) in *Radioactive Isotopes in Physiology, Diagnostics and Therapy* (Schwiegk, H. and Turba, F.,eds), pp. 705–751, Springer-Verlag, Berlin
10 Marks, P. A. and Feigelson, P. (1957) *J. Clin. Invest.* 36, 1279–1284
11 Siu, P. M. L. and Wood, H. G. (1959) *J. Biol. Chem.* 234, 2223–2226
12 Longenecker, J. P. and Williams, J. F. (1980) *Biochem. J.* 188, 859–865

13 Katz, J. (1981) *Trends Biochem. Sci.* 6, XIV–XV

14 Rognstad, R., Wals, P. and Katz, J. (1982) *Biochem. J.* 208, 851–855

15 Longenecker, J. P. and Williams, J. F. (1980) *Biochem. J.* 188, 847–857

16 Grunnet, N. and Katz, J. (1978) *Biochem. J.* 172, 595–603

17 Williams, J. F. (1981) *Trends Biochem. Sci.* 6, XVI–XVII

18 Bernstein, I. A., Lentz, K., Malm, M., Schambye, P. and Wood, H. G. (1955) *J. Biol. Chem.* 215, 137–152

19 Marks, P. A. and Horecker, B. L. (1956) *J. Biol. Chem.* 218, 327–333

20 Muntz, J. A. and Murphy, J. R. (1957) *J. Biol. Chem.* 224, 971–986

21 Hostetler, K. Y. and Landau, B. R. (1967) *Biochemistry* 6, 2961–2964

22 Williams, J. F., Rienits, K. G., Schofield, P. J. and Clark, M. G. (1971) *Biochem. J.* 123, 923–943

23 Cohen, S. M., Rognstad, R., Shulman, R. G. and Katz, J. (1981) *J. Biol. Chem.* 256, 3428–3432

K. Arora and John F. Williams are at the Australian National University, PO Box 4, Canberra ACT 2600, Australia; J. P. Longenecker is now at California Biotechnology Inc., PO Box 51650, Palo Alto, CA 94303, USA.

Evidence against the L-type pathway

Bernard R. Landau and Harland G. Wood

We hope that readers will consider the following when assessing the response of Williams *et al.* (p. 128) to our article (p. 119).

(1) The pentose cycle varies as a function of the physiological status of the animal and the tissue being studied. In the experiments of Table A (p. 128), the pentose cycle contributions are relatively small. In other conditions, as in regenerating liver (Table I, p. 124) this is not the case. The question being addressed is whether the 'L-type pathway' exists in liver (and other tissues) and not the relative contribution of the classical pathway.

In Refs 6 and 7 of the response, ^{14}C from [1-^{14}C]ribose was incorporated into carbons 1 and 3 of glucose units. Differing ratios of C-1/C-3 were a function of the experimental conditions and in keeping with the transaldolase–transketolase reactions of the classical pentose cycle (see discussion in Ref. 7 and the paper by Katz and Rognstad (*Biochemistry* (1967) 6, 2227). Furthermore, there was negligible ^{14}C in C-2 (Refs 6 and 7) which should have been labeled if the 'L-type pathway' was present (see Fig. 2, p. 121).

(2) Neither in Ref. 8 of the response nor in Table III (p. 125) is there evidence for a *direct* exchange between glucose and glycogen. Furthermore, there need not be a net synthesis of glycogen from glucose for the glucose units of glycogen to reflect the distribution of ^{14}C in glucose 6-P, so long as glucose 6-P is the precursor of the glucose units.

(3) Our Table I, as we stated, is a summary of data in the literature on the distributions of ^{14}C from [2-^{14}C]glucose in the glucose units of glycogen. We may have missed one or possibly more publications, but this was not intentional. As we also stated, where two or more experiments were done (this was the case for many of these studies), their average is recorded. The first distribution recorded in the Table is the average of two experiments. No experiments differed more in any study than in this one. In one experiment, the distribution of ^{14}C in carbons 1, 2 and 3 was 7.2, 80.5, 3.8 (C-1/C-3=1.8) and in the other 13.5, 68.2, 1.3 (C-1/C-3=11.3) giving the average, setting C-2=100, of 13.9, 100, 3.3 (C-1/C-3=4). In Ref. 10 of the response, the C-1/C-3 ratio averaged 3.8 for fasted rats as Professor Williams states, but was 1.7 for fed rats. The explanations for these ratios are discussed in Ref. 10 in terms of the classical cycle and its transketolase and transaldolase catalysed reactions. A C-1/C-3 ratio is predicted of 2 only for the theoretical model which requires that conditions are such that there is no reversal of the non-oxidative portion of the cycle.

(4) Futile ^{14}C exchange via oxalacetate might cause dilution of ^{14}C of C-1 of the triose-P, but it would not cause preferential dilution of C-3 relative to C-2. Thus, even if this exchange occurs, ^{14}C from [4,5,6-^{14}C]glucose should be converted both to C-1 and C-2 of the fructose 6-P by the 'L-type pathway'. We continue to believe that neither the 'L-type pathway' nor any other known or postulated pathway can account for the fact that Williams finds essentially ^{14}C only in carbon 2 of glucose 6-P, whether formed from [5-^{14}C]glucose or [4,5,6-^{14}C]glucose.

(5) Williams has proposed a series of reactions to account for the formation of [6-^{14}C]glucose-6-P from [2-^{14}C]glucose. We attempted (*footnote, p. 122) to

illustrate how this might occur, but our second reaction is in error, as Williams has noted. His proposed series of reactions (*Search* (1971) 2, 80) involves a transaldolase exchange of [3-^{14}C] glyceraldehyde 3-P with unlabeled fructose 6-P, but he does not show how unlabeled fructose 6-P could be formed from glucose 2-[14]C. For this to occur, there would need to be a remarkable compartmentation of intermediates.

In any event, the formation of [6-^{14}C]glucose 6-P from [2-^{14}C]glucose is not a consideration in support of the 'L-type pathway' and should not distract the reader from the basic issues, i.e. (1) the pathway does not account for that formation; (2) the incorporation of ^{14}C into carbon 6 was observed only at early time point in the studies of Williams; and (3) under the conditions of his incubations with [5-^{14}C]glucose and [4,5,6-^{14}C]glucose, he did not observe incorporation of ^{14}C from [2-^{14}C]glucose into carbon 6 of the glucose 6-P (also ^{14}C in carbon 6 was not found in the glucose unit of glycogen in the study in Ref. 10 of his response).

(6) Williams states that our footnote† (p. 123) 'only shows that Landau and Wood have arithmetically discovered the difference between the quoted theoretical limits of our model and the reality of the results'. The readers should recognize how very large this difference is as indicated in the footnote. Williams states that the critics 'are more preoccupied with the diagram (Fig. 2) than the narrative and data of Refs 12 and 15'. We believe we have thoroughly considered his interpretations and data and presented his data (including Table II), so that readers can draw their own conclusions.

B. R. Landau and H. G. Wood are at the Departments of Medicine and Biochemistry, Case Western Reserve University, Cleveland, Ohio, USA.

Fat and phosphorylation — the role of covalent enzyme modification in lipid synthesis

Grahame Hardie

The rapid effects of certain hormones on lipid synthesis can be explained by changes in the phosphorylation state of several key regulatory enzymes. This system provides an elegant example of the interplay between covalent modification and allosteric regulation.

The fatty acid and sterol components of triacylglycerols and membrane lipids can be derived either by interconversions of dietary fat, or by *de novo* synthesis. The pathways of conversion of carbohydrate into lipid in mammals are summarised in Fig. 1. The liver plays the major role in this process although adipose tissue is also very active in triacylglycerol synthesis and, in some species, fatty acid synthesis. Since the synthesis of one molecule of triacylglycerol from acetyl-CoA and glycerol-3-phosphate requires the consumption of around 50 molecules of ATP and 50 molecules of NADPH, it should come as no surprise that the pathway is stringently regulated. The lipogenic enzymes are subject to reversible control at the level of protein synthesis, a phenomenon which is well-documented, though poorly understood. However, since these enzymes generally have half-lives of 24 h or more, there is clearly a need for acute regulation of enzyme activity. The synthesis of fatty acids is stimulated within minutes by insulin, and inhibited by adrenaline or glucagon. These controls ensure that lipids are synthesized in times of plenty (when insulin levels are high) but not during times of stress or starvation (when catecholamines and/or glucagon are released).

Most biochemistry textbooks state that the rate of fatty acid synthesis is controlled entirely by allosteric effectors. However, recent studies have shown that this view is, at best, only part of the story. It is now clear that fatty acid synthesis, and the other pathways of lipid synthesis, are controlled by covalent enzyme modification as well as allosteric regulation. The purpose of the present review is to discuss these new findings on covalent modification and rationalize them with earlier views on the allosteric regulation of lipid synthesis.

I will now consider the role of protein phosphorylation in each of the pathways involved in the conversion of carbohydrate to lipid (Fig. 1).

The regulation of lipid synthesis by protein phosphorylation

Conversion of glucose-6-phosphate to mitochondrial acetyl-CoA

This pathway, which supplies a proportion of the precursor for fatty acid synthesis, is inhibited by hormones which raise the concentration of cyclic AMP in the liver. Measurements of intermediates in isolated hepatocytes show that dibutyryl cyclic AMP decreases the accumulation of lactate and pyruvate while increasing the cell contents of hexose phosphates and phosphoenolpyruvate[1]. This suggests that the steps catalysed by phosphofructokinase and pyruvate kinase are the sites of inhibition. Glucagon treatment also produces changes in the kinetic properties of phosphofructokinase[2] and pyruvate kinase[3] which survive homogenization and gel filtration, conditions which would remove normal allosteric effectors. In both cases glucagon decreases the apparent affinity for substrate (fructose 6-phosphate or phosphoenolpyruvate), while V_{max} is unaffected. Pyruvate kinase also becomes more susceptible to inhibition by ATP or alanine, and less sensitive to activation by fructose 1,6-bisphosphate. These effects cannot be ascribed to changes in the concentration of any of the 'classical' allosteric effectors. For pyruvate kinase, it is now well established that the effects of glucagon are the result of increased cyclic AMP leading to phosphorylation of pyruvate kinase by cyclic AMP-dependent protein kinase[4]. The picture is less clear for phosphofructokinase. While the liver enzyme does become phosphorylated in vivo after injection of glucagon[5], recent work has suggested that the effect of glucagon on the activity of the enzyme is the result of a decrease in the concentration of a novel allosteric activator, fructose-2,6-bisphosphate, which is effective in the micromolar range[6].

In the liver, glucose is a poor precursor for fatty acid synthesis, and lactate and glycogen are the major sources of carbon for this pathway in non-ruminants. While fatty acid synthesis from lactate may not be affected by inhibition of glycolysis, synthesis from glycogen clearly would be[7]. Inhibition of phosphofructokinase and pyruvate kinase by glucagon would therefore have a dual role of activating net gluconeogenesis and inhibiting fatty acid synthesis.

The isoenzymes of phosphofructokinase and pyruvate kinase found in adipose tissue are different from those found in the liver, and in this tissue hormones which activate adenylate cyclase do not inhibit glycolysis. In this case stimulatory effects of insulin appear to be more important. At least two sites of action of insulin have been recognized, other than its well-known stimulation of glucose uptake, namely the activation of pyruvate kinase and pyruvate dehydrogenase. The effect on pyruvate kinase cannot be explained by changes in known allosteric activators of the enzyme, and

covalent modification of the enzyme would be an attractive alternative hypothesis[8]. In the case of pyruvate dehydrogenase it is now well established that the stimulatory effect of insulin is due to a net dephosphorylation of the enzyme[9].

Conversion of mitochondrial acetyl-CoA to cytoplasmic acetyl-CoA

As the inner mitochondrial membrane is impermeable to acetyl-CoA a sequence of three steps are necessary to circumvent the barrier (Fig. 1). There is little evidence that this pathway is regulated in vivo, although the final enzyme, ATP-citrate lyase, is subject to reversible phosphorylation. The purified rat liver[10] and rat mammary gland[10] enzymes contain acid-stable phosphate, and the rat mammary enzyme can be phosphorylated stoichiometrically by cyclic AMP-dependent protein kinase[11]. This latter observation explains the increased phosphorylation of ATP-citrate lyase observed in isolated hepatocytes treated with glucagon[12,13] or isolated adipocytes treated with adrenaline[14], since these hormones cause increases in cyclic AMP in their respective target cells. An intriguing and still unexplained observation is the apparent increase in phosphorylation of ATP-citrate lyase observed after treating isolated hepatocytes[12] or adipocytes[14] with insulin. As yet no effect of phosphorylation on the activity of ATP-citrate lyase has been reported, and the function of this covalent modification remains unknown.

Cytoplasmic acetyl-CoA to fatty acid

It is generally agreed that acetyl-CoA carboxylase catalyses the rate-limiting step for fatty acid synthesis under most conditions. The regulation of the enzyme by reversible phosphorylation is well established. Acetyl-CoA carboxylase purified from rat mammary gland is phosphoryl-

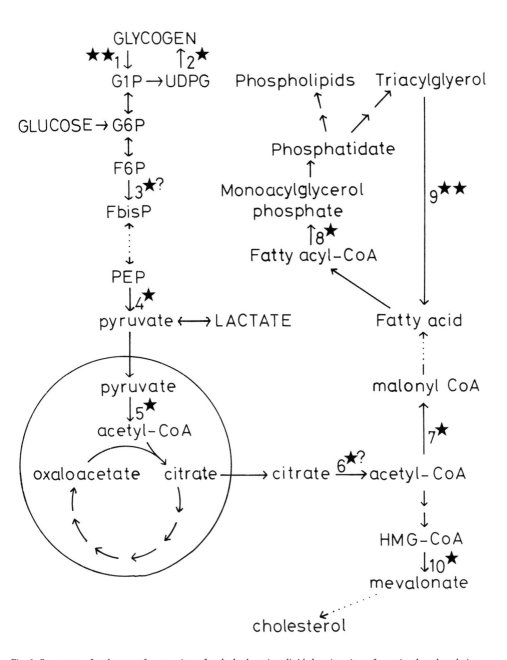

Fig. 1. Summary of pathways of conversion of carbohydrate into lipid showing sites of protein phosphorylation.
KEY: ★ enzyme inactivated by phosphorylation; ★★ enzyme activated by phosphorylation; ★? enzyme phosphorylated but function unknown.
ENZYMES: (1) phosphorylase, (2) glycogen synthase, (3) phosphofructokinase, (4) pyruvate kinase, (5) pyruvate dehydrogenase, (6) ATP-citrate lyase, (7) acetyl-CoA carboxylase, (8) glycerol phosphate acyl transferase, (9) hormone-sensitive lipase, (10) hydroxymethylglutaryl-CoA reductase.
INTERMEDIATES: GIP; F bis P etc.: glucose 1-phosphate, fructose 1,6-bisphosphate etc., PEP: phosphoenolpyruvate; HMG-CoA: hydroxymethylglutaryl-CoA.
The major precursors for lipogenesis are shown in capital letters.

ated and inactivated reversibly by cyclic AMP-dependent protein kinase[15]. Phosphorylation does not change the apparent K_m values for substrates, but reduces V_{max} two-fold and also brings about a two-fold decrease in the apparent affinity for the allosteric activator, citrate. The activity of the purified enzyme during phosphorylation by cyclic AMP-dependent protein kinase correlates with the state of phosphorylation of a serine residue located in a neutral tryptic peptide[15], and the phosphorylation of this same peptide is increased six-fold by adrenaline in intact fat cells[16]. Since adrenaline raises the concentration of cyclic AMP in fat cells, the inactivation of acetyl-CoA carboxylase by adrenaline in adipose tissue may be ascribed to phosphorylation by cyclic AMP-dependent protein kinase. It seems likely that the same mechanism will explain the inactivation and increased phosphorylation of acetyl-CoA carboxylase observed when isolated hepatocytes are treated with glucagon[17].

Other hormones, such as insulin and vasopressin, can affect the activity of acetyl-CoA carboxylase in the absence of changes in cyclic AMP concentration[18]. There is evidence for cyclic AMP-independent protein kinases which can phosphorylate and inactivate acetyl-CoA carboxylase[15, 19] and it is tempting to speculate that these may be involved in the actions of hormones which do not act via cyclic AMP.

Triacylglycerol synthesis

The effects of hormones on the enzymes of triacylglycerol synthesis were considered in a previous *TIBS* review[20]. At least one of these enzymes, glycerol phosphate acyl transferase, may be regulated by phosphorylation. The activity of this enzyme is decreased acutely by adrenaline treatment of adipose tissue *in vitro*[21] or by treatment of microsomal preparations with cyclic AMP-dependent protein kinase[22]. In the latter case the inactivation is reversed by treatment with alkaline phosphatase. This represents convincing evidence that a protein phosphorylation inhibits the enzyme, although further work is required to show that the glycerol phosphate acyl transferase itself is modified.

Cholesterol synthesis

The regulation of hydroxymethylglutaryl (HMG)-CoA reductase by protein phosphorylation is now well established[23]. This is a 'bicyclic' system in which HMG-CoA reductase is inactivated by a reductase kinase, which is itself activated by a reductase kinase kinase. While HMG-CoA reductase is generally believed to be rate-limiting for cholesterol synthesis, the physiological significance of its phosphorylation has not been clear. Recently, however, it has been shown that the decrease in the proportion of HMG-CoA reductase in the phosphorylated form that occurs on incubation of isolated hepatocytes, is accentuated by insulin and prevented by glucagon. These changes can be ascribed to alterations in the activity of HMG-CoA reductase kinase which occur in the reciprocal direction[24]. Neither reductase kinase nor reductase kinase kinase appear to be cyclic AMP-dependent, and the mechanism for the glucagon effect remains uncertain.

Relationship of protein phosphorylation and allosteric regulation

In the past, the proponents of allosteric regulation have sometimes argued vehemently against protein phosphorylation as if the two regulatory devices were mutually exclusive. In fact the two mechanisms fulfil roles that are different, although complementary. This is well illustrated in the case of acetyl-CoA carboxylase. The enzyme is allosterically activated by a precursor of fatty acid synthesis, citrate, and inhibited by an end product, long-chain fatty acyl-CoA. These effectors are competitive with each other and are believed to act by changing the state of polymerisation of the enzyme. The inhibition of fatty acid synthesis in the liver during short-term fasting has been ascribed both to a decrease of intracellular citrate produced by inhibition of glycolysis[25] and to an increase in intracellular fatty acyl-CoA[26]. While citrate does not decrease in the livers of fed rats treated with glucagon[27], probably because of the presence of circulating lactate which circumvents the inhibition of glycolysis[28], these allosteric mechanisms may play a role in inhibiting fatty acid synthesis during fasting. However, since phosphorylation of acetyl-CoA carboxylase by cyclic AMP-dependent protein kinase decreases the apparent affinity for citrate as well as decreasing V_{max}[15], the effect of changes in allosteric effectors will be greatly accentuated. Thus, in response to a signal from elsewhere in the body (release of glucagon from the pancreas), the response of the liver to changes in local conditions can be modified. It is also worth noting that the changes in the concentrations of allosteric effectors are the result of covalent modification in other pathways. The decrease in citrate is probably due in part to glucagon-stimulated phosphorylation of liver pyruvate kinase, while the increase in fatty acyl-CoA is due to fatty acid release from adipose tissue caused by increased phosphorylation, and hence activation, of hormone-sensitive lipase[29].

The 1970s were to covalent modification what the 1960s were to allosteric regulation. A glance at the asterisks in Fig. 1 should convince the reader that protein phosphorylation is a regulatory mechanism of widespread, if not universal, significance in mammalian cells[30]. Allosteric regulation is an intracellular homeostatic mechanism which also allows the cell to respond to changes in substrate concentration in its immediate environment. Covalent modification in response to a hormone can modulate this internal control in order to meet the needs of the body as a whole. As such it is an essential means of integration of function in a multicellular organism.

References

1 Harris, R. A. (1975) *Arch. Biochem. Biophys.* 169, 168–180
2 Castano, J. G., Nicto, A. and Felfu, J. E. (1979) *J. Biol. Chem.* 254, 5576–5579
3 Felfu, J. E., Hue, L. and Hers, H. G. (1976) *Proc. Natl Acad. Sci. USA* 73, 2762–2766
4 Engstram, L. (1980) in *Molecular Aspects of Cellular Regulation* (Cohen, P., ed.), Vol. 1, pp. 11–31, Elsevier/North-Holland
5 Kagimoto, T. and Uyeda, K. (1979) *J. Biol. Chem.* 254, 5584–5587
6 Van Schaftingen, E., Hue, L. and Hers, H. G. (1980) *Biochem. J.* 192, 897–901
7 Hopkirk, T. J. and Bloxham, D. P. (1979) *Biochem. J.* 182, 383–397
8 Denton, R. M., Edgell, N. J., Bridges, B. J. and Poole, G. P. (1979) *Biochem. J.* 180, 523–531
9 Hughes, W. A., Brownsey, R. W. and Denton, R. M. (1980) *Biochem. J.* 192, 469–481
10 Linn, T. C. and Srere, P. A. (1979) *J. Biol. Chem.* 254, 1691–1698
11 Guy, P. S., Cohen, P. and Hardie, D. G. (1979) *FEBS Lett.* 109, 205–208
12 Alexander, M. C., Kowaloff, E. M., Witters, L. A., Dennihy, D. T. and Avruch, J. (1979) *J. Biol. Chem.* 254, 8052–8056
13 Janski, A. M., Srere, P. A., Cornell, N. W. and Veech, R. L. (1979) *J. Biol. Chem.* 254, 9365–9368
14 Ramakrishna, S. and Benjamin, W. B. (1979) *J. Biol. Chem.* 254, 9232–9236
15 Hardie, D. G. and Guy, P. S. (1980) *Eur. J. Biochem.* 110, 167–177
16 Brownsey, R. W. and Hardie, D. G. (1980) *FEBS Lett.* 120, 67–70
17 Witters, L. A., Kowaloff, E. M. and Avruch, J. (1979) *J. Biol. Chem.* 254, 245–248
18 Hardie, D. G. (1980) in *Molecular Aspects of Cellular Regulation* (Cohen, P., ed.), Vol. 1, pp. 33–62, Elsevier/North-Holland
19 Carlson, C. A. and Kim, K. H. (1973) *J. Biol. Chem.* 248, 378–380
20 Saggerson, D. (1979) *Trends Biochem. Sci.* 4, 33–35
21 Sooranna, S. R. and Saggerson, E. D. (1978) *FEBS Lett.* 96, 141–144
22 Nimmo, H. G. and Houston, B. (1978) *Biochem. J.* 176, 607–610
23 Ingebritsen, T. S. and Gibson, D. M. (1980) in *Molecular Aspects of Cellular Regulation* (Cohen, P., ed.), Vol. 1, pp. 63–93, Elsevier/North-Holland
24 Ingebritsen, T. S., Geelen, M. J. H., Parker, R. A., Evenson, K. J. and Gibson, D. M. (1979) *J. Biol.*

Chem. 254, 9986–9989

25 Watkins, P. S., Tarlow, D. M. and Lane, M. D. (1977) *Proc. Natl Acad. Sci. USA* 74, 1497–1501

26 Seitz, J. H., Müller, M. J., Krone, W., Tarnowski, W., Carsten, D., Dunkelmann, B. and Harneit, A. (1977) *Arch. Biochem. Biophys.* 183, 647–663

27 Cook, G. A., Nielsen, R. C., Hawkins, R. A., Mehlman, M. A., Lakshmanan, M. R. and Veech, R. L. (1977) *J. Biol. Chem.* 252, 4421–4424

28 McGarry, J. D., Takabayashi, Y. and Foster, D. W.

(1978) *J. Biol. Chem.* 253, 8294–8300

29 Khoo, J. C., Steinberg, D., Huang, J. J. and Vagelos, P. R. (1976) *J. Biol. Chem.* 251, 2882–2890

30 Cohen, P. (ed.) (1980) *Molecular Aspects of Cellular Regulation*, Vol. 1

Grahame Hardie is at the Biochemistry Department, Medical Sciences Institute, University of Dundee, Dundee DD1 4HN, Scotland, UK.

Addendum

The most spectacular progress since the writing of the original review has been in our understanding of the regulation of phosphofructokinase by the novel allosteric effector discovered by van Schaftingen, Hue and Hers, i.e. fructose 2,6-bisphosphate. This molecule is now known to be a potent inhibitor of fructose-1,6-bisphosphatase as well as an activator of phosphofructokinase[31], so that depression of its concentration by glucagon in hepatocytes from fed rats switches the substrate cycle catalysed by these two enzymes away from glycolysis (and hence, fatty acid synthesis) in favour of gluconeogenesis. Fructose 2,6-bisphosphate is now known to be formed from fructose 6-phosphate and ATP via a specific enzyme, 6-phospho-fructo-2-kinase, and to be broken down to fructose 6-phosphate by a fructose-2,6-bisphosphatase. Purification of these two activities by Pilkis' group[32] has led to the remarkable observation that they are catalysed by distinct regions of the same polypeptide. This bifunctional protein is phosphorylated at a single site by cAMP-dependent protein kinase, which inactivates the kinase and activates the phosphatase. These observations elegantly explain the potent depression of fructose 2,6-bisphosphate concentrations in rat hepatocytes by glucagon.

If we turn to fatty acid synthesis itself, the role of cAMP-dependent protein kinase in the effects of glucagon in rat hepatocytes is now well established. The hormone causes phosphorylation of acetyl-CoA carboxylase in isolated cells at the same site as that phosphorylated (*in vitro*) by this protein kinase on the purified enzyme[33]. Acetyl-CoA carboxylase is also phosphorylated at several other sites (at least five) in unstimulated cells. The function of these sites is not clear, but some of them must be regulatory since dephosphorylation results in dramatic activation of the enzyme[33].

Although insulin has opposite effects to those of glucagon or catecholamines on the rate of fatty acid synthesis, all of these hormones increase the phosphorylation of both ATP-citrate lyase and acetyl-CoA carboxylase in isolated hepatocytes and adipocytes. On ATP-citrate lyase the insulin-stimulated phosphorylation occurs at the same serine residue phosphorylated by cAMP-dependent protein kinase, and phosphorylation is not stoichiometric[34], suggesting that it is unlikely that it has any real function. Although phosphorylation of acetyl-CoA carboxylase in response to insulin occurs at a site distinct from that phosphorylated by cAMP-dependent protein kinase[35], current evidence suggests that this phosphorylation does not change the kinetic parameters of the enzyme[36]. The relationship between stimulation of fatty acid synthesis and stimulation of protein phosphorylation by insulin is therefore not clear. Recent results do, however, suggest that insulin stimulates phosphorylation by activation of a protein (serine/threonine) kinase[37], and these lipogenic enzymes may still represent a useful system with which to identify insulin-stimulated kinases.

The tentative proposals in the review that both pyruvate kinase and glycerol phosphate acyl transferase may be regulated by phosphorylation in adipocytes have not been substantiated. Direct ^{32}P-labelling experiments have failed to demonstrate phosphorylation of the enzyme protein[38,39], and the original reports of hormone-induced changes in activity remain unconfirmed.

Although our knowledge of the structure of (HMG)CoA reductase has increased enormously[40], our understanding of its regulation has not increased at quite the same pace. In 1981, the regulation of the enzyme by phosphorylation had been amply demonstrated in cell-free systems and in isolated hepatocytes, but its physiological importance was disputed because attempts to demonstrate changes in phosphorylation state *in vivo* had not been successful. However Easom and Zammit have recently reported that the conditions used for the preparation of tissue prior to enzyme assay are critical[41], and have been able to demonstrate a diurnal rhythm in the degree of phosphorylation of the rat liver enzyme *in vivo* which correlates inversely with feeding patterns and hence, presumably with insulin/glucagon ratios[42].

In summary, the central role of pro-tein phosphorylation in hormonal regulation of lipid synthesis is as clear today as it was in 1981. However, in at least one case, protein phosphorylation operates less directly than originally anticipated, i.e. by regulating the enzymes controlling the concentration of the allosteric signal molecule, fructose 2,6-bisphosphate.

References

31 Van Schaftingen, E. and Hers, H., G. (1981) *Proc. Natl Acad. Sci. USA* 78, 2861–2863

32 El-Maghrabi, M. R., Claus, T. H., Pilkis, J., Fox, E. and Pilkis, S. J. (1982) *J. Biol. Chem.* 257, 7603–7607

33 Holland, R., Witters, L. A. and Hardie, D. G. (1984) *Eur. J. Biochem.* 140, 325–333

34 Pierce, M. W., Palmer, J. L., Keutmann, H. T., Hall, T. A. and Avruch, J. (1982) *J. Biol. Chem.* 257, 10681–10686

35 Brownsey, R. W. and Denton, R. M. (1982) *Biochem. J.* 202, 77–86

36 Witters, L. A., Tipper, J. P. and Bacon, G. W. (1983) *J. Biol. Chem.* 258, 5643–5648

37 Brownsey, R. W., Edgell, N. J., Hopkirk, T. J. and Denton, R. M. (1984) *Biochem J.* 218, 733–743

38 Denton, R. M. and Brownsey, R. W. (1983) *Phil. Trans. Roy. Soc. Lond. B* 302, 33–45

39 Nimmo, G. A. and Nimmo, H. G. *Biochem. J.* (in press)

40 Chin, D. J., Gil, G., Russell, D. W., Liscum, L., Luskey, K. L., Basu, S. K., Okayama, H., Berg, P., Goldstein, J. L. and Brown, M. S. (1984) *Nature* 308, 613–617

41 Eason, R. A. and Zammit, V. A. (1984) *Biochem. J.* 220, 733–738

42 Eason, R. A. and Zammit, V. A. (1984) *Biochem. J.* 220, 739–745

Two long-chain acyl coenzyme A synthetases: their different roles in fatty acid metabolism and its regulation

Shosaku Numa

A puzzling phenotype of mutants of a hydrocarbon-utilizing yeast has led to the discovery of two functionally different long-chain acyl-CoA synthetases. One is responsible for the production of long-chain acyl-CoA to be utilized exclusively for the synthesis of cellular lipids, whereas the other provides long-chain acyl-CoA destined exclusively for degradation via β-oxidation. The long-chain acyl-CoA for lipid synthesis, but not that for degradation, is involved in the repression of acetyl-CoA carboxylase, the key enzyme for the regulation of fatty acid synthesis.

Acetyl-CoA carboxylase [acetyl-CoA: carbon-dioxide ligase (ADP-forming), EC 6.4.1.2] plays a critical role in the regulation of fatty acid synthesis[1] and is repressed by exogenous fatty acid in mammalian[2,3] and yeast cells[4,5]. The decrease in the cellular content of acetyl-CoA carboxylase is due to diminished synthesis of the enzyme[3,5], caused by a reduction in the mRNA coding for the enzyme[6]. The hydrocarbon-utilizing yeast *Candida lipolytica* is used as a eukaryotic system to study the mechanism responsible for the repression of acetyl-CoA carboxylase. This yeast can use fatty acid (or *n*-alkane) or glucose as a sole carbon source and thus exhibits large variations in enzyme content[5]. In an attempt to determine whether the repressive effect is mediated by fatty acid itself or by a metabolite derived from it, we isolated mutant strains of *C. lipolytica* with apparently no long-chain acyl-CoA synthetase [acid:CoA ligase (AMP-forming), EC 6.2.1.3] activity[7]. The mutants were selected by their inability to grow in the presence of exogenous fatty acid under conditions where the cellular synthesis *de novo* of fatty acids was blocked by cerulenin[8], an antibiotic known to inhibit fatty acid synthetase. Because the activation of exogenous fatty acid is obligatory for its further metabolism, it was unexpected and surprising that these mutants were able to grow normally on fatty acid (or *n*-alkane) as a sole carbon source. This puzzling phenotype has been analysed as described below.

Fatty acid metabolism in the mutants

To elucidate the mechanism by which fatty acid is metabolized to support the growth of the mutant strains we cultivated them on pentadecanoic acid (a fatty acid with an odd number of carbons in its chain), and then analysed the composition of cellular fatty acids[7]. Whereas the fatty acids of wild-type cells (or cells of a spontaneous revertant obtained from a mutant) grown under the same conditions were almost all odd-numbered chain lengths (17:1, 15:0, 17:2, etc.), nearly all the fatty acids of the mutant cells were even-numbered (18:1, 18:2, 16:1, 16:0, etc.). In a control experiment, in which cells were grown on an even-chain-length fatty acid, the cellular fatty acids of all strains were even-numbered. Thus, the mutant strains, unlike the wild-type strain (or the revertant strain), cannot incorporate whole exogenous fatty acid into cellular lipids, but utilize the fatty acids synthesized *de novo* from acetyl-CoA produced by degradation of the exogenous fatty acid. This exogenous fatty acid must somehow be activated in the mutant strains prior to its degradation.

Four possible mechanisms of fatty acid activation were considered. First, thioesterification of fatty acid catalysed by an additional, hypothetical acyl-CoA synthetase; second, ω-oxidation to dicarboxylic acid followed by thioesterification at either carboxyl group; third, ω-oxidation to semi-aldehyde followed by CoA-dependent dehydrogenation; and finally, α-oxidation to an α-keto acid followed by CoA-dependent oxidative decarboxylation. We could distinguish between these possibilities by cultivating cells on either [1-^{14}C]- or [10-^{14}C]oleic acid and then determining the incorporation of radioactivity into cellular lipids as well as the ^{14}C content of the carboxyl carbon relative to that of the total carbons of the fatty acids liberated from the lipids. The results obtained have unambiguously shown that the first mechanism is valid[7], thus predicting the presence of an additional long-chain acyl-CoA synthetase, which would operate even in the mutant strains and which exhibits no apparent activity under normal assay conditions.

Two functionally different long-chain acyl-CoA synthetases

Our prediction has been verified by the discovery of a second long-chain acyl-CoA synthetase, the activity of which can be measured in the particulate fraction when phosphatidylcholine is added to the assay mixture[9]. This enzyme, designated as acyl-CoA synthetase II, occurs both in the mutant and wild-type strains. The enzyme missing in the mutant strains, designated as acyl-CoA synthetase I, is measurable in the particulate fraction without added phosphatidylcholine. The two enzymes have been separated from each other[9]; when the particulate fraction from wild-type cells grown on oleic acid, which possess both enzymes, is treated with 5 mM Triton X-100, a non-ionic detergent, and then subjected to high-speed centrifugation, acyl-CoA synthetase I is recovered in the supernatant, whereas acyl-CoA synthetase II is found in the precipitate. Acyl-CoA synthetase I has been purified to homogeneity[10]. Studies with antibody to the purified enzyme indicate that the two acyl-CoA synthetases are immunochemically distinguishable[10].

Further evidence for the presence of the two distinct long-chain acyl-CoA synthetases has been provided by the isolation of mutant strains that, in contrast to those already discussed, are defective in acyl-CoA synthetase II but possess intact acyl-CoA synthetase I[11]. The mutants lacking acyl-CoA synthetase II cannot grow at all on fatty acid as a sole carbon source, but are able to incorporate exogenous fatty acid as a whole into cellular lipids.

Biochemical, immunochemical and genetic evidence firmly established the existence of two distinct long-chain acyl-CoA synthetases. The phenotypes of the mutants defective in either of the two enzymes showed that acyl-CoA synthetase I produces long-chain acyl-CoA that is utilized exclusively for the synthesis of cellular lipids, whereas acyl-CoA synthetase II provides long-chain acyl-CoA that is exclusively degraded via β-oxidation (see Fig. 2). Thus, there are two independent long-chain acyl-CoA pools, one for lipid synthesis and one for β-oxidation, and they cannot take the place of each other.

Consistent with the different physiological roles of the two long-chain acyl-CoA synthetases are the following findings. Acyl-CoA synthetase II, in contrast to acyl-CoA synthetase I, is induced by fatty acid and exhibits a broad substrate specificity with respect to fatty acid[9]. Acyl-CoA synthetase I is distributed among various

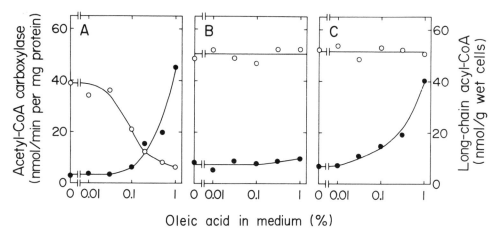

Fig. 1. *Effect of the two long-chain acyl-CoA pools on acetyl-CoA carboxylase. Cells of* C. lipolytica *strains A-633-7 (A), LA-633 (B) and LB-742 (C) (for specification of the mutants, see the text) were grown in media containing oleic acid at the indicated concentrations and 2% glucose. The cells harvested were divided into two portions for determination of the levels of long-chain acyl-CoA (●) and acetyl-CoA carboxylase (○). Data taken from Ref. 11.*

subcellular fractions, including microsomes and mitochondria where glycerophosphate acyltransferase, the enzyme responsible for the initial step of glycerolipid synthesis, is located, while acyl-CoA synthetase II is localized in microbodies where the acyl-CoA-oxidizing system is located[12].

It is noteworthy that the cellular lipids of *C. lipolytica* mutants which lack acyl-CoA synthetase I contain, almost exclusively, even-chain-length fatty acids, even when they are grown on odd-chain-length hydrocarbons. In view of the fact that naturally occurring fatty acids are generally even-numbered, these mutant cells seem to be more useful for the production of single-cell protein than wild-type cells.

Long-chain acyl-CoA for lipid synthesis is involved in the repression of acetyl-CoA carboxylase

As described above, the acetyl-CoA carboxylase content of wild-type *C. lipolytica* cells is markedly reduced when they are grown in the presence of fatty acid. In contrast, repression of acetyl-CoA carboxylase hardly occurs in the mutants defective in acyl-CoA synthetase I[11]. The

mutants defective in acyl-CoA synthetase II as well as the revertants derived from an acyl-CoA synthetase I mutant exhibit a normal repression of acetyl-CoA carboxylase by exogenous fatty acid[11]. Thus, the activation of exogenous fatty acid by acyl-CoA synthetase I, but not that by acyl-CoA synthetase II, is required for the repression of acetyl-CoA carboxylase.

In the experiment presented in Fig. 1, we have attempted to measure separately the two independent long-chain acyl-CoA pools generated by acyl-CoA synthetase I and acyl-CoA synthetase II, using appropriate mutant strains. When fatty acid is added to the culture medium in increasing concentrations, the mutant defective in acyl-CoA synthetase II (Fig. 1A) should accumulate the long-chain acyl-CoA to be utilized exclusively for lipid synthesis, whereas the mutant lacking acyl-CoA synthetase I (and also the acyl-CoA-oxidizing system) (Fig. 1C) should accumulate the long-chain acyl-CoA destined exclusively for β-oxidation. On the other hand, the mutant defective in both acyl-CoA synthetases (Fig. 1B) should produce no long-chain acyl-CoA from exogenous fatty acid. Repression of acetyl-CoA carboxylase is observed only in the mutant defective in acyl-CoA synthetase II. Thus, the long-chain acyl-CoA destined for lipid synthesis is causally related to the repression of acetyl-CoA carboxylase, whereas the long-chain acyl-CoA destined for degradation via β-oxidation is not involved.

This regulatory mechanism is obviously of teleological significance in view of the homeostasis of lipid synthesis, as schematically shown in Fig. 2. The long-chain acyl-CoA destined for lipid synthesis is supplied both by fatty acid synthesis *de novo*, the rate of which is regulated by acetyl-CoA carboxylase, and by the activation of exogenous fatty acid catalysed by acyl-CoA synthetase I. In view of our finding that the decrease in the content of acetyl-CoA carboxylase in fatty acid-grown cells is associated with a corresponding reduction in the level of the mRNA coding for the enzyme[6], it seems probable that the long-chain acyl-CoA destined for lipid synthesis, or a compound metabolically related to it, acts as a co-repressor or its eukaryotic equivalent to suppress the expression of the gene coding for acetyl-CoA carboxylase.

Also worthy of note is the fact that long-chain acyl-CoA is a specific allosteric inhibitor of acetyl-CoA carboxylase[13]. We have demonstrated that palmitoyl-CoA binds tightly and reversibly to mammalian acetyl-CoA carboxylase in an equimolar ratio to completely inhibit the enzyme[14]; the inhibition constant (K_i) is as low as 6 nM, about three orders of magnitude smaller than the critical micellar concentration of palmitoyl-CoA. Comparison of the K_i values for various structural analogues of palmitoyl-CoA indicates that the 3' phosphate of the CoA moiety and the long-chain acyl residue are essential for the inhibition of the enzyme[15]. The reversible formation of the equimolar enzyme–inhibitor complex, together with the rather strict structural requirement for the inhibitor, strongly supports the idea that long-chain acyl-CoA is a physiological regulator of the catalytic efficiency of acetyl-CoA carboxylase. Thus, long-chain acyl-CoA has a dual role in the regulation of acetyl-CoA carboxylase, acting not only as a putative co-repressor but also as a specific inhibitor.

References

1 Numa, S. and Yamashita, S. (1974) *Curr. Top. Cell. Regul.* 8, 197–246

2 Jacobs, R. A., Sly, W. S. and Majerus, P. W. (1973) *J. Biol. Chem.* 248, 1268–1276

3 Kitajima, K., Tashiro, S. and Numa, S. (1975) *Eur. J. Biochem.* 54, 373–383

4 Kamiryo, T. and Numa, S. (1973) *FEBS Lett.* 38, 29–32

5 Mishina, M., Kamiryo, T., Tanaka, A., Fukui, S. and Numa, S. (1976) *Eur. J. Biochem.* 71, 301–308

6 Horikawa, S., Kamiryo, T., Nakanishi, S. and Numa, S. (1980) *Eur. J. Biochem.* 104, 191–198

7 Kamiryo, T., Mishina, M., Tashiro, S. and Numa, S. (1977) *Proc. Natl. Acad. Sci. U.S.A.* 74, 4947–4950

8 Ōmura, S. (1976) *Bacteriol. Rev.* 40, 681–697

9 Mishina, M., Kamiryo, T., Tashiro, S. and Numa, S. (1978) *Eur. J. Biochem.* 82, 347–354

10 Hosaka, K., Mishina, M., Tanaka, T., Kamiryo, T. and Numa, S. (1979) *Eur. J. Biochem.* 93, 197–203

11 Kamiryo, T., Nishikawa, Y., Mishina, M., Terao, M. and Numa, S. (1979) *Proc. Natl. Acad. Sci. U.S.A.* 76, 4390–4394

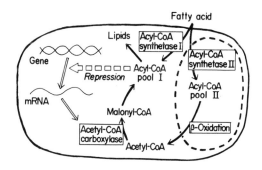

Fig. 2. Functions of the two long-chain acyl-CoA synthetases and the mechanism of repression of acetyl-CoA carboxylase.

12 Mishina, M., Kamiryo, T., Tashiro, S., Hagihara, T., Tanaka, A., Fukui, S., Osumi, M. and Numa, S. (1978) *Eur. J. Biochem.* 89, 321–328

13 Numa, S., Bortz, W. M. and Lynen, F. (1965) *Adv. Enzyme Regul.* 3, 407–423

14 Ogiwara, H., Tanabe, T., Nikawa, J. and Numa, S. (1978) *Eur. J. Biochem.* 89, 33–41

15 Nikawa, J., Tanabe, T., Ogiwara, H., Shiba, T. and Numa, S. (1979) *FEBS Lett.* 102, 223–226

Shosaku Numa is at the Department of Medical Chemistry, Kyoto University Faculty of Medicine, Yoshida, Sakyo-ku, Kyoto 606, Japan.

Brown fat mitochondria

David G. Nicholls and Eduardo Rial

Brown fat mitochondria possess a unique protein in their inner membranes which can short-circuit their respiratory chain to generate heat.

Our normal response to cold is to shiver. There is, however, an alternative means of generating heat under certain conditions which has been termed 'non-shivering thermogenesis' (NST). NST is important at birth, as well as being vital for the cold-adaptation of a variety of small mammals, and for the arousal of hibernators[1]. A closely related phenomenon – 'diet-induced thermogenesis' (DIT) has been described, whereby the ability of the body to burn off the excess calories resulting from over-eating may function as a mechanism for weight regulation[2].

Animals which have been adapted to a cold environment have a greatly increased capacity for NST. When cold-adapted rats are infused with noradrenaline (the hormone which switches on NST) there is a 3-fold increase in their respiration, and a study of the oxygen uptake by the different tissues attributed at least 60% of the increase to brown fat, which accounts for less than 2% of body weight[3]. This specificity is remarkable in view of the number of organs which possess receptors for noradrenaline, and indicates that the tissue must possess very specialized mechanisms for heat production.

The brown adipocyte can be distinguished from a white fat cell by its high content of very invaginated mitochondria and, usually, by the presence of many small fat droplets rather than a single large droplet. Noradrenaline, released from sympathetic nerve terminals, binds to distinctive β-receptors[4], activating adenyl cyclase, thereby elevating cyclic AMP, which in turn activates a hormone-sensitive lipase. This mobil-izes the triacylglycerol stores, releasing fatty acids which are the predominant substrate of the tissue under thermogenic conditions (for review see Ref. 5).

The major questions facing the biochemist are: (1) How are the mitochondria adapted to allow such a spectacular rate of respiration and heat production? (2) How does noradrenaline switch on this respiration? (3) Why do cold-adapted animals have an increased capacity for NST?

The proton short-circuit

The chemiosmotic theory provides three mechanisms by which, in principle, a mitochondrion could increase its respiration beyond that required to maintain the normal energy requirements of the cell. (1) ATP turnover can be accelerated by an activation of ATP hydrolysis within the cell. (2) The respiratory chain can be modified such that it no longer pumps protons and respiration is no longer linked to ATP synthesis. (3) The normal proton impermeability of the membrane can be modified such that protons extruded by the respiratory chain can re-enter the mitochondrion without passing through the ATP synthase – again uncoupling respiration from ATP turnover.

A significant early discovery with isolated brown fat mitochondria was that they showed no respiratory control until certain purine nucleotides were added to the incubation mixture[6]. The initial lack of respiratory control is not a consequence of accelerated ATP turnover, since the ATP synthase inhibitor oligomycin fails to induce respiratory control. The uncontrolled mitochondria show a normal extrusion of protons in an oxygen-pulse experiment, indicating that the respiratory chain is not modified; however the decay of the pH gradient is unusually fast, and can be slowed down by the 'recoupling' purine nucleotides, suggesting that the energetic lesion is nucleotide-regulated proton permeability[7]. Two independent approaches confirm the presence of this 'short-circuit': (1) Non-respiring mitochondria swell in media which demand free permeation of protons across the inner membrane for charge and pH neutralization (such as potassium acetate in the presence of valinomycin)[8]; purine nucleotides inhibit this swelling. (2) The uncontrolled mitochondria maintain a low proton electrochemical potential ($\Delta\mu H^+$) despite their high respiration, indicating a high proton conductance of the membrane; purine nucleotide addition is accompanied by a 10-fold decrease in this conductance, with a consequent elevation of $\Delta\mu H^+$ and inhibition of respiration[7].

The uncoupling protein

The purine nucleotides act by binding to a specific site on the outer face of the inner mitochondrial membrane with an affinity constant of 1 μM for GDP at pH 7[9]. The nature of the binding site was revealed by photoaffinity labelling with radioactive 8-azido ATP[10]; binding occurred to a 32 000 mol. wt protein and could be prevented by allowing GDP to compete with the nucleotide prior to photoreaction. This 32 000 uncoupling protein has been isolated and purified using techniques similar to those for the adenine nucleotide translocator; hydrodynamic and cross-linking studies indicate that the protein functions as a dimer[11].

The uncoupling protein is inducible

The uncoupling protein may be quantified by its ability to bind purine nucleotide[9], by radio-immunoassay

using antibodies raised against the purified protein[12] and, less accurately, by inspection of the polyacrylamide gel pattern of the membrane proteins[13]. The amount of the protein in the membrane relates to the thermogenic state of the animal (reviewed in Ref. 5), being high at birth, falling during development at thermoneutral temperature and rising again when the animal is cold-adapted. In addition, over-feeding increases the uncoupling protein relative to controls maintained at the same temperature on a normal diet. The genetically obese (*ob/ob*) mouse has a defective NST, and a somewhat decreased content of uncoupling protein, while the protein appears to be depressed also during pregnancy and lactation (conditions under which the animal needs to conserve metabolic energy). Thus in every case there appears to be a correlation between the thermogenic capacity of the tissue and the amount of the uncoupling protein in the mitochondrial inner membrane.

The hormonal control of the induction of the uncoupling protein has been a matter of some controversy. However, recently, Mory et al.[14] have shown that they can mimick cold adaptation in rats by implanting a mini-osmotic pump to give a continuously elevated concentration of circulating noradrenaline. The uncoupling protein is coded by a nuclear gene, and cell-free synthesis of the protein has been achieved using mRNA from brown fat in a reticulocyte lysate[15].

The acute regulation of the uncoupling protein

The acute stimulation of respiration by noradrenaline can be seen with isolated brown adipocytes, which increase their respiration rate by an order of magnitude within a few minutes of the addition of noradrenaline. Prior to noradrenaline addition the mitochondria within the cells are coupled, since the basal cell respiration rate can be increased by addition of protonophores[16]. This implies that the uncoupling protein is inhibited under these non-thermogenic conditions. Since noradrenaline acts at the plasma membrane, some form of cytosolic messenger must exist to activate the uncoupling protein in synchrony with the arrival of substrate from lipolysis. Although changes in purine nucleotide concentration can mimick this transition in isolated mitochondria, there is no evidence for any change in cytosolic purine nucleotides which could cause, rather than merely be the effect, of mitochondrial uncoupling.

The simplest messenger would be a normal intermediate of the lipolytic sequence, since its concentration would rise at the initiation of lipolysis, and fall when the thermogenic phase is terminated. At various times, free fatty acids[6] and acyl-CoA[17] have been proposed for this role. Although fatty acids are nonspecific uncouplers of a variety of mitochondria, there are compelling reasons for believing that the fatty acids released by lipolysis is brown fat activate the uncoupling protein in a highly specific way. First, brown fat mitochondria from cold-adapted animals can be uncoupled by sub-micromolar concentrations of free fatty acids[18]. Second, brown fat mitochondria from warm-adapted animals, which have a greatly decreased complement of uncoupling protein, are an order of magnitude less sensitive to fatty acid uncoupling, as are mitochondria from liver[19]. Third, the ability of fatty acids to induce proton permeability in non-respiring mitochondria can be regulated by purine nucleotides, indicating that the fatty acids act at a locus which is within the influence of the nucleotide binding site, i.e. on the uncoupling protein[20]. The alternative proposal that the CoA esters are the actual messenger[17], is attractive because the purine rings of CoA and purine nucleotides show structural homology, but fails to show either the sensitivity or dependence on the presence of the uncoupling protein shown by the free fatty acid[5,19].

Fatty acids act by altering the current-voltage relationship of the uncoupling protein[20]. In the presence of the millimolar purine nucleotide concentrations expected within the cell, the mitochondria maintain a low proton conductance until $\Delta\mu H^+$ rises above 220 mV, after which the conductance increases rapidly. This 'non-ohmic' conductance is also seen in liver mitochondria[21]. Addition of low concentrations of fatty acids to the brown fat mitochondria lowers by some 50 mV the 'break-point' potential at which the conductance increases, and thus prevents $\Delta\mu H^+$ from achieving a level sufficient for respiratory control[20].

Chloride permeability

Brown fat mitochondria have a high electrogenic permeability to halide anions such as chloride which can be monitored by the rate of chloride-limited swelling in KCl in the presence of valinomycin[3] or by Cl^-/Cl^- exchange[22]. Swelling in this medium, as well as the proton-limited swelling in K-acetate plus valinomycin[7] are inhibited by GDP at concentrations which correlate with the nucleotide binding to the uncoupling protein[23] indicating that the protein provides the pathway for halide permeation. There are however a number of complications with halide permeation which still remain to be resolved. First, fatty acids are without effect on chloride conductance, in contrast to their modulatory action on proton conductance[8]. Second, the conditions required for Cl^- to compete with protons for transport are the subject of some debate[8,20,22,24]. Resolution of these problems may well provide clues to the molecular mechanism of this unusual transport protein.

Future trends

Despite the advances which have been made in the last few years in understanding the regulation of the uncoupling protein, there is virtually no information on its molecular mechanism – the nature of the ion-conducting pathway, the way in which the purine nucleotides and fatty acids regulate the conductance, etc. It is also important to establish both the means by which a chronically elevated noradrenaline concentration activates the expression of the protein, and the mechanism by which is is inserted into and removed from the inner membrane. Finally, the extent to which the weight-regulating function of the tissue, which has been shown for other animals, can be extrapolated to man is a burning and controversial issue which remains to be resolved.

References

1 Girardier, L. and Stock, M. J. (eds) (1983) *Mammalian Thermogenesis,* Chapman and Hall

2 Rothwell, N. J. and Stock, M. J. (1979) *Nature* 281, 31–35

3 Foster, D. O. and Frydman, M. L. (1978) *Can. J. Physiol. Pharmacol.* 56, 110–122

4 Arch, J. R. S., Ainsworth, A. T., Cawthorne, M. A., Piercy, V., Sennitt, M. V., Thody, V. E., Wilson, C. and Wilson, S. (1984) *Nature* 309, 163–165

5 Nicholls, D. G. and Locke, R. M. (1984) *Physiol. Rev.* 64, 1–64

6 Rafael, J., Ludolph, H. J. and Hohorst, H. J. (1969) *Hoppe-Seyler's Z. Physiol. Chem.* 350, 1121–1131

7 Nicholls, D. G. (1974) *Eur. J. Biochem.* 49, 573–583

8 Nicholls, D. G. and Lindberg, O. (1973) *Eur. J. Biochem.* 37, 523–530

9 Nicholls, D. G. (1976) *Eur. J. Biochem.* 62, 223–228

10 Heaton, G. M., Wagenvoord, R. J., Kemp, A. and Nicholls, D. G. (1978) *Eur. J. Biochem.* 82, 515–521

11 Lin, C. S. and Klingenberg, M. (1982) *Biochem.* 21, 2950–2956

12 Cannon, B., Hedin, A. and Nedergaard, J. (1982) *FEBS Lett.* 150, 129–132

13 Ricquier, D. and Kader, J. C. (1976) *Biochim. Biophys. Res. Commun.* 106, 582–589

14 Mory, G., Bouillaud, F., Combes-George, M. and Ricquier, D. (1984) *FEBS Lett.* 166, 393–396

15 Ricquier, D., Thibault, J., Bouillaud, F. and Kuster, Y. (1983) *J. Biol. Chem.* 258, 6675–6677

16 Prusiner, S. B., Cannon, B., Ching, T. M. and Lindberg, O. (1968) *Eur. J. Biochem.* 7, 51–57

17 Cannon, B., Sundin, U. and Romert, L. (1977) *FEBS Lett.* 74, 43–46

18 Heaton, G. M. and Nicholls, D. G. (1976) *Eur. J. Biochem.* 67, 511–517

19 Locke, R. M., Rial, E. and Nicholls, D. G. (1982) *Eur. J. Biochem.* 129, 381–387

20 Rial, E., Poustie, A. and Nicholls, D. G. (1983) *Eur. J. Biochem.* 137, 197–203

21 Nicholls, D. G. (1974) *Eur. J. Biochem.* 50, 305–315

22 Nicholls, D. G. (1974) *Eur. J. Biochem.* 49, 585–593

23 Rial, E. and Nicholls, D. G. (1983) *FEBS Lett.* 161, 284–288

24 Kopecky, J., Guerrieri, F., Jezek, P., Drahota, Z. and Houstek, J. (1984) *FEBS Lett.* 170, 186–190

David G. Nicholls and Eduardo Rial are at the Dept of Psychiatry, Ninewells Medical School, University of Dundee, Dundee DD1 9SY, UK.

Does brown adipose tissue have a metabolic role in the rat?

Gregory J. Cooney and Eric A. Newsholme

Brown adipose tissue is thought to be an important organ for thermogenesis in cold acclimation and dietary stress in mice and rats. However, some of the metabolic characteristics of the tissue suggest that it may play a much wider role in homeostatis than simply as a thermogenic tissue.

Brown adipose tissue (BAT) consists of small cells which contain many mitochondria and many lipid droplets, in contrast to white adipose tissue which contains large cells with few mitochondria and a single lipid droplet. BAT was presumably called adipose tissue because of its high lipid content, but as well as being structurally distinct it is metabolically and functionally different from white adipose tissue.

There is no doubt BAT is involved in heat production, particularly in hibernating animals during arousal and in very young animals which do not shiver. The biochemical mechanism for the formation of heat is now well established[1]. As with mitochondria from other tissues the oxidation of fuels leads to the generation of a proton-motive force, but BAT mitochondria possess a specific protein in the inner membrane that transfers protons from outside to inside the inner mitochondrial membrane without concomitant ATP formation. The proton-carrier activity of this protein can be regulated by adenine nucleotides and fatty acids of specific chain-length[2]. In contrast to the detailed and systematic studies into the mechanism of thermogenesis in BAT mitochondria[3], the metabolic work with this tissue has involved studies mainly on lipogenesis. Furthermore, the metabolic studies have been largely restricted to the physiological conditions of cold acclimation or diet-induced thermogenesis[4–6]. In this article some questions concerning the metabolic role of this tissue are posed and speculative or preliminary answers provided. We hope that this will provide a stimulus for further work on BAT in situations when thermogenesis is not the prime concern of the animal.

Can the oxidative capacity of BAT be assessed biochemically?

It is generally accepted that BAT can utilize oxygen at a high rate. This view is based largely on physiological measurements: blood-flow is measured by the accumulation of radiolabelled microspheres in the tissue after they are injected into the arterial circulation, and the oxygen consumption is determined by arterio–venous concentration differences across the interscapular BAT. However, the usual physiological means of obtaining blood samples – via indwelling catheters in vessels immediately supplying and draining BAT – have not been employed. The arterial oxygen content is measured at a site removed from BAT and venous oxygen content in a sample taken after the Sulzers vein is severed and blood allowed to accumulate in the interscapular space[7,8]. From these measurements a rate of utilization of oxygen is obtained. It has been shown that in the cold-acclimated rat stimulated with a maximum dose of noradrenaline, 60% of the *increased* oxygen consumption is due to brown adipose tissue[7]. Such studies are, how-

Table I. Calculated fluxes through the Krebs cycle in brown adipose tissue from rats and mice

Animal	Rate of O_2 uptake *in vivo* (μmol/min/g fresh weight)	Calculated Krebs cycle flux (μmol/min/g fresh weight)	
		From O_2 uptake	From oxoglutarate dehydrogenase activity
Cold-acclimated rat	66.9	22.3	29.7
Lean (*ob/+*) mouse	44.9	16.1	24.9

Rates of *in vivo* oxygen uptake were taken from data in Refs 7 and 8. Flux through the Krebs cycle was calculated assuming that during oxidation of palmitate 2.875 molecules of oxygen are consumed for each turn of the cycle and that for a rise in temperature of 10°C the activity of oxoglutarate dehydrogenase would increase by a factor of 2.0.

ever, not easy and they are restricted to sites of BAT where it is possible to measure arterio–venous differences. Can such physiological findings be confirmed biochemically and is there a biochemically easier means of measuring the maximum rate of oxygen consumption (and therefore the maximum capacity of thermogenesis in this tissue)?

One of the problems for biochemical studies is that a satisfactory *in vitro* tissue preparation has not been established. Some preparations of individual cells of BAT have been calculated to have a similar oxygen consumption to the *in vivo* tissue[9], but the same reviewers point out that there is great variability between preparations of brown adipocytes.

In some instances quantitative information about the maximum capacity of metabolic pathways can be obtained from measurement of the maximum *in vitro* catalytic activities of certain key enzymes in these pathways. In muscle the maximal activity of the enzyme oxoglutarate dehydrogenase has been shown to provide a quantitative index of the maximum flux throughout the Krebs cycle[10,11]. Could this measurement be used also for BAT? This would also provide an indication of the maximum capacity for thermogenesis, since the Krebs cycle is the final common pathway for fuel oxidation.

The highest rate of oxygen consumption for interscapular BAT was measured by Foster and Frydman in noradrenaline-stimulated, cold-acclimated animals[7]. From these results the rate of the Krebs cycle is calculated to be 22.3 μmol/min per g fresh wt (Table I). The maximum rate of the Krebs cycle predicted from the activity of oxoglutarate dehydrogenase in extracts of BAT from cold-acclimated rats of the same age and weight is 29.7 μmol/min per g fresh wt (Table I). The agreement between the two values is within 25%. A similar level of agreement is found when rates of oxygen consumption of BAT in lean (*Ob/+*) mice[8] is compared to the calculated value (Table I). These results demonstrate that a simple biochemical measurement provides data which are in reasonable agreement with those provided by the considerably more complex physiological experiments. Hence, the activity of this enzyme could be used to indicate the maximal aerobic, and therefore the maximum thermogenic capacity, of BAT in other depots and in biopsy samples of the tissue from animals that are less amenable to physiological study.

Does BAT use fuels other than fatty acids for thermogenesis?

The obvious availability of triglyceride in BAT, the release of fatty acids and glycerol from this tissue during the warming up of hibernating animals, the decrease in triglyceride content of BAT during exposure to the cold, and the hypothesis that the raised intracellular concentration of fatty acids is responsible for initiating thermogenesis (by increasing the activity of the proton-transporting protein in the mitochondrial membrane)[3], have all led to the proposal that triglyceride is the main, if not the only, fuel for oxidation and thermogenesis in this tissue. However, other fuels, such as glucose or amino acids have not been eliminated as substrates to provide energy for thermogenesis by oxidation in BAT. Unfortunately, there are no reported studies on the arterio–venous concentration differences of such fuels across the tissue. Nonetheless, there is considerable indirect evidence that BAT could use glucose, ketone bodies or acetate for thermogenesis[12–14]: the tissue in rat possesses a high glycolytic capacity[12] (though this is apparently not the case in hamster[15]); and the activities of two key glycolytic enzymes, hexokinase and 6-phosphofructokinase, are increased 2-fold by cold acclimation (Table II). Indeed, during cold acclimation BAT possesses the highest activity of hexokinase of any of the major glucose-utilizing tissues of the body[12]. Since high activities of pyruvate dehydrogenase have also been reported for this tissue[5], the possibility must exist that this tissue oxidizes at least some of the pyruvate produced from glycolysis and the energy released is used for thermogenesis.

Is BAT important in the regulation of the blood glucose concentration?

Since BAT has a high capacity for glucose utilization, and since this pathway may be sensitive to insulin, could BAT play a quantitatively important role in the removal of glucose after a carbohydrate load and hence in the control of blood glucose concentration? If it is assumed that interscapular BAT represents approximately 25% of the total BAT in the rat and that the maximum activities of hexokinase in Table II represent the maximal capacity for gly-

colysis, the total tissue *could* utilize 5 and 19 μmol per min of glucose in normal and cold-acclimated animals, respectively. It is known that after feeding, much of the glucose removed by the liver is converted to glycogen at the rate of about 1 μmol per min[16]. Hence BAT could play a quantitatively important role in removal of glucose after a meal. If this is the case, then an impaired ability of this tissue to respond to insulin or a decreased glycolytic capacity could play a role in the impaired glucose tolerance observed in conditions such as obesity or type-II diabetes. This possibility is supported by findings that during cold-acclimation of the rat, which increases the amount of brown adipose tissue and its glycolytic capacity (Table II) the insulin sensitivity *in vivo* is increased[17].

There are several physiological conditions when the rate of lipogenesis in BAT is known to change: it is decreased during starvation[14] and lactation[18] (in comparison to the rate during pregnancy) but is increased during cold acclimation[6]. During these conditions the maximal activities of hexokinase in BAT change in parallel to the changes in rates of lipogenesis (Table II). These findings support the view that BAT has an important metabolic role in the rat in addition to that of thermogenesis.

Is there a metabolic relationship between lipogenesis and thermogenesis in BAT?

The major metabolic characteristics of BAT can be summarized as follows: it has a high capacity for glucose utilization; it has the unique capacity for uncoupling oxidative phosphorylation from electron transport to allow fuels to be oxidized without generation of ATP; it has a high capacity for oxidation of fatty acid; and it has a high capacity for lipogenesis. Are these characteristics metabolically related?

It is at first surprising that the biosynthesis of palmitate from glucose results

Table II. Effect of cold-acclimation, starvation, pregnancy and lactation on the maximal activity of hexokinase in brown adipose tissue of the rat

Condition	Weight of interscepular brown adipose tissue (g)	Hexokinase activity	
		μmol/min/g fresh weight	nmol/min/mg protein
Control	0.21 ± 0.02	6.0 ± 0.4 (8)	72 ± 6
Cold-acclimated	0.40 ± 0.03	12.2 ± 0.7 (8)	104 ± 7
48 h starved	0.11 ± 0.01	4.1 ± 0.5 (8)	34 ± 3
Pregnant	0.35 ± 0.03	8.7 ± 1.1 (4)	53 ± 10
Lactating	0.16 ± 0.02	2.3 ± 0.4 (5)	23 ± 4

Hexokinase activity was measured by a radiochemical method described in Ref. 12. Results are presented as means ± SEM and the number of animals is given in parenthesis.

in the formation of ATP. Lipogenesis generates NADH which, when oxidized by the electron transfer chain results in the conversion of ADP to ATP: for each molecule of palmitate synthesized from glucose, a net production of five molecules of ATP can result[19]. Consequently, high rates of lipogenesis might be limited by the accumulation of ATP. If BAT is important in the removal of glucose from the bloodstream for conversion to and storage as triglyceride, it is tempting to speculate that the physiological uncoupling process, which appears to be unique to this tissue, is necessary to permit such high rates of lipogenesis. Other tissues known to synthesize triglyceride from glucose may be able to utilize ATP in other ways; in white adipose tissue the rate of lipogenesis is much lower than that in BAT so that sufficient ATP utilization may occur via substrate ('futile') cycling especially the triglyceride/fatty acid cycle[20]. In other tissues that have a more varied metabolism, such as liver and mammary gland, the extra ATP generated during lipogenesis could be used by this metabolism. The heat formation in BAT due to mitochondrial uncoupling during lipogenesis might have been important in maintenance of body temperature in homoiothermic animals when the environmental temperature fell below the thermoneutral. The advantage of the 'addition' of the complete oxidative system (β-oxidation and the Krebs cycle with the corresponding electron transfer process) to this uncoupling system would be the potential for much higher rates of thermogenesis and therefore a greater ability to maintain the body temperature. This may have had considerable survival value. Of course the complete oxidative system can produce heat without concomitant lipogenesis but there are many conditions in which lipogenesis and thermogenesis are increased in parallel, suggesting an evolutionary link.

References

1 Nicholls, D. G. (1979) *Biochim. Biophys. Acta* 549, 1–29
2 Rial, E., Poustie, A. and Nicholls, D. G. (1983) *Eur. J. Biochem.* 137, 197–203
3 Nicholls, D. G. (1983) *Biosci. Rep.* 3, 431–441
4 Trayhurn, P. (1979) *FEBS Lett.* 104, 13–16
5 McCormack, J. G. and Denton, R. M. (1977) *Biochem. J.* 166, 627–630
6 Trayhurn, P. (1981) *Biochim. Biophys. Acta* 664, 549–560
7 Foster, D. O. and Frydman M. L. (1978) *Can. J. Physiol. Pharmacol.* 56, 110–122
8 Thurlby, P. L. and Trayhurn, P. (1980) *Pflugers. Arch.* 385, 193–201
9 Nedergaard, J. and Lindberg, O. (1982) *Int. Rev. Cytol.* 74, 187–286
10 Read, G., Crabtree, B. and Smith, G. H. (1977) *Biochem, J.* 164, 349–355
11 Cooney, G. J., Taegtmeyer, H. and Newsholme, E. A. (1981) *Biochem. J.* 200, 701–703
12 Cooney, G. J. and Newsholme, E. A. (1982) *FEBS Lett.* 148, 198–200

13 Agius, L. and Williamson, D. H. (1981) *Biochim. Biophys. Acta* 666, 127–132
14 Sugden, M. C., Watts, D. I. and Marshall, C. E. (1981) *Biosci. Rep.* 1, 469–476
15 Williamson, J. R., Pusiner, S., Olson, H. S. and Fukami, H. (1970) *Lipids* 5, 1–14
16 Hems, D. A., Whitton, P. A. and Taylor, E. A. (1972) *Biochem. J.* 129, 529–538
17 Baker, D. G. and Sellers, E. A. (1953) *Annu. J. Physiol.* 174, 459–461
18 Agius, L. and Williamson, D. H. (1980) *Biochem. J.* 190, 477–480
19 Flatt, J. P. (1970) *J. Lip. Res.* 11, 131–143
20 Brooks, B. S., Arch, J. R. S. and Newsholme, E. A. (1983) *Biosci. Rep.* 3, 263–267

Gregory J. Cooney and Eric A. Newsholme are at the Department of Biochemistry, University of Oxford, South Parks Road, Oxford OX1 3QU, UK.

The role of peroxisomes in lipid metabolism

Colin Masters and Denis Crane

Recent studies of lipid turnover in living mammals support the concept that peroxisomes have a significant physiological role in the metabolism of neutral lipids. These findings also raise intriguing questions about the influence of peroxisomes on phospholipid catabolism, the biosynthesis of complex lipids, and inter-tissue and inter-compartmental communication.

An earlier review discussed the broad scope of peroxisomal metabolism in mammalian tissues[1], and referred briefly to the involvement of peroxisomes in lipid metabolism. This latter topic has since been further investigated both *in vitro* and *in vivo*, and a far more complete picture of peroxisomal oxidation and its regulatory significance is now available[2-5].

In broad terms, peroxisomes are respiratory organelles which can catabolize a number of common substrates via the component flavin oxidases and catalase (Fig. 1)[5]. These substrates include hydroxy acids, amino acids, urates, alcohols and fatty acids, and their oxidation in this organelle may contribute significantly to total cellular respiration.

Despite the increased knowledge of the influence of peroxisomes on lipid metabolism[6-11] several significant questions remain unanswered. Most previous studies, for example, used isolated tissue preparations, and hence provided little insight into the communication and interaction between tissues which may be significant in lipid metabolism in the whole animal. This review focusses on experiments which perturb peroxisomes in live animals. These experiments[12-15] are based on the simultaneous assay of two isotopes which have been incorporated into specific classes of lipids. This allows both degradation and synthesis of the individual lipid fractions to be studied[16,17] and indicates that a number

of significant alterations in turnover characteristics of tissue lipids take place in response to treatment with compounds such as clofibrate and glycolate (Table I).

Effects of peroxisomal agents on lipid metabolism

Table I shows similarities associated with the common involvement of the perturbing agents with the peroxisomal pathway of lipid oxidation (see Fig. 1). The actions of all the agents can be viewed in terms of an effect on the overall flux through the pathways indicated; clofibrate through induction of

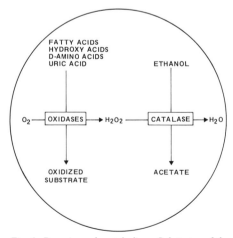

Fig. 1. Peroxisomal metabolism. Substrates of the peroxisomal oxidases may be metabolized with the production of hydrogen peroxide. Hydrogen peroxide in turn may be catalytically decomposed, with or without the attendant oxidation of substrates such as ethanol.

Table I. Turnover response of lipid fractions in animal tissues following treatment with peroxisomal agents

Treatment	Lipid fraction	Liver	Kidney	Heart	Adipose tissue	Carcass
Clofibrate	TL	0	0	0	↑	↑
	TG	↑	↑	↑	↑	↑
	NL	↑	↑	↑	↑	↑
	TP	0	0	0	0	0
	PE	0	↓	0	0	0
	PC	↑	0	0	0	0
	PS & I	↑	0	0	0	0
Glycolate	TL	↑	0	0	0	↑
	TG	↑	0	0	↑	↑
	NL	↑	↑	↓	↑	↑
	TP	↑	0	↓	0	↓
	PE	↑	0	↓	0	0
	PC	↑	0	↓	0	↓
	PS & I	↑	0	0	0	0
Ethanol	TL	↑	0	↓	↑	0
	TG	↑	0	0	↑	0
	NL	↑	0	↓	↑	0
	TP	↑	0	0	0	0
	PE	0	0	0	0	0
	PC	↑	0	0	0	0
	PS & I	↑	0	0	0	0
Aminotriazole	TL	0	0	0	↑	↑
	TG	↑	0	0	↑	0
	NL	0	0	0	↑	0
	TP	↑	0	↓	↑	0
	PE	0	0	↓	0	0
	PC	↑	0	0	0	0
	PS & I	0	↓	↓	0	↑

↑ = significant increase in turnover; ↓ = significant decrease in turnover; 0 = no change; TL = total lipid; TG = triacylglycerol; TP = total phospholipid; PE = phosphatidyl ethanolamine; PC = phosphatidyl choline; PS & I = phosphatidyl serine and inositol; NL = neutral lipid. For further experimental details see Refs 13–15.

the peroxisomal pathways of β-oxidation by means of an increase in oxidase and catalase[13]; glycolate and ethanol through activation of this pathway, albeit at different loci[14,15]; and aminotriazole through inhibition of the pathway at the catalase step[12,18].

It may first be noted that the clofibrate treatment is associated with an increased metabolic flux in most tissues, but with a preference to degradation and mobilization of acyl glycerols (Table I)[13]. It may also be noted that the glycolate and ethanol treatments caused significant and widespread changes in lipid flux (Table I)[14,15]. All these treatments provide a strong indication of the significant variability of peroxisomal metabolism, and the cell's ability to increase activities to cope with abnormal substrate concentrations. Furthermore, this 'inducibility' may be an important aspect of the metabolism of peroxisomes and the metabolic relationships between peroxisomes, mitochondria and other subcellular compartments[5].

At the same time, the results with aminotriazole (which indicate its significant influence on lipid turnover) suggest that peroxisomes have an appreciable role in lipid metabolism under normal conditions *in vivo* (Table I). In this case, inhibition of the peroxisomal pathway of oxidation at the catalase step, led to widespread variation in the turnover characteristics of tissue lipids and, in particular, decreased the oxidation of fatty acids[12].

Peroxisomal versus mitochondrial oxidation

The relative contribution of peroxisomes and other organelles to lipid metabolism is a contentious question when viewed only from the perspective of *in vitro* results[10,19]. While some studies *in vitro* indicate that peroxisomal oxidation of lipids represents a relatively small proportion of total lipid oxidation, and may be subservient to the process occurring in mitochondria under normal steady state conditions[10,20], other data support the substantial nature of the peroxisomal contribution[6,8,9]. However, the extensive nature of the tissue lipid changes seen in these experiments *in vivo* do provide substantial support for an important contributory and regulatory role of peroxisomes in the overall balance of lipid metabolism. Indeed the results indicate that, under certain conditions, peroxisomal oxidation may become more significant than mitochondrial oxidation in some tissues. These data also relate to the widely accepted suggestion that the major physiological role of peroxisomal β-oxidation be regarded as a mechanism for eliminating fatty acids that are poorly oxidized by mitochondria (e.g. rare long chain and trans fatty acids[8]). While peroxisomes may well be specially suitable for this type of process in many cells and tissues, these results emphasize that these organelles also play a significant role in the oxidation of the more common fatty acid substrates.

A further point of interest is that all of the experimental treatments were associated with increased turnover of the major phospholipid classes. The fatty acids released by this process apparently become available for oxidation and energy production under these conditions.

The relationship between peroxisomes and phospholipid metabolism is reinforced by Parthasarathy *et al.*[21] who showed that drugs induce peroxisomal proliferation (e.g. clofibrate) also inhibit phospholipid synthesis. Again, it has also been noted that peroxisomes play a significant role in the degradation of phospholipid components in yeasts[22], and that phospholipid degradation is often an indication of transmembrane control of cellular functions[23].

Communication between metabolic compartments

The *in vivo* data also indicate that these peroxisomal agents often induce a greater alteration in turnover in tissues which are not especially rich in peroxisomes. For example, the changes in the double isotope ratios are often greater in adipose and cardiac tissue than in liver and kidney. Results such as these emphasize that intertissue effects may assume a major role in considerations of peroxisomal metabolism.

How is tissue–tissue communication achieved in such cases? One possibility is the existence of a chemical messenger related to peroxisomal metabolism. It is observed, for example, that turnover in extra-hepatic lipid is often significantly higher in animals treated with aminotriazole than in normal animals[12]. It may be that peroxisomal metabolism of fatty acids restrains lipid turnover in peripheral tissues, and that inactivation of the peroxisomal pathway at the catalase step tends to diminish this restraining influence. Given the known substrate specificity of the separate organellar β-oxidation sequences (preference of peroxisomes for long chain fatty acid substrates and incomplete oxidation; mitochondrial preference for medium chain fatty acids and complete oxidation to two carbon units) the data suggest that fatty acids of medium chain length may moderate intercompartmental communication.

It is known that long chain fatty acids control lipid metabolism and their role as characteristic end products provides appropriate feed-back or feed-forward regulation in relation to lipid synthesis and degradation[24]. In a similar manner, fatty acids of medium chain length may be regarded as characteristic products of peroxisomal metabolism, acting in the translation of peroxisomal influences on lipid metabolism. Recent reports indicate that the chain length of fatty acids is a major discriminating factor in such regulation. For example, citrate efflux from mitochondria represents one prime control point in lipid biosynthesis which is differentially affected in this manner. Whereas citrate transport is inhibited strongly by fatty acyl CoA esters with chain lengths of 14–18 carbons, fatty acyl CoA esters of medium chain length (C8-12) invoke a markedly different response, being comparatively ineffective in this regard[25]. Similarly, not only the rate of synthesis of complex lipids, but also the direction of this synthesis has been reported to be sensitive to the chain length of fatty acids[26,27].

If medium chain length fatty acids are peroxisomal messengers, it follows that communication between tissues would be facilitated by the predominant occurrence of peroxisomes in such prime sites of lipid oxidation as liver and kidney. The potential for synergistic regulation by peroxisomes and mitochondria through chemical messengers becomes clearer by considering the following

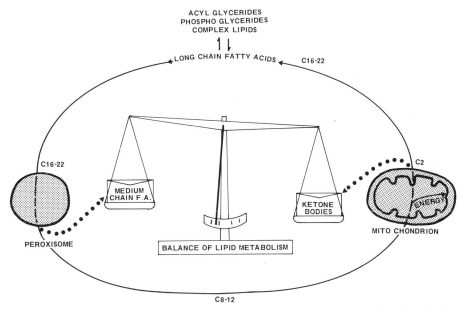

Fig. 2. Peroxisomal and mitochondrial oxidation of fatty acids in relation to overall lipid metabolism. Long chain fatty acids (C16 and longer), derived from lipolysis of complex lipids, may undergo initial oxidation in peroxisomes to fatty acids of medium chain length (C8-12). These medium chain fatty acids are then oxidized to completion in the mitochondria, with the production of two-carbon units, which may, in turn, be converted to ketone bodies. The balance of lipid metabolism in the individual tissues of the whole animal, and the distinctive role of the peroxisomes and mitochondria, may be effected through the relative concentration of their end products, namely fatty acids and ketone bodies.

facts. (1) The substrate specificities and extent of cycling of fatty acids differs markedly between these two oxidative compartments. (2) As a result medium chain fatty acids and ketone bodies emerge as distinctive end products of fatty acid oxidation in these compartments (Fig. 2). (3) Ketone bodies act as a mitochondrial messenger which plays a significant role in lipolysis and the overall balance of lipid metabolism in the animal body[28]. Utilizing both signals feedback regulation could extend beyond fatty acid degradation and energy production in the tissue of location, and into communication between different compartments and tissues, and the relative direction and emphasis of lipid turnover in all major tissues of the organism. This would provide a far more subtle and appropriate regulation of whole body metabolism than could be provided by either organelle singly. Recent reports of a linear correlation between peroxisomal and mitochondrial oxidation in rat liver support the concept of simultaneous, sequential control as illustrated in Fig. 2[29]; The emerging emphasis on the role of peroxisomes in the biosynthesis of complex lipids also supports the overall relationships in this figure[30].

Acknowledgements

The authors wish to acknowledge the contributions of Roger Holmes to this series of investigations, and the financial assistance of the Australian Research Grants Scheme.

References

1 Masters, C. J. and Holmes, R. S. (1979) *Trends Biochem. Sci.* 4, 233–236
2 Tolbert, N. E. (1981) *Annu. Rev. Biochem.* 50, 133–157
3 De Duve, C. (1982) *Ann. N.Y. Acad. Sci.* 386, 1–4
4 Masters, C. J. (1982) *Ann. N.Y. Acad. Sci.* 386, 301–313
5 Osumi, T. and Hashimoto, T. (1984) *Trends Biochem. Sci.* 103, 317–319
6 Kondrup, J. and Lazarow, P. B. (1982) *Ann. N.Y. Acad. Sci.* 386, 404–405
7 Mannaerts, G. P. and Debeer, L. J. (1982) *Ann. N.Y. Acad. Sci.* 386, 30–39
8 Osmundsen, H. (1982) *Ann. N.Y. Acad. Sci.* 386, 13–27
9 Cannon, B., Alexson, S. and Nedergaard, J. (1982) *Ann. N.Y. Acad. Sci.* 386, 40–61
10 Mannaerts, G. P., Debeer, L. J., Thomas, J. and de Schepper, P. J. (1979) *J. Biol. Chem.* 254, 4585–4595
11 Thurman, R. G. and McKenna, W. (1974) *Hoppe-Seyler's Z. Physiol. Chem.* 355, 336–340
12 Crane, D. I. and Masters, C. J. (1984) *Arch. Biochem. Biophys.* 229, 104–111
13 Crane, D. I., Holmes, R. S. and Masters, C. J. (1980) *Biochem. Biophys. Res. Commun.* 93, 258–263
14 Crane, D. I., Holmes, R. S. and Masters, C. J. (1980) *Biochem. Int.* 1, 133–138
15 Crane, D. I., Holmes, R. S. and Masters, C. J. (1981) *Int. J. Biochem.* 13, 395–399
16 Lee, T. C. and Snyder, F. (1973) *Biochim. Biophys. Acta* 291, 71–82
17 Arias, I. M., Doyle, D. and Schimke, R. T. (1969) *J. Biol. Chem.* 244, 3303–3315
18 Price, V. E., Sterling, W. R., Tarantola, V. A., Hartley, R. W. Jr and Rechcigl, M. Jr (1962) *J. Biol. Chem.* 237, 3468–3475
19 Lazarow, R. P. (1978) *J. Biol. Chem.* 253, 1522–1528
20 Foerster, E. C., Fahrenkemper, T., Rabe, U., Graf, P. and Sies, H. (1981) *Biochem. J.* 196, 705–712
21 Parthasarathy, S., Kritchevsky, D. and Baumann, W. J. (1982) *Proc. Natl Acad. Sci. USA* 79, 6890–6893
22 Zwart, K. and Harder, W. (1982) *Ann. N.Y. Acad. Sci.* 386, 414–416
23 Nishizuka, Y. (1983) *Trends Biochem. Sci.* 8, 13–16
24 Block, K. and Vance, D. E. (1977) *Annu. Rev. Biochem.* 46, 263–298
25 Evans, C. T., Scraff, A. H. and Ratledge, C. (1983) *Eur. J. Biochem.* 132, 617–622
26 Mayorek, N. and Bar-Tana, J. (1983) *J. Biol. Chem.* 258, 6789–6792
27 Pelech, S. L., Pritchard, P. H., Brindley, D. N. and Vance, D. E. (1983) *J. Biol. Chem.* 258, 6782–6788
28 Stryer, L. (1981) in *Biochemistry*, pp. 395, W. H. Freeman and Co.
29 Brady, P. S. and Hoppel, C. L. (1983) *Biochem. J.* 212, 891–894
30 Borst, P. (1983) *Trends Biochem. Sci.* 8, 269–272

Colin Masters and Denis Crane are at the School of Science, Griffith University, Nathan, Brisbane, Q.4111, Australia.

Metabolism and functions of glutathione

Alton Meister

The reactions of the γ-glutamyl cycle account for the synthesis of glutathione and much of its utilization, which involves membrane transport of glutathione and γ-glutamyl amino acids, and inter-organ translocation of glutathione. Glutathione functions in an impressive number and variety of cellular phenomena.

Glutathione (L-γ-glutamyl-L-cysteinyl-glycine; GSH) was first detected in yeast in 1888, and its structure proved by synthesis in 1935. It is probably the most abundant natural low molecular weight thiol. It is found in virtually all cells (except perhaps certain bacteria) often in millimolar concentrations, and at much lower concentrations in extracellular fluids such as blood plasma. Many roles have been ascribed to this ubiquitous tripeptide, and recent studies have begun to delineate its metabolism and physiological function[1–5]. This article attempts to summarize the current status of our knowledge; (Fig. 1).

GSH as an intracellular reductant

It has long been known that GSH participates in transhydrogenation reactions. Thiol–disulfide transhydrogenations involving GSH were first observed with homocysteine and cysteine and later with compounds such as CoA and proteins. Mixed disulfides between GSH and other thiols, including proteins, have also been observed. GSH functions to form or maintain protein thiol groups which may be required for catalysis, and involved in protein assembly and degradation. It also provides reducing capacity for other reactions, e.g. formation of deoxyribonucleotides by ribonucleotide reductase; reduced glutaredoxin, formed by reaction with glutaredoxin with GSH, interacts with ribonucleoside diphosphate to form deoxyribonucleoside diphosphate and glutaredoxin[6].

GSH protects proteins and cell membranes against peroxides and free radicals and GSH peroxidase catalyses the reaction of GSH with H_2O_2 and organic peroxides to yield glutathione disulfide (GSSG). Reduction of GSSG to GSH is catalysed by the widely distributed enzyme GSH reductase, which uses NADPH. Normally, the intracellular concentration of GSH far exceeds that of GSSG. In the erythrocyte, oxidation of glucose-6-phosphate and 6-phosphogluconate provides NADPH. In the diseases characterized by glucose-6-phosphate dehydrogenase deficiency, inefficient reduction of GSSG is associated with the denaturation of hemoglobin and the destruction of erythrocyte membranes.

Formation of S-substituted GSH derivatives

The discovery, in 1879, that giving bromobenzene or chlorobenzene to dogs leads to urinary excretion of mercapturic acids (*N*-acetylated *S*-substituted cysteine derivatives) began a century of investigation which ultimately showed that many 'foreign' compounds could react with GSH. This process, often mediated by enzymes (GSH S-transferases), leads to the formation of *S*-substituted GSH derivatives[2]. The γ-glutamyl and glycine moieties of these derivatives are removed and the resulting cysteine derivatives are acetylated to form mercapturic acids. Removal of the γ-glutamyl moiety is facilitated by γ-glutamyl amino acid formation (see below). GSH derivatives are also formed in endogenous metabolism. Thus, formation of leukotriene D, a 'slow reacting substance' of anaphylaxis, involves the addition of GSH to leukotriene A, an epoxide derived from arachidonic acid. Removal of the glutamyl moiety of the adduct, leukotriene C, yields leukotriene D (Ref. 7). Similar reactions occur in the metabolism of steroids and prostaglandins. 'Foreign' compounds metabolized by this pathway are usually excreted in the urine or feces as the corresponding N-acetyl-S-substituted cysteines. The exact pathways taken by endogeneous compounds metabolized in this way are not yet known: some such GSH derivatives may have important physiological functions. Thus, 5-S-gluta-thione-DOPA, formed in melanocytes, is an intermediate in the incorporation of cysteine sulfur into melanin pigments[8]

Coenzymatic functions

GSH serves as a coenzyme for several enzymes including glyoxylase, maleyl-acetoacetate isomerase, formaldehyde dehydrogenase, and DDT dehydrochlorinase; GSH seems also to function in the de-iodination of thyroxine.

Metabolism of glutathione; the γ-glutamyl cycle

The synthesis and degradation of GSH take place by reactions of the γ-glutamyl cycle[4,5]. Most of the studies on the cycle, formulated about 10 years ago, have been done on mammals, but there is increasing evidence that the cycle also functions in other organisms including insects, bacteria, phytoplanktons, and *Hydra*. There is now

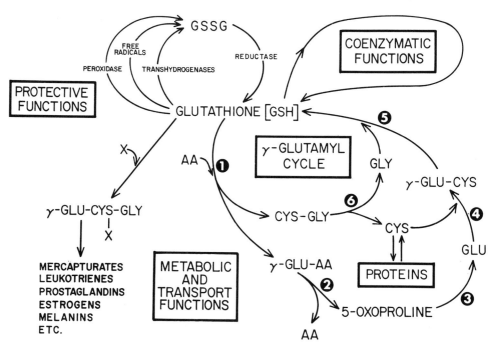

Fig. 1. Overall scheme of GSH metabolism and function. Enzymes: (1) γ-glutamyl transpeptidase; (2) γ-glutamyl cyclotransferase; (3) 5-oxoprolinase; ATP; (4) γ-glutamylcysteine synthetase; ATP; (5) GSH synthetase; ATP; (6) dipeptidase; AA, amino acids. X, compounds that react with GSH to yield adducts involved in the formation of mercapturic acids, leukotrienes, and melanin and in the metabolism of estrogens, prostaglandins and other compounds.

substantial evidence that the cycle functions *in vivo* and that it is one of the systems that mediates amino acid transport. Since the cycle involves GSH synthesis, its functions are closely connected with the other roles of GSH.

GSH is synthesized by successive actions of γ-glutamylcysteine and GSH synthetases (Fig. 1). Utilization of GSH is initiated by γ-glutamyl transpeptidase, a membrane-bound enzyme that catalyses the transfer of the γ-glutamyl moiety to amino acid acceptors to form γ-glutamyl amino acids. According to the cycle hypothesis, γ-glutamyl amino acids, formed in close association with the cell membrane, are translocated into the cell; thus, the γ-glutamyl group serves as carrier for the transported amino acid. The transport of such a dipeptide is perhaps analogous to that of other dipeptides which are transported across cell membranes[9]. Kidney, and probably other cells have a separate transport system for γ-glutamyl amino acids that is not shared by free amino acids[10]. The intracellular enzyme γ-glutamyl cyclotransferase catalyses conversion of γ-glutamyl amino acids to 5-oxoproline (pyroglutamate) and amino acids. 5-Oxoproline is converted by 5-oxoprolinase to glutamate in a reaction coupled to cleavage of ATP. Cysteinylglycine, formed in the transpeptidation reaction, is split by dipeptidase to cysteine and glycine. The research that has been stimulated by the cycle hypothesis has led to many new findings about GSH metabolism, to modifications and elaborations of the original concept, and to major revisions in our understanding of GSH metabolism[4,5].

γ-Glutamyl transpeptidase

γ-Glutamyl transpeptidase is localized at sites extensively involved in transport, e.g. renal and intestinal brush-borders, epithelia of the ciliary body and choroid plexus; activity is also found in endo-plasmic reticulum and the Golgi apparatus. The enzyme is present in many other locations including, interestingly, certain neurons of the central nervous system[11]. It has also been found in microorganisms, plants, and insects[12]. In the kidney, the enzyme is concentrated on the external surface of proximal tubule cells; it also occurs elsewhere in the kidney.

The transpeptidase catalyses transfer of the γ-glutamyl moiety of GSH; cystine and glutamine are among the most active acceptors. Although the enzyme can catalyse hydrolysis of γ-glutamyl compounds, transpeptidation is a significant function *in vivo*. When catalytic amounts of the enzyme are incubated at pH 7.4 with levels of GSH and amino acids that occur in blood plasma, transpeptidation accounts for at least 50% of the GSH used[13]. The extent of transpeptidation, relative to hydrolysis, may be even higher *in vivo*. Transpeptidation increases as the concentrations of amino acids increase. γ-Glutamyl amino acids have been found in tissues and body fluids. When animals are given moderate doses of amino acids, the amount of GSH in the kidney decreases, an effect prevented by giving transpeptidase inhibitors. Similar findings were made on isolated renal cells suspended in media containing amino acids, and in kidneys perfused with solutions containing amino acids[14].

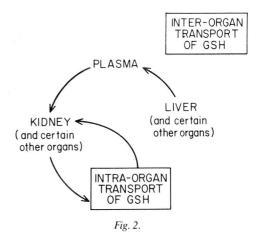

Fig. 2.

Transport of GSH; intra-organ and inter-organ cycles of GSH metabolism (Fig. 2)

Early work suggested that GSH and GSSG were transported out of cells, but it could not be excluded that the results were related to oxidative or other types of cell damage. However, the finding of an enzyme on one side of a membrane, and of its substrate on the other led to the postulate that there is a mechanism for the transport of intracellular GSH to membrane-bound transpeptidase. When transpeptidase is inhibited in vivo by injecting animals with inhibitors, large amounts of GSH appear in the urine[15]; levels as high as 30 mM have been found in the urine of mice treated with such an inhibitor (normal, 2–5 μM). These and other studies indicate that transported renal GSH is normally a substrate of the transpeptidase; such transport to the enzyme undoubtedly also occurs at other anatomical locations, e.g. choroid plexus. Transport of GSH is thus a discrete step in the γ-glutamyl cycle. Transport of GSH has been observed in perfused isolated liver preparations[16] and in human lymphoid cells[17] and fibroblasts grown in culture[18]. Studies on cells that have different amounts of transpeptidase show that transport of GSH is a general phenomenon. In kidney and at other sites with high concentrations of transpeptidase, intracellular GSH is transported to the membrane-bound enzyme, and the products of enzyme action are taken up by the cell. Tissues that have low transpeptidase levels, e.g. liver and muscle, transport GSH to the blood plasma; rat blood plasma contains about 25 μM (85% GSH). Plasma GSH is rapidly converted to GSSG and mixed disulfides[19]. When an inhibitor of GSH synthesis (e.g. buthionine sulfoximine) is given, there is a prompt decrease in tissue concentrations of GSH, and consequently the amount of GSH in the plasma falls. GSH is removed from plasma by the action of transpeptidase, much of

which is in the kidney. When a transpeptidase inhibitor is given, the level of GSH in the plasma increases. Thus, kidney uses GSH that is transported from renal cells, as well as GSH present in plasma. Studies on anephric animals treated with transpeptidase inhibitors show that about 67% of plasma GSH is used by the kidney and the remainder by extrarenal transpeptidase[20,21].

That hepatic vein plasma has much more GSH than arterial plasma is consistent with such an inter-organ cycle of GSH metabolism[22]. About 80% of arterial plasma GSH is removed during passage through the kidney showing that there is a mechanism, in addition to glomerular filtration, for removing GSH[21,22]. After inhibitors of transpeptidase were given to rats, removal of plasma GSH during passage through the kidney approached values anticipated for filtration alone suggesting that transpeptidase not located in the tubule is also involved in the renal utilization of GSH[22]. O_2-dependent conversion of GSH to GSSG occurs with kidney (but not liver) preparations; purified transpeptidase also exhibits 'GSH oxidase activity'. Such 'activity' is mediated by cysteinylglycine (formed by transpeptidation) which reacts rapidly and non-enzymatically with O_2 to form cystinylbis-glycine; non-enzymatic transhydrogenation between the latter and GSH yields GSSG[23]. These and similar reactions are important contributors to the extracellular formation of the disulfide forms of cysteine, γ-glutamylcysteine, and GSH. GSSG metabolism is analogous to that of GSH; thus, GSSG is converted to cystine.

Consequences of enzyme deficiency and inhibition

Animals treated with transpeptidase inhibitors, as well as patients with γ-glutamyl transpeptidase deficiency excrete, in addition to GSH and GSSG, large amounts of γ-glutamylcysteine and cysteine moieties in their urine[24]. This indicates that the function of transpeptidase is associated with the metabolism or transport (or both) of cyst(e)ine and γ-glutamylcyst(e)ine. Recent work indicates that urinary γ-glutamylcystine, in animals treated with transpeptidase inhibitors, is formed by the action of residual transpeptidase, which catalyses transpeptidation between GSH and cystine to form γ-glutamylcystine; transport of the latter into cells is inhibited by the high levels of GSH which accompany inhibition of transpeptidase. Little if any γ-glutamylcyst(e)ine arises by cleavage of the Cys–Gly bond of GSH[25]. The finding of urinary γ-glutamylcysteine and cysteine moieties in transpeptidase deficiency or inhibition is in accord with the fact that cystine is an excellent acceptor substrate of transpeptidase[26]. γ-Glutamylcystine, after transport into the cell, may be reduced to γ-glutamylcysteine and cysteine, both of which are substrates for GSH synthesis.

Other blocks of the cycle have also been found in nature or achieved by use of inhibitors[4,5]. Thus, giving a competitive inhibitor of 5-oxoprolinase to mice decreases the metabolism of 5-oxoproline, which accumulates. Accumulation is greater after giving both the inhibitor and amino acids, especially those which are good acceptor substrates of transpeptidase. Giving amino acids increases transpeptidation and thus the amount of 5-oxoproline formed by the cyclotransferase. Similar results were obtained even when animals were also given inhibitors of γ-glutamylcysteine synthetase. The formation of 5-oxoproline by the combined activities of γ-glutamylcysteine synthetase and γ-glutamyl cyclotransferase is not a major pathway for normal formation of 5-oxoproline. However, such a pathway is prominent in 5-oxoprolinuria (see below).

Administration of a competitive inhibitor of γ-glutamyl cyclotransferase to animals leads to a marked decrease in the amount of 5-oxoproline in the kidney, and studies with a model substrate show that this results from *in vivo* inhibition of cyclotransferase[27]. Blockage of the cycle at the γ-glutamylcysteine synthetase step occurs in patients deficient in this enzyme; they have GSH deficiency, hemolysis, disturbances of the central nervous system and aminoaciduria[28].

In 5-oxoprolinuria, an inborn error marked by mental deficiency, acidosis and a deficiency of GSH synthetase, there is GSH deficiency, massive urinary excretion of 5-oxoproline and increased amounts of this compound in the blood leading to acidosis[28]. GSH normally regulates its own biosynthesis by feedback inhibition of γ-glutamylcysteine synthetase[29]. Thus, when the concentrations of GSH are low, γ-glutamylcysteine is overproduced and converted to 5-oxoproline and cysteine by γ-glutamyl cyclotransferase. 5-Oxoproline formation exceeds the capacity of 5-oxoprolinase. Thus, there is a futile cycle of γ-glutamylcysteine synthesis followed by its conversion to 5-oxoproline and cysteine.

Concluding remarks

It seems significant that aminoaciduria occurs in γ-glutamylcysteine synthetase deficiency, and that cystinuria and perhaps other defects in re-absorption of amino acids are found in γ-glutamyl transpeptidase deficiency. That dramatic defects in amino acid transport have not been observed in blocks of 5-oxoprolinase, GSH synthetase, and γ-glutamyl cyclotransferase is not surprising since the inhibitions achieved so far are far from complete, and also because there are multiple amino acid transport systems which overlap in specificity. Since transport of amino acids is a crucially important cellular activity, a number of mechanisms have probably evolved to insure that this process takes place efficiently at various stages of development and under different environmental conditions. Amino acids are thought to be transported by several different 'systems', but little is now known about the mechanisms involved. Certain metabolic reactions were probably modified through evolution to serve as transport mechanisms; the available data support the thesis that one of the functions of GSH, through its metabolism, is intimately connected with a pathway of amino acid transport. This pathway probably does not function in all cells, or in a given cell for all amino acids. Presently available data indicate that cyst(e)ine and glutamine are the most likely amino acids to be transported as γ-glutamyl derivatives.

With regard to the energy requirements of the γ-glutamyl cycle, it is notable that the transport of GSH out of cells (which seems to be an obligatory step in GSH turnover), followed by its extracellular or membranous breakdown, must require minimally the equivalent of the cleavage of two molecules of ATP. For the process to include formation of 5-oxoproline, an additional molecule of ATP (for 5-oxoprolinase) would be needed; less energy than this would be needed if intracellular or membranous hydrolysis of the γ-glutamyl amino acid occurs.

It is remarkable that GSH, with its two characteristic structural features (SH group, γ-glutamyl moiety), has been adapted to perform a wide variety of functions. The intracellular stability of GSH is favored by its γ-glutamyl linkage, which is not split by α-peptidases, and which protects the SH-group from rapid oxidation. The glycine moiety of GSH protects it from the action of cyclotransferase. GSH· thus functions as a storage form of cysteine, which is incorporated into and released from GSH by reactions of the γ-glutamyl cycle. The intracellular concentrations of GSH far exceed those of cysteine, which is rapidly utilized for protein synthesis or degraded.

The recent work on GSH emphasizes the metabolic significance of the γ-glutamyl moiety, the several cycles of GSH metabolism (interconversion between GSH and GSSG, γ-glutamyl cycle, intra-organ and inter-organ cycles), and the transport of GSH across cell membranes. These phenomena are intimately connected with an impressive number of cellular processes. Hopefully these new developments in GSH metabolism may help to elucidate some intriguing and unsolved problems. What is the mechanism of GSH transport? Is it connected with the transport of γ-glutamyl amino acids, a process that is inhibited by inhibitors of GSH synthesis and of transpeptidase? What is the significance of the finding that certain tumors (e.g. of liver, skin, colon) have very high γ-glutamyl transpeptidase activities? What is the role of GSH in the central nervous system? Why do GSH levels decrease in aging tissues? Can GSH analogs or modification of the amounts of GSH, or of the enzyme activities involved in GSH metabolism, be useful in treating or preventing disease?

References

1 Sies, H. and Wendel, A., eds (1978) *Proceedings in Life Sciences*, Springer-Verlag

2 Arias, I. M. and Jakoby, W. B., eds (1976) *GSH, Metabolism and Function*, Raven Press

3 Meister, A. (1975) in *Metabolism of Sulfur-Compounds*, third edition, 7, 101–188, Academic Press

4 Meister, A. and Tate, S. S. (1976) *Annu. Rev. Biochem.* 45, 559–604

5 Meister, A. (1981) in *Current Topics in Cellular Regulation* (Horecker, B. and Stadtman, E., eds), 18, 21–57

6 Holmgren, A. (1981) *Trends Biochem. Sci.* 6, 26–29

7 Örning, L., Hammarström, S. and Samuelson, B. (1980) *Proc. Natl Acad. Sci. USA* 77, 2014–2017

8 Prota, G. (1980) in *Natural Sulfur Compounds* (Cavallini, D. *et al.*, eds), pp. 391–398, Plenum

9 Peptide Transport and Hydrolysis (1977) *Ciba Foundation Symposium*, 50, Elsevier, Exerpta Medica, North Holland

10 Griffith, O. W., Bridges, R. J., Meister, A. (1979) *Proc. Natl Acad. Sci. USA* 76, 6319–6322

11 Meister, A., Tate, S. S., Ross, L. L. (1976) in *The Enzymes of Biological Membranes* (Martinosi, A., ed.), 3, 315–347, Plenum

12 Meister, A. (1980) in *Microorganisms and Nitrogen Sources*, (Payne, J. W., ed.), 493–509, John Wiley and Sons

13 Allison, R. D. and Meister, A. (1981) *J. Biol. Chem.* 256, 2988–2992

14 Ormstad, K., Lastbom, T. and Orrenius, S. (1980) *FEBS Lett.* 112, 55–59

15 Griffith, O. W. and Meister, A. (1979) *Proc. Natl Acad. Sci. USA* 76, 268–272

16 Bartoli, G. M. and Sies, H. (1978) *FEBS Lett.* 86, 89–91

17 Griffith, O. W., Novogrodsky, A. and Meister, A. (1979) *Proc. Natl Acad. Sci. USA* 76, 2249–2252

18 Bannai, S. and Tsukeda, H. (1979) *J. Biol. Chem.* 254, 3444–3450

19 Anderson, M. E. and Meister, A. (1980) *J. Biol. Chem.* 255, 9530–9533

20 Griffith, O. W. and Meister, A. (1979) *Proc. Natl Acad. Sci. USA* 76, 5606–5610

21 Haberle, D., Wahllander, A. and Sies, H. (1979) *FEBS Lett.* 108, 335–340

22 Anderson, M. E., Bridges, R. J. and Meister, A. (1980) *Biochem. Biophys. Commun.* 96, 848–853

23 Griffith, O. W. and Tate, S. S. (1980) *J. Biol. Chem.* 255, 5011–5014

24 Griffith, O. W. and Meister, A. (1980) *Proc. Natl Acad. Sci. USA* 77, 3384–3387

25 Griffith, O. W., Bridges, R. J. and Meister, A. (1981) *Proc. Natl Acad. Sci. USA* 78, 2777–2781

26 Thompson, G. A. and Meister, A. (1975) *Proc. Natl Acad. Sci. USA* 72, 1985–1988

27 Bridges, R. J., Griffith, O. W. and Meister, A. (1980) *J. Biol. Chem.* 255, 10, 787–792

28 Meister, A. (1978) in *The Metabolic Basis of Inherited Diseases* (4th edition) (Stanbury, J. B., Wyngaarden, J. B. and Frederickson, D. S., eds) Ch. 16, pp. 328–336, McGraw-Hill

29 Richman, P. and Meister, A. (1975) *J. Biol. Chem.* 250, 1422–1426

Alton Meister is at the Department of Biochemistry, Cornell University Medical College, 1300 York Avenue, New York, NY 10021, USA.

Addendum

Recent work on GSH has been advancing on several fronts; see Refs 30–32 for reviews. An updated review on 5-oxoprolinuria and other disorders affecting the γ-glutamyl cycle has been published[33]. The hypothesis that the γ-glutamyl moiety may serve as an amino acid carrier in one pathway of amino acid transport (previously indicated by data which show that γ-glutamyl amino acids are formed *in vivo*[25,31] and under *in vitro* conditions that closely resemble physiological conditions[13], and also that they are transported) is further supported by the finding that administration of γ-glutamylcystine to mice leads to significantly increased levels of GSH in the kidney as compared to controls. Studies with γ-glutamylcystine selectively labeled with ^{35}S in either the internal or external ^{35}S atom indicate preferential utilization of the γ-glutamylcysteine moiety of this compound for GSH synthesis. The findings suggest a pathway in which γ-glutamylcystine formed by transpeptidation between GSH and cystine, is transported and reduced to form cysteine and γ-glutamylcysteine; the latter is used directly for GSH synthesis. The findings thus show transport of γ-glutamyl amino acids and indicate an alternative pathway for GSH synthesis[34].

GSH is transported out of cultured human lymphoid cells at rates proportional to the intracellular GSH concentrations[35]; further evidence has been obtained that cellular export of GSH is a general process[30,31]. In contrast, cellular uptake of GSH (although it may occur in some cells) has not yet been observed. The apparent uptake of GSH by human lymphoid cells is due to γ-glutamyl transpeptidase-dependent breakdown of GSH, transport of the products, and intracellular resynthesis[36]. Although GSH disappears in the basolateral circulation of rat kidney[21,22], the apparent 'uptake' is the result of cleavage of GSH to its constituent amino acids[37]. This finding is in accord with the observation[38] that there is significant transpeptidase on the basolateral side of renal cells. The report[39] that rat kidney vesicles prepared in the presence of an inhibitor of γ-glutamyl transpeptidase apparently transport GSH by a Na^+-dependent mechanism, if confirmed, suggests that transport phenomena observed with isolated vesicle systems do not always accurately reflect *in vivo* processes.

Reversible conversion of leukotriene C_4 to leukotriene D_4 and of the latter to leukotriene E_4 have been studied with homogeneous preparations of γ-glutamyl transpeptidase, dipeptidase and aminopeptidase M. Transpeptidase-dependent conversion of leukotriene C_4 to leukotriene D_4 is significantly faster in the presence of an amino acid mixture and is accompanied by γ-glutamyl amino acid formation. Incubation of leukotriene E_4 with γ-glutamyl transpeptidase and GSH leads to formation of a new leukotriene[40], which appears to be γ-glutamyl leukotriene E_4 (later named leukotriene F_4)[41]; this reaction is analogous to that in which γ-glutamylcystine is formed by transpeptidation between GSH and cystine[26,34].

The question raised above about the possibility that modification of the amounts of GSH or of the enzyme activities involved in GSH metabolism might be useful in the treatment or prevention of human disease has now been substantially elucidated[42]. GSH synthesis can be effectively inhibited by administering buthionine sulfoximine[43,44], a compound which evolved from earlier studies on methionine sulfoximine[45-48]. The latter compound inhibits both glutamine synthetase and γ-glutamylcysteine synthetase.

Replacement of the methyl group of methionine sulfoximine by an *n*-butyl group gives buthionine sulfoximine, which is a selective inhibitor of γ-glutamylcysteine synthetase and therefore of GSH synthesis. The idea that depletion of cellular GSH by treatment with sulfoximine inhibitors of γ-glutamylcysteine synthetase might make tumor cells more susceptible to radiation and certain chemotherapeutic agents[49] is currently being investigated[42]. GSH depletion may be effective in situations in which the cells to be killed and the cells to be spared have different quantitative requirements for GSH. Although many normal cells probably have an excess of GSH, certain tumors and parasites may have GSH concentrations which are close to the minimum required for cell survival. The destructive effects of reactive oxygen compounds (which may be produced by irradiation) such as superoxide and peroxide, free radicals and various chemical agents might thus be used advantageously in the selective destruction of cells.

There is good evidence that buthionine sulfoximine-induced depletion of GSH increases sensitivity of cells to radiation[35]. In some cells there is selective sensitization under hypoxic conditions and therefore a decrease in the oxygen enhancement ratio[42]. Selective sensitization of hypoxic cells is considered to be important in radiation therapy of tumors since hypoxic cells are less sensitive to radiation than are oxic cells. The development of drug resistance in some cases appears to be associated with an increase in cellular GSH concentrations. Certain parasites and some tumors have relatively low concentrations of catalase and superoxide dismutase. Decreasing the GSH concentrations of such cells, which would lead to decreased function of GSH peroxidase, would be expected to have deleterious effects, but would not be anticipated to affect normal cells significantly[42]. It has been found that mouse leukemia cells that became resistant to therapy with phenylalanine mustard developed GSH concentrations about twice those of the corresponding sensitive cells. Treatment of the resistant cells *in vitro* and *in vivo* with buthionine sulfoximine restored sensitivity to the chemotherapeutic agent and increased the longevity of experimental animals bearing such tumors[50].

Procedures that increase cellular GSH concentrations may be beneficial under certain conditions, especially in the detoxication of certain drugs and in the protection of cells against radiation[42]. Although the upper concentration of GSH is controlled by feedback inhibition by GSH[29], cellular GSH concentrations also depend on the supply of its constituent amino acids. Cysteine is often the limiting component, but administration of cysteine is usually not an ideal way to increase GSH concentrations because this amino acid is rapidly metabolized and its administration is often followed by toxicity. In studies on purified 5-oxoprolinase it was found that the 5-oxoproline analog in which the 4-methylene moiety of 5-oxo-L-proline is replaced by a sulfur atom (i.e. L-2-oxothiazolidine-4-carboxylate) is a good substrate for the enzyme[51–54]. The enzyme converts the thiazolidine to L-cysteine. The thiazolidine is effectively transported and converted to cysteine intracellularly; this leads to a substantial increase in GSH in the liver. Thus, the thiazolidine is an effective intracellular cysteine delivery agent and can be used effectively to combat certain types of drug toxicity. Administration of a cysteine precursor that is well transported has limitations, however, because GSH concentrations higher than those regulated by feedback inhibition of γ-glutamylcysteine synthetase can probably not be achieved in this manner. It is possible to bypass the feedback regulated step of GSH synthesis by administering a substrate of GSH synthetase. Thus, giving γ-glutamylcystine (or similar compounds) leads to a substantial increase in the GSH concentration in the kidney[34].

Another way of increasing cellular GSH concentrations would be to administer a GSH derivative which is well transported and which, after transport, is readily converted to GSH within the cell[55,56]. Promising derivatives having such properties include the monoesters of GSH in which the glycine carboxyl group is esterified. For example, the monoethyl ester of GSH is effectively transported into several types of cells (including liver and kidney) and is rapidly de-esterified intracellularly. Administration of the monoethyl (or methyl) ester of GSH to mice was followed by considerable increases in the GSH concentrations in the liver and kidney[55]. Similar results have been obtained in human lymphoid cells grown in tissue culture and in human skin fibroblasts[56]. In the experiments on these cells, cellular concentrations of GSH were achieved that are in considerable excess of those usually found. It was found that such cells could be effectively protected against radiation by administering GSH ester. Similarly, GSH ester effectively protected mice against lethal doses of paracetamol. The studies summarized above and discussed elsewhere[32,42] indicate that modification of cellular GSH concentrations and of the activities of enzymes involved in GSH metabolism can produce useful and selective effects on cells, and can thus be valuable in therapy and in prevention of toxicity.

References

30 Larsson, A., Orrenius, S., Holmgren, A. and Mannervik, B., eds (1983) *Functions of Glutathione – Biochemical, Physiological and Toxicological Aspects*, Raven Press

31 Meister, A. and Anderson, M. E. (1983) *Annu. Rev. Biochem.* 52, 711–760

32 Meister, A. *Federation Proceedings*, 43 (William Rose Award Lecture) (in press)

33 Meister, A. (1983) in *Metabolic Basis of Inherited Diseases* (J. B. Stanbury *et al.*, eds), pp. 348–359

34 Anderson, M. E. and Meister, A. (1983) *Proc. Natl Acad. Sci. USA* 80, 707–711

35 Dethmers, J. K. and Meister, A. (1981) *Proc. Natl Acad. Sci. USA* 78, 7492–7496

36 Jensen, G. L. and Meister, A. (1983) *Proc.*

Natl Acad. Sci. USA 80, 4714–4717

37 Abbott, W. A., Bridges, R. J. and Meister, A. *J. Biol. Chem.* 260 (in press)

38 Spater, H. W., Poruchynsky, M. S., Quintana, N., Inoue, M. and Novikoff, A. B. (1982) *Proc. Natl Acad. Sci. USA* 79, 3547–3550

39 Lash, L. H. and Jones, D. P. (1983) *Biochem. Biophys. Res. Commun.* 112, 55–60

40 Anderson, M. E., Allison, R. D. and Meister, A. (1982) *Proc. Natl Acad. Sci. USA* 78, 7492–7496

41 Hammarstrom, S. (1983) *Annu. Rev. Biochem.* 52, 355–377

42 Meister, A. (1983) *Science* 220, 471–477

43 Griffith, O. W., Anderson, M. E. and Meister, A. (1979) *J. Biol. Chem.* 254, 1205–1210

44 Griffith, O. W. and Meister, A. (1979) *J. Biol. Chem.* 254, 7558–7560

45 Ronzio, R. and Meister, A. (1968) *Proc. Natl Acad. Sci. USA* 59, 164–170

46 Ronzio, R. A., Rowe, W. B. and Meister, A. (1969) *Biochemistry* 8, 1066–1075

47 Rowe, W. B. and Meister, A. (1970) *Proc.*

Natl Acad. Sci. USA 66, 500–506

48 Meister, A. (1978) in *Enzyme-Activated Irreversible Inhibitors* (Seiler, N., Jung, M. J. and Koch-Weser, J., eds), pp. 187–211, Elsevier-North Holland Biomedical Press

49 Meister, A. and Griffith, O. W. (1979) *Cancer Treat. Rep.* 63, 1115–1121

50 Suzkake, K., Petro, B. J. and Vistica, D. T. (1983) *Biochem. Pharmacol.* 32, 165

51 Williamson, J. M. and Meister, A. (1981) *Proc. Natl Acad. Sci. USA* 78, 936–939

52 Williamson, J. M., Boettcher, B. and Meister, A. (1982) *Proc. Natl Acad. Sci. USA* 79, 6246–6249

53 Williamson, J. M. and Meister, A. (1982) *J. Biol. Chem.* 257, 12039–12042

54 Boettcher, B. and Meister, A. (1984) *Analyt. Biochem.* 138, 449–450

55 Puri, R. N. and Meister, A. (1983) *Proc. Natl Acad. Sci. USA* 80, 5258–5260

56 Wellner, V. P., Anderson, M. E., Puri, R. N., Jensen, G. L. and Meister, A. *Proc. Natl Acad. Sci. USA* (in press)

Regulation of carbamoyl-phosphate synthase (ammonia) in liver in relation to urea cycle activity

Alfred J. Meijer

The properties of carbamoyl-phosphate synthase (ammonia) are extremely interesting from the point of view of metabolic regulation and make the enzyme the main candidate for the rate-controlling step in urea synthesis.

Carbamoyl-phosphate synthase (ammonia) (CPS), which is localized in the mitochondria in the livers of ureotelic animals, has an absolute requirement for N-acetylglutamate (AGA) as activator[1]. Activation of the enzyme by AGA (K_m is about 0.1 mM for rat-liver CPS)[2] is associated with changes in the conformation and subunit structure of the enzyme protein[3]. In addition, the activity of the enzyme is fully dependent on the presence of Mg^{2+}: both MgATP and free Mg^{2+} ions are required, the former as substrate and the latter for maximal activity[1,2]. The kinetic properties of enzyme are fairly complex because of the large number of variables involved in the enzymic reaction (see Ref. 2).

The total amount of CPS protein increases with increasing protein content of the diet[4]. This long-term adaptation to the increased demands on the body to dispose of excess nitrogen under these conditions is similar to that of the other urea cycle enzymes[4]. However, as we will see, the enzyme is also subject to short-term regulation. Rapid inactivation of CPS under certain conditions is essential in order to prevent a complete drain of all NH_2 present in liver cells into the urea cycle, since NH_2 is a precursor of pyrimidines, of glutamate and, through glutamate, of non-essential amino acids[5].

It has been shown[6-9] that about 20% of the total mitochondrial matrix protein is comprised of CPS. It is estimated that the concentration of CPS in the matrix is 0.4 mM[7-8] or even higher[9]. This concentration is of the same order of magnitude as the concentration of substrates (NH_3, bicarbonate, MgATP) and effectors (AGA, Mg^{2+}) in the mitochondrial matrix and it can easily be calculated that CPS in normal liver mitochondria does not function at maximal capacity[7,8]. Because of the high concentration of CPS *in vivo* a re-evaluation of the kinetic properties of CPS, at high enzyme concentrations, is required[7,8].

Synthesis of N-acetylglutamate

The important work of Shigesada and Tatibana[10-12] has stressed the importance of AGA in the control of urea cycle flux and the role of AGA synthesis in this respect (see Krebs *et al.* (Ref. 5) for discussion). AGA is synthesized in the mitochondria from acetyl-CoA and glutamate[10,11]. AGA synthase is markedly stimulated by arginine in an allosteric manner[10-12], although enzyme activity is not completely dependent on the presence of this activator. The activating effect is specific for arginine; it is not given by any other amino acid or intermediate of the urea cycle[10]. Arginine increases the V_{max} of AGA synthase but has no effect on the K_m values for the substrates[12].

The amount of AGA synthase increases with increasing protein content of the diet[13], similar to the behaviour of CPS and the other urea cycle enzymes.

Synthesis of AGA has been demonstrated directly in intact liver mitochondria isolated from mouse[10,11] and rat[14] and indirectly in rabbit-liver mitochondria[15]. From the data of Shigesada and Tatibana[11] a minimal rate of AGA synthesis from glutamate and acetate in mouse-liver mitochondria of 0.006 nmol/min per mg mitochondrial protein at 37°C can be calculated. With arginine also present, this rate increased to up to 0.04 nmol/min per mg protein (calculated from Ref. 10). AGA synthesis occurs more rapidly in isolated mitochondria from rat liver than in those from mouse liver: in the presence of glutamate alone, AGA is produced at a rate of about 0.15 nmol/min per mg protein at 25°C[14] and increases to up to 0.5 nmol/min per mg protein when acetylcarnitine and arginine are also present[16].

According to Shigesada and Tatibana[12] isolated rat-liver AGA synthase is subject to product inhibition by AGA with a K_i of 0.07 mM. This may be the explanation for the observation that AGA production by intact isolated rat-liver mitochondria declines when the mitochondrial AGA concentration increases above 1 nmol/mg protein[14].

Relationship between the rate of citrulline synthesis and the mitochondrial AGA content

As anticipated by Charles and co-workers[17], synthesis of AGA by mitochondrial suspensions explains a number of hitherto puzzling observations with regard to the synthesis of citrulline by isolated liver mitochondria. First, the lag period of about 5 min in citrulline synthesis by rat-liver mitochondria incubated with glutamate, HCO_3^-, and NH_3 and ornithine[17,18], can, at least in part, be explained by synthesis

of AGA[14]. Secondly, maximal stimulation of citrulline synthesis from bicarbonate, NH_3 and ornithine by glutamate occurs at a concentration of glutamate of 10 mM, which is higher than that required for maximal ATP production[17]. This value is in agreement with the rather high K_m (3 mM) of glutamate for AGA synthase[12]. Thirdly, different oxidizable substrates stimulate citrulline synthesis to different degrees[17]. This effect, too, appears to be related to synthesis of AGA which occurs efficiently only with those substrates capable of producing intramitochondrial glutamate[14].

Of importance for the interpretation of studies on citrulline synthesis in isolated mitochondria is the amount of AGA present in the mitochondria immediately after isolation. As shown by McGivan and co-workers[13] the endogenous AGA content of isolated liver mitochondria increases with increasing protein content of the diet of the rats used. They showed that this phenomenon is directly responsible for the variations they observed in the initial rate of citrulline synthesis upon subsequent incubation of these mitochondria.

Permeability of the mitochondrial membrane for N-acetylglutamate

The exclusive mitochondrial localization of AGA synthase and of CPS facilitates an efficient interaction between the positive effector and its target enzyme[10]. On the other hand, breakdown of AGA to acetate and glutamate occurs in the cytosol only[5,13,19]. Since AGA measured in total liver extracts represents mainly mitochondrial AGA[11], it can be concluded that the cytosolic degradation of AGA is an active process relative to its synthesis. Because of the mitochondrial localization of its synthesis and the cytosolic localization of its breakdown, transport of AGA from mitochondria to cytosol is an obligatory step in the degradation of this compound.

Studies on the permeability properties of the mitochondrial membrane for AGA are scanty. Efflux of AGA has been demonstrated in isolated rat-liver mitochondria synthesizing AGA, but the mechanism by which this occurs is not clear[14]. The effect of added AGA on citrulline synthesis in intact liver mitochondria has been reported to be stimulatory[15,20,21] or negligible[17]. According to Charles and co-workers[17] added AGA may not penetrate the mitochondrial membrane under certain conditions.

Recently we have re-examined this problem and found that added AGA stimulates citrulline synthesis only when the mitochondria are in a low-energy state or when the incubation temperature of the mitochondria is raised to 37°C[16]. Curiously enough, however, when the uptake of [14C]AGA was studied under these conditions, no detectable entry of label into the mitochondrial matrix space was observed[16]. No explanation for this phenomenon is at present available.

Synthesis of N-acetylglutamate *in vivo* and its relationship to urea cycle flux

The level of AGA in the liver of mice and rats changes with the protein content of the diet[11,22-24] and shows a positive correlation with the urea[11,24], ornithine[22,24], arginine and glutamate content of the liver[22]. In both species the AGA content of the liver was found to vary from 10–20 nmol/g wet weight at low protein intake to up to 100–150 nmol/g wet weight at high protein[22-24]. Assuming that 1 g wet weight of liver contains 60 mg mitochondrial protein and assuming that under all conditions the measured AGA is mainly mitochondrial[11], it can be calculated that the mitochondrial AGA concentration increased from about 0.2 to 2 nmol per mg mitochondrial protein upon increasing the protein content of the diet (up to 60–70% casein diet). Intramitochondrial AGA concentrations of this magnitude have been observed after prolonged incubation of isolated rat-liver mitochondria with glutamate, acetylcarnitine and arginine[16].

According to Tatibana and Shigesada[22] the arginine concentration in mouse liver increases from 26 nmol/g wet weight when the protein content of the diet is low to 170 nmol/g wet weight when it is high. These values are higher than the concentration of arginine (5–10 μM) required for half-maximal stimulation of isolated AGA synthase, suggesting at first sight that the enzyme is always maximally activated by arginine *in vivo*. However, nothing is known about the distribution of arginine across the mitochondrial membrane. Since arginine is a basic amino acid, and since the pH of the mitochondrial matrix is slightly more alkaline than that of the cytosol, it may be expected that the intramitochondrial arginine concentration is lower than that in the cytosol. Thus when the protein content of the diet is low the mitochondrial arginine concentration may be below saturation for its activating effect on AGA synthase. A good indication in this direction is the fact that intraperitoneal injection of mice with arginine greatly increased the AGA content of the liver (up to 6-fold under certain conditions)[22,23].

The changes in the concentration of AGA following dietary transitions are relatively fast since they precede the activity changes of the urea cycle enzymes due to synthesis/degradation of enzyme protein[24]. Tatibana and co-workers have directly measured the rate of AGA synthesis and degradation in mouse liver *in vivo*[23]. After injection of mice with a mixture of arginine and glutamine the AGA content of the liver increased from 20 nmol/g wet weight to a peak value of 125 nmol/g wet weight in 30 min[23]. This *in vivo* rate agrees nicely with the rate of AGA synthesis observed in isolated mouse-liver mitochondria incubated with glutamate, acetate and arginine[10]. It would be interesting to follow the synthesis of AGA in rats *in vivo*, since rat-liver mitochondria appear to have a higher capacity for AGA synthesis[13,14], so that the *in vivo* fluctuations in AGA may be even faster in this animal.

The half-life of AGA degradation in mouse liver *in vivo* is about 20 min[23]. Since AGA is degraded in the cytosol only, this indicates that *in vivo* AGA leaves the mitochondria at a rate that is about equal to the rate of its synthesis.

In addition to the *in vivo* studies described above, an excellent correlation between the intracellular content of AGA and flux through CPS has also been demonstrated in isolated hepatocytes under various experimental conditions[13,23]. This once again stresses the key role of AGA in regulation of flux through the urea cycle.

Regulation of carbamoyl-phosphate synthase activity by factors other than N-acetylglutamate

Evidence has been brought forward that CPS activity in mitochondria may be controlled under certain conditions by changes in the mitochondrial free Mg^{2+} concentration, for example via changes in mitochondrial citrate[25]. In this context it is of interest that the K_m for free Mg^{2+} of isolated CPS is decreased when AGA is increased and vice versa[2]. If this is also true for CPS in the intact mitochondrion the effects of changes in AGA and free Mg^{2+} may reinforce each other and will make CPS activity extremely sensitive to these parameters.

Recently we have found that Ca^{2+} is able to antagonize the activation of isolated CPS by Mg^{2+} [16]. Furthermore, in intact rat-liver mitochondria citrulline synthesis was found to be accelerated by EGTA and strongly inhibited by addition of small amounts of Ca^{2+} [16]. When mitochondria were incubated with bicarbonate, NH_3, ornithine, glutamate and EGTA, intramitochondrial Ca^{2+} was slowly lost to the medium in about 5 min at 25°C; this loss of Ca^{2+} coincided with the lag in citrulline synthesis[16]. Thus it appears that the increase in citrulline synthesis with time[17] is caused by two factors: an increase in mitochondrial AGA[14] and a decrease in mitochondrial Ca^{2+}.

Several groups have reported that glucagon treatment of rats results in an increased capacity of liver mitochondria to synthesize citrulline[26-28]. This may be due to a stimulation by glucagon of the rate of ATP formation in the mitochondria leading to a higher steady-state concentration of mitochondrial ATP[26,27] or to an increased mitochondrial AGA content[28]. Unfortunately, no information on the latter point is available. Alternatively, it is possible that the observed differences are due to differences in the mitochondrial Ca^{2+} content, since evidence has been presented that glucagon causes a release of mitochondrial Ca^{2+} [29,30]. A similar mechanism, mediated by Ca^{2+}, has been proposed for hormonal regulation of pyruvate carboxylase[31].

Besides the involvement of AGA, Mg^{2+} and Ca^{2+}, it is possible that other factors are involved in the regulation of CPS as well. Krebs and co-workers[5] failed to observe any accumulation of carbamoyl phosphate during perfusion of rat liver with alanine in the absence of ornithine, despite the fact that NH_3 accumulated in the perfusate. Addition of ornithine resulted in a prompt acceleration of urea synthesis. It therefore seems that at sub-optimal concentration of ornithine some regulatory mechanism controls CPS activity[5]. Tatibana and Shigesada[22,23] showed that the concentration of carbamoyl phosphate in mouse liver is remarkably low and constant (1–2 nmol/g wet weight), in spite of wide variations in the protein content of the diet of the animals used. They concluded that this constancy is attributable, at least in part, to coordinated variations in the levels of AGA and ornithine. Reported values for the concentration of carbamoyl phosphate in rat liver are about 100-fold higher[8]. The reason for this quantitative difference in results is not clear (see discussion in Ref. 22).

Several explanations have been proposed for the activating effect of ornithine on CPS[5,22]. None, however, seems to be satisfactory. A direct effect of ornithine on CPS is ruled out[7]. Feedback inhibition by carbamoyl phosphate is unlikely because of the high K_i for carbamoyl phosphate (10–20 mM) of CPS[32], although it must be kept in mind that this K_i was determined with very dilute enzyme solutions. Activation by the arginine–AGA system is unlikely since AGA synthesis is too slow to account for the fast response to ornithine of flux through CPS[5,22]. Moreover, also in intact isolated mitochondria

where arginine synthesis does not occur, strong inhibition of CPS has been observed in the absence of ornithine under certain conditions[16,18]. Raijman[8] proposed that CPS and ornithine transcarbamoylase may form a complex *in vivo*. Perhaps the formation of such a complex is promoted by ornithine[8].

Problems to be solved

Fig. 1 gives a summary of the factors controlling CPS activity in mitochondria. From the foregoing discussion it is clear that there are many unsolved problems. What are the kinetic properties of CPS at high enzyme concentrations? What is the precise role of Ca^{2+} and Mg^{2+}? What is the mechanism of transport of AGA out of the mitochondria? Is it subject to metabolic control? What factors govern the distribution of arginine across the mitochondrial membrane? What is the mechanism responsible for inactivation of CPS when the concentration of ornithine falls?

It is to be hoped that answers to these

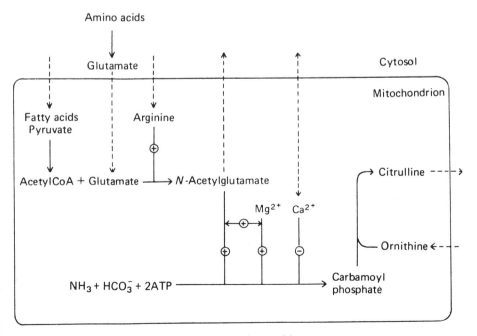

Fig. 1. Regulation of carbamoyl-phosphate synthase (ammonia).

questions will be found in the near future.

Acknowledgements

The studies by the author described in this review were supported by a grant from The Netherlands Organization for the Advancement of Pure Research (Z.W.O), under the auspices of The Netherlands Foundation for Chemical Research (S.O.N.).

References

1 Marshall, M., Metzenberg, R. L. and Cohen, P. P. (1961) *J. Biol. Chem.* 236, 2229–2237
2 Elliott, K. R. F. and Tipton, K. F. (1974) *Biochem. J.* 141, 807–816
3 Guthöhrlein, G. and Knappe, J. (1968) *Eur. J. Biochem.* 7, 119–127
4 Schimke, R. T. (1962) *J. Biol. Chem.* 237, 459–468
5 Krebs, H. A., Hems, R. and Lund, P. (1973) *Adv. Enz. Regul.* 11, 361–377
6 Clarke, S. (1976) *J. Biol. Chem.* 251, 950–961
7 Raijman, L. and Jones, M. E. (1976) *Arch. Biochem. Biophys.* 175, 270–278
8 Raijman, L. (1976) in *The Urea Cycle* (Grisolia, S., Báguena, R. and Mayor, F., eds), pp. 243–254, John Wiley and Sons
9 Lusty, C. J. (1978) *Eur. J. Biochem.* 85, 373–383
10 Shigesada, K. and Tatibana, M. (1971) *Biochem. Biophys. Res. Commun.* 44, 1117–1124
11 Shigesada, K. and Tatibana, M. (1971) *J. Biol. Chem.* 246, 5588–5595
12 Shigesada, K. and Tatibana, M. (1978) *Eur. J. Biochem.* 84, 285–291
13 McGivan, J. D., Bradford, N. M. and Mendes-Mourão, J. (1976) *Biochem. J.* 154, 415–421
14 Meijer, A. J. and van Woerkom, G. M. (1978) *FEBS Lett.* 86, 117–121
15 Bryla, J. (1974) *FEBS Lett.* 47, 60–65
16 Meijer, A. J., van Woerkom, G. M. and Hensgens, H. E. S. J. (1978) (unpublished observations)
17 Charles, R., Tager, J. M. and Slater, E. C. (1967) *Biochim. Biophys. Acta* 131, 29–41
18 Glasgow, A. M. and Chase, H. P. (1976) *Biochem. J.* 156, 301–307
19 Reglero, A., Rivas, J., Mendelson, J., Wallace, R. and Grisolia, S. (1977) *FEBS Lett.* 81, 13–17
20 Caravaca, J. and Grisolia, S. (1960) *J. Biol. Chem.* 235, 684–693
21 Natale, P. J. and Tremblay, G. C. (1969) *Biochem. Biophys. Res. Commun.* 37, 512–517
22 Tatibana, M. and Shigesada, K. (1976) in *The Urea Cycle* (Grisolia, S., Báguena, R. and Mayor, F., eds), pp. 301–313, John Wiley and Sons
23 Shigesada, K., Aoyagi, K. and Tatibana, M. (1978) *Eur. J. Biochem.* 85, 385–391
24 Saheki, T., Katsunuma, T. and Sase, M. (1977) *J. Biochem.* 82, 551–558
25 Meijer, A. J. and van Woerkom, G. M. (1977) *Biochim. Biophys. Acta* 500, 13–26
26 Yamazaki, R. K. and Gratz, G. S. (1977) *Arch. Biochem. Biophys.* 178, 19–25
27 Bryla, J., Harris, E. J. and Plumb, J. A. (1977) *FEBS Lett.* 80, 443–448
28 Triebwasser, K. C. and Freedland, R. A. (1977) *Biochem. Biophys. Res. Commun.* 76, 1159–1165
29 Foden, S. and Randle, P. J. (1978) *Biochem. J.* 170, 615–625
30 Chen, J.-L. J., Babcock, D. F. and Lardy, H. A. (1978) *Proc. Natl Acad. Sci. USA* 75, 2234–2238
31 Foldes, M. and Barritt, G. J. (1977) *J. Biol. Chem.* 252, 5372–5380
32 Elliott, K. R. F. and Tipton, K. F. (1974) *Biochem. J.* 141, 817–824

Alfred J. Meijer is at the Laboratory of Biochemistry, B.C.P. Jansen Institute, University of Amsterdam, Plantage Muidergracht 12, 1018 TV Amsterdam, The Netherlands.

Addendum

In reviewing the progress that has been made since 1979 concerning the regulation of CPS activity and the importance of CPS in the short-term control of urea synthesis, it is appropriate to consider the questions raised at that time.

Studies with permeabilized rat-liver mitochondria have indicated that the kinetic properties of CPS, in the macromolecular environment of the mitochondrial matrix, are very similar to those of the enzyme in solution[33].

No information has become available on whether or not variations in mitochondrial Ca^{2+} or Mg^{2+} can affect CPS activity in the intact hepatocyte. According to Cerdan *et al.*[34], Ca^{2+} is unlikely to be involved because in the hepatocyte the intramitochondrial concentration of free Ca^{2+} may always be too low to affect the activity of CPS.

Transport of AGA across the mitochondrial membrane is slow, unidirectional (out of the mitochondria only) and requires energy. As yet, there is no evidence that a specific translocator is involved. Apart from the concentration of intramitochondrial AGA no other factors have been found so far that affect the rate of mitochondrial AGA efflux[35]. It has been suggested that this process is under hormonal control[37].

The role of arginine in controlling AGA synthesis is controversial. In rats injected with mixtures of 20 amino acids (with arginine either absent or present) there is no relationship between intrahepatic arginine and AGA[37]. The intramitochondrial content of arginine in hepatocytes suggests that AGA synthase is always saturated with its activator[38]. However, it was recently shown that the response of AGA synthase to arginine activation varies with the time after feeding; the activation increases from 1.6-fold at the start of the feeding to almost 6-fold, 9 h after feeding[39]. Thus it appears that AGA synthase is not regulated by changes in the concentration of arginine itself but by variations in the V_{max} of the enzyme in the presence of the activator which are caused by other factors.

The mechanism responsible for inactivation of CPS when the concentration of ornithine falls is still not known. The effect must be indirect because ornithine does not activate CPS in mitochondria in which ornithine transcarbamoylase is specifically inhibited[40]. Feedback inhibition of carbonic anhydrase by carbamoyl phosphate[41] is unlikely, because flux through CPS during citrulline synthesis in isolated mitochondria is not very sensitive to concentrations of carbamoyl phosphate in the mitochondrial matrix[40]

which cause powerful inhibition of carbonic anhydrase *in vitro*[41]. A problem not considered so far is that accumulation of intramitochondrial carbamoyl phosphate requires a stoichiometric mitochondrial influx of P_i^- and H^+ ions which may cause local acidification. Exchange of ornithine$^+$ against H^+ and (uncharged) citrulline would then release these protons.

The kinetics of the changes in AGA and in CPS activity have been studied both *in vivo*[37] and in isolated hepatocytes[36,38]. Large increases in the two parameters (4–10-fold) have been observed within 10 minutes of administering nitrogen loads. Half-maximal activation of CPS is observed at 0.8–1 nmol AGA per mg mitochondrial protein[37]. From these studies it has become clear that glutamate is an important determinant of intramitochondrial AGA. Whether variations in mitochondrial acetyl CoA can also control AGA concentration under normal conditions is not known. However, it is certain that severe depletion of intrahepatic acetyl CoA under pathological conditions, such as occurs in organic acidurias, leads to a large decrease in AGA with resulting hyperammonemia.

The rapid increase in the capacity of liver mitochondria to synthesize citrulline after treatment of rats with glucagon is largely caused by an increase in AGA[38,42]. Under these conditions, an increase in glutamate concentration is not responsible for this effect, because intrahepatic glutamate falls after glucagon administration[42].

In a recent study the amount of control that CPS exerts on urea cycle flux has been quantified (Meijer, A. J., Lof, C., Ramós, I. and Verhoeven, A. J., unpublished results). From this study we concluded that *in vivo* urea cycle flux is entirely controlled by the concentration of ammonia in the mitochondria and the activity of CPS. Activation of CPS by AGA will help the enzyme in buffering the intrahepatic ammonia concentration (see Ref. 5), so that an increase in urea production rate (following an increased supply of amino acids to the liver) can be obtained at almost constant concentration of ammonia in the mitochondria.

The role of AGA as a short-term regulator of urea synthesis has recently been questioned by Lund and Wiggins[43]. According to these authors, CPS is always saturated with AGA, regardless of the nitrogen supply. This conclusion is based on the fact that a new method for the measurement of intracellular AGA yields much higher values for AGA than those published in the literature so far. (For a discussion of this controversy the reader is referred to Ref. 44.)

Finally, reference should be made to an entirely different view of the function of the urea cycle. According to Atkinson and Camien, the primary function of the urea cycle is not the removal of excess ammonia but rather the removal of excess bicarbonate. They consider the urea cycle to be a mechanism for the maintenance of pH homeostasis; this is discussed in this book in the following two articles.

References

33 Lof, C., Cohen, M., Vermeulen, L. P., Van Roermund, C. W. T., Wanders, R. J. A. and Meijer, A. J. (1983) *Eur. J. Biochem.* 135, 251–258

34 Cerdan, S., Lusty, C. J., Davis, K. N., Jacobsohn, J. A. and Williamson, J. R. (1984) *J. Biol. Chem.* 259, 323–331

35 Meijer, A. J. and Van Woerkom, G. M. (1982) *Biochim. Biophys. Acta* 721, 240–246

36 Morita, T., Mori, M. and Tatibana, M. (1982) *J. Biochem.* 91, 563–569

37 Stewart, P. M. and Walser, M. (1980) *J. Biol. Chem.* 255, 5270–5280

38 Hensgens, H. E. S. J., Verhoeven, A. J. and Meijer, A. J. (1980) *Eur. J. Biochem.* 107, 197–205

39 Kawamoto, S., Ishida, H., Mori, M. and Tatibana, M. (1982) *Eur. J. Biochem.* 123, 637–641

40 Cohen, N. S., Cheung, C. W., Kyan, F. S., Jones, E. E. and Raijman, L. (1982) *J. Biol. Chem.* 257, 6898–6907

41 Carter, N. D., Chegwidden, W. R., Hewett-Emmett, D., Jeffery, S., Shiels, A. and Tashian, R. E. (1984) *FEBS Lett.* 165, 197–200

42 Staddon, J. M., Bradford, N. M. and McGivan, J. D. (1984) *Biochem. J.* 217, 855–857

43 Lund, P. and Wiggins, D. (1984) *Biochem. J.* 218, 991–994

44 Meijer, A. J. and Verhoeven, A. J. *Biochem. J.* (in press)

The role of ureagenesis in pH homeostasis

Daniel E. Atkinson and Edmund Bourke

Catabolism of protein liberates HCO_3^-, which cannot be eliminated in the necessary amounts through the lungs, kidneys, or intestines, and thus poses a threat of alkalosis to air-breathing animals. That threat is met by biosynthetic sequences that consume the weak acid NH_4^+ and liberate its proton for reaction with HCO_3^-. Different kinds of air-breathing animals use different syntheses for this purpose; mammals utilize ureagenesis. Modulation of the rate of urea synthesis in response to pH is an important part of the interacting regulatory systems by which pH homeostasis is maintained in mammals.

Because of the profound effects of pH on the stability and conformation of macromolecules, reaction rates and transfers through membranes, it is essential that intracellular pH be maintained within rather narrow limits. In vertebrates this control has become systemic, and the pH of blood and interstitial fluid is closely regulated. The HCO_3^-/CO_2 system provides most of the buffering capacity of vertebrate blood and nearly all of the buffering of the interstitial fluid. Thus the extracellular pH in vertebrates may appropriately be discussed in terms of the HCO_3^-/CO_2 ratio, to which it is related by the Henderson–Hasselbach equation:

$$pH = 6.1 + \log (HCO_3^-/CO_2) \quad (1)$$

Need for disposal of bicarbonate

Total oxidation of dietary carbohydrates and fats yields only CO_2 (and water), but oxidation of compounds containing carboxylate ions yields an amount of HCO_3^- equimolar with the carboxylate. Carnivores and omnivores encounter carboxylates mainly in the amino acids derived from dietary protein. Hydrolysis of protein yields dipolar amino acids without net consumption or liberation of proton, and hence without effect on body buffers. In the complete oxidation of a simple amino acid illustrated here by alanine, the substituted

ammonium ion ($R\text{-}NH_3^+$) is converted to free ammonium ion. Consumption of proton from the body buffer (equation 2) leads to stoichiometric production of bicarbonate (equation 3). Net CO_2 production is then proportional to the number of other carbon atoms in the amino acid (equation 4). These same amounts

$$\begin{array}{c} NH_3^+ \\ | \\ CH_3\text{–}CH\text{–}COO^- + 3\,O_2 + H^+ \\ \rightarrow 3\,CO_2 + 2\,H_2O + NH_4^+ \quad (2) \end{array}$$

$$CO_2 + H_2O \rightleftharpoons HCO_3^- + H^+ \quad (3)$$

$$\begin{array}{c} NH_3^+ \\ | \\ CH_3\text{–}CH\text{–}COO^- + 3\,O_2 \rightarrow 2\,CO_2 \\ + HCO_3^- + H_2O + NH_4^+ \quad (4) \end{array}$$

of NH_4^+ and HCO_3^- are produced also if the amino acid is converted either wholly or in part to fat or carbohydrate. Metabolism of a typical daily human intake of 100 g of protein yields about one mol of bicarbonate[1]. Part of the sulfur of cysteine and methionine is converted to sulfuric acid, but even total conversion would liberate only enough protons to titrate about 7% of the HCO_3^- produced from the same amount of protein. It is therefore evident that metabolism of protein produces a large net amount of bicarbonate, the conjugate base of the predominant buffer system, and a consequent threat of alkalosis. Herbivores face an especially serious potential alkalosis because of the large amounts of salts of carboxylic acids in the vacuolar sap of leaves. Their special adaptations will not be discussed in this article.

The need to dispose of CO_2, NH_4^+, and HCO_3^- is common to all heterotrophs. Gill-breathing vertebrates encounter no difficulty in eliminating all three waste products into the water flowing through the gills. The situation is quite different for air-breathing vertebrates: carbon dioxide can be eliminated through the lungs, but the ionic waste products cannot. Development of a means of disposing of HCO_3^- in a regulated way so as to stabilize pH was essential to the evolution of air-breathing animals.

Some bicarbonate is eliminated in feces, and under some conditions a relatively small amount of bicarbonate may be lost in the urine. But neither of these routes can handle more than a small fraction of the bicarbonate that is generated in protein metabolism – the feces in part because of the large amount of balancing cations that would be required, and the urine because of problems of back-diffusion at the high concentrations that would be necessary and especially because calcium carbonate would precipitate in the tubules. Thus the only means that we can envisage whereby bicarbonate can be disposed of and pH homeostasis maintained is by protonation, either directly to yield CO_2 or in the course of conversion to some other uncharged carbon compound. No acid strong enough to protonate HCO_3^- directly is available at anywhere near the necessary amount.

Ammonium ion bears a dissociable proton and is produced in metabolism at about the same rate as bicarbonate. It is indeed the only potential source of the protons needed for disposal of bicarbo-

nate. However, NH_4^+ is too weak an acid by a factor of over 1 000 to protonate HCO_3^- (the pK_a values are about 9.25 and 6.1 respectively). Thus adaptation to air-breathing life was possible only if the weakly acidic ammonium ion could be converted to a compound in which the nitrogen function is strongly acidic and hence will donate a proton to the body buffer system.

In the evolution of amphibians the pre-existing pathway for synthesis of arginine was supplemented by the enzyme arginase, which splits off urea and regenerates ornithine, a precursor of arginine, thus permitting cyclic synthesis of urea. This synthesis, previously used by sharks and other elasmobranchs that accumulate urea to balance the osmolarity of seawater, took on a new and vital significance in air-breathing vertebrates. Protonated amido groups are strong acids; hence two protons are liberated from NH_4^+ ions in the synthesis of each molecule of urea. One in effect titrates the HCO_3^- that is incorporated into urea and the other is liberated (equation 5) to react with the body buffers (equation 6). The net result (equation 7) is the removal of two

$$HCO_3^- + 2\,NH_4^+$$
$$\rightarrow H_2NCONH_2 + 2\,H_2O + H^+ \quad (5)$$

$$H^+ + HCO_3^- \rightleftharpoons CO_2 + H_2O \quad (6)$$

$$2HCO_3^- + 2\,NH_4^+$$
$$\rightarrow H_2NCONH_2 + CO_2 + 3\,H_2O \,(7)$$

bicarbonate ions for each molecule of urea synthesized. Four molecules of ATP are used for each molecule of urea formed; thus it is functionally meaningful to consider the urea cycle to be a means by which protons can be pumped from the weak acid NH_4^+ against an energy gradient to protonate HCO_3^-, with the hydrolysis of 2 ATP's per proton supplying the necessary energy.

The problem of disposal of bicarbonate and the evolutionary strategy by which it was solved are general. Virtually all air-breathing animals use ATP to convert NH_4^+ into an organic compound in which the nitrogen functions are sufficiently acidic to ensure that the protons needed for disposal of HCO_3^- will be released in the course of the synthesis. Amphibian eggs and larvae live in water and can eliminate bicarbonate as such. The enzymes of the urea cycle develop during metamorphosis, and the adults dispose of HCO_3^- by ureagenesis. Reptiles achieved independence of an aqueous stage in the life cycle by development of an egg with a covering sufficiently impervious to water to allow incubation in air. This development would have been hindered or prevented by the accumulation of urea during incubation; thus an alternative way of disposing of HCO_3^- was necessary. In this case a different preexisting pathway, that for synthesis of purines, was turned to a new use, with ammonium nitrogen being incorporated into insoluble uric acid. Again the nitrogen functions in the product are strongly acidic and a proton from each NH_4^+ ion is liberated to prevent alkalosis. Birds, which also pass the embryonic stage in an impervious egg, have retained the use of uric acid as the means of obtaining protons from NH_4^+. (Insects independently evolved the ability to obtain protons from the conversion of NH_4^+ to uric acid, and spiders and other arachnids similarly use purine synthesis, but stop at guanine as the disposal product.) The evolution of a life cycle in which the embryo develops within the body of the mother allowed mammals to revert to the use of ureagenesis for this purpose.

In summary, we propose that: (1) Protein metabolism liberates HCO_3^- in amounts much larger than the sum of available metabolic acids. (2) Bicarbonate cannot be eliminated as such in the necessary amounts through the lungs, kidneys, or intestines. (3) The air-breath-

ing way of life therefore appears to be possible only if metabolic energy is used to incorporate NH_4^+ ion into a compound in which a proton is obtained from each nitrogen function for titration of HCO_3^-. (4) The choice of which synthesis to use depends on the life cycle and life style of the organism, but all or nearly all air-breathing animals use ATP energy in specific disposal syntheses that have the result that proton is derived from NH_4^+ ion for use in the disposal of metabolic HCO_3^-. Most of these concepts are discussed in greater detail in an earlier article[1].*

Man, like other omnivores and carnivores, excretes a small amount of NH_4^+ in the urine, typically about 2–5% as much as the nitrogen excreted as urea. This apparent slight excess of NH_4^+ is surprising, since it seems clear that the

---

*Some of the points in that article are reiterated in a recent paper by Halperin and Jungas[2]. We feel, however, that they obscure a major point by following the common practice of writing an overall equation for conversion of amino acids to urea as if that were an integrated pathway. A metabolic pathway is a sequence of reactions that together effect a conversion that is advantageous for the cell or organism. Examples are regeneration of ATP, synthesis of an amino acid, storage of carbon and energy as fat or glycogen, and disposal of a waste product. The concept of a pathway is, we feel, meaningful only in terms of function. The functionally useful products of amino acid catabolism are ATP and intermediates for biosyntheses such as lipogenesis and glycogenesis. Ureagenesis is functionally useful not because it furnishes urea, but because it disposes of bicarbonate (and ammonium). It is not meaningful to treat two such different sequences, with such disparate functions, as if they were a single pathway. Aerobic protein metabolism necessarily produces HCO_3^- and NH_4^+ in all organisms capable of such metabolism. In a separate and discrete pathway these degradation products are removed by conversion to urea in some air-breathing species. Other conversions serve the same function in other species. Treating ureagenesis as if it were an integral and necessary aspect of protein metabolism obscures important physiological relationships and ignores an important chapter of evolutionary metabolic adaptation.

primary rate of metabolic production of bicarbonate in the metabolism of almost any normal human diet will be greater than the rate of production of ammonium ion. Ammonium and bicarbonate are produced in almost exactly equal amounts in protein metabolism, and that is by far the major source of NH_4^+. But the salts of carboxylic acids that are abundant in most kinds of plant materials will lead to bicarbonate. It appears that mammals are able to deal with a larger amount of HCO_3^- than the amount of NH_4^+ that is available directly from catabolism. We propose that part of the available NH_4^+ is recycled and used twice in the disposal of HCO_3^-. A recent review[3], comparing results from several laboratories, estimates that about one-quarter of the urea produced is excreted into the gut, where it is quantitatively hydrolysed to NH_4^+ and HCO_3^-. Nearly all of the liberated NH_4^+ is taken back into the blood, presumably at least in part by an active process[4] since the pH gradient would not favor passive diffusion. How much of the liberated HCO_3^- is reabsorbed remains to be established. To the extent that NH_4^+ is absorbed in larger amount than HCO_3^-, the excess is available to supply the protons needed for the disposal of additional HCO_3^-. The obvious importance of this process suggests the possibility that the secretion of urea into the gut or the reabsorption of NH_4^+ or HCO_3^- is regulated so as to provide an adequate amount of recycled NH_4^+ for pH homeostasis.

Regulation of bicarbonate disposal

In order to stabilize body pH it is not enough to dispose of CO_2 and HCO_3^-; the rates of removal of these waste products must be regulated so as to maintain a constant ratio of their concentrations. Regulation of respiration to hold the concentration of CO_2 in blood at 1.2 mM has been much studied and will not be discussed here. Equally important is the coordinate control of the rate of ureagenesis, by which HCO_3^- is disposed of in the liver. Urea is the disposal product that is formed as a means of making the protons of NH_4^+ available for removal of HCO_3^-; glutamine is the form into which nitrogen is packaged for transport, for example to the kidney. From the concepts discussed in the preceding section, it follows that much of the control of the rate of disposal of HCO_3^- may be considered to depend on the partitioning of the nitrogen that is available to the liver between urea and glutamine. As much NH_4^+ as is needed for pH homeostasis will be converted to urea and the remainder converted to (or left as) glutamine. Thus as the pH rises, the incorporation of NH_4^+ into urea should increase in order to remove HCO_3^- from the blood buffer. The rate of glutamine synthesis should decrease and may become negative; that is, there may be net removal of glutamine from the blood. When the pH tends to fall, less urea need be made, and the excess NH_4^+, in the form of glutamine, can be diverted to the kidney where some of the nitrogen will be excreted as NH_4^+ in the urine. As discussed below, ammonium ion in the urine does not represent excretion of acid[1,2,5].

The changes in relative rates of ureagenesis and net synthesis of glutamine that are to be expected on the basis of these concepts have been observed in several laboratories. A decrease in the rate of urea synthesis in rat liver resulted from conditions simulating respiratory acidosis[6], with the concentration of HCO_3^- held constant. The net rate of glutamine synthesis by perfused rat liver decreased with an increase in pH (Ref. 7). Perfused rat liver supplied glutamine to the perfusate at pH 7.15 but not at 7.45, and the rate of urea synthesis was greater at the higher pH (Ref. 8). In perfused rat muscle a decrease in pH caused an increase in glutamine release[6].

Normalizing these results and those obtained with perfused liver to the whole body, it was calculated that the values for the increase in glutamine synthesis and the decrease in urea synthesis resulting from decreased pH were within about 10% of each other. When HCl, NH_4Cl and NH_4HCO_3 were administered to man[9] and rat[10], the results were in general agreement with the concepts presented here: HCl caused reduction in urea excretion and increase in NH_4^+, as expected because removal of HCO_3^- by titration leaves less to be disposed of by urea synthesis; NH_4Cl caused an increase in NH_4^+ excretion with little effect on urea production; and NH_4HCO_3 caused an increase in urea synthesis with little effect on NH_4^+ excretion, as expected because this salt mimics protein in supplying both a bicarbonate load and the amount of ammonium ion needed for its disposal. The rate of urea synthesis by perfused liver and by hepatocytes increased with increased pH but was not affected by the absolute concentrations of HCO_3^- and CO_2 (Ref. 11). As previously observed, the rate of urea synthesis increased with an increase in the concentration of NH_4^+ when lactate (a bicarbonate-producing substrate) was supplied. Remarkably, however, the rate decreased with increased ammonium concentration when glucose or no exogenous substrate was supplied[11]. This result seems incompatible with the accepted view that the primary function of ureagenesis is elimination of NH_4^+.

The functional relationships discussed here are reflected in the histological localization of enzymes in the liver (see Ref. 12 and next article in this book).

Relation to accepted views

The concepts expressed here differ in several respects from the views that are presented in most textbooks and monographs. In their most condensed form, the accepted views consist of two assertions about stoichiometry – that metabolism of protein produces acid and that ammonium ion in the urine represents excretion of acid – and the regulatory corollary that the kidneys control the urinary excretion of ammonium to remove the necessary number of protons from the blood buffers and maintain pH homeostasis. In this view the concentration of bicarbonate ion is regulated primarily by the kidney, and it is therefore the kidney that, in cooperation with the respiratory control system, is responsible for pH homeostasis. We disagree with each of these points.

The belief that metabolism of protein yields acid is usually supported by the fact that part of the sulfur from cysteine and methionine is oxidized to sulfuric acid. However, as pointed out earlier in this article and in more detail in Appendix A of a previous paper[1], the protons liberated in the metabolism of protein can titrate only a small fraction of the HCO_3^- that is produced from the same protein. Consideration of balanced ionic equations, such as equation 4, shows that metabolism of protein necessarily produces a large net yield of HCO_3^-, and hence a threat of alkalosis.

The prevailing view with regard to urinary NH_4^+ was expressed clearly by Hills[13]:

> Every urinary NH_4^+ contains a proton which was detached from combination with some base in extracellular fluid; and since virtually all urinary ammonia is present as NH_4^+, urinary total ammonium excretion represents, to a very near approximation, protons transferred out of extracellular fluid . . .

This belief evidently stems from the fact that NH_4^+ is the conjugate acid of the NH_4^+/NH_3 system. Hills' comment would be true if NH_3 were injected or otherwise introduced into the body. Being a relatively strong base, it would abstract protons from body buffers. But most metabolic NH_4^+ arises from metabolism of protein. Hydrolysis of protein yields dipolar amino acids without net consumption or liberation of protons.

The nitrogen is already protonated; from the standpoint of nitrogen chemistry, the amino acid is an alkyl-substituted ammonium ion. The proton is retained when the C–N bond is cleaved. Thus nitrogen is liberated in protein metabolism almost entirely as NH_4^+ ion, and if it appears as NH_4^+ ion in urine it cannot have gained any protons along the way or have had any effect on acid–base balance.

Since protein metabolism does not lead to a net yield of protons that must be excreted to maintain pH homeostasis, and since excretion of NH_4^+ does not represent excretion of proton, the accepted role of the kidney in acid-base balance seems to be impossible. We propose that regulation of the rate of disposal of HCO_3^- by the liver is coordinate with regulation of the rate of CO_2 elimination through the lungs, and that the response of each primarily to pH underlies the well-established phenomena of metabolic compensation (adjustment of the HCO_3^- concentration up or down from its normal level as needed if the CO_2 concentration varies from 1.2 mM) and respiratory compensation (similar adjustment of CO_2 concentration if the level of HCO_3^- varies from 24 mM), which minimize the variations in pH if the system regulating the concentration of either CO_2 or HCO_3^- is stressed beyond its capacity.

It is generally believed that the function of ureagenesis is the disposal of ammonia, and that the rate of urea synthesis responds primarily to the amount of ammonia that must be eliminated. It is clear that urea synthesis does remove NH_4^+. It should, however, be noted that, although the daily excretion of one mol of HCO_3^-, as such, in urine would be impossible, no such bar exists in the case of NH_4^+. At a urine pH of 4.4, the concentration of NH_4^+ in urine would be 1 000 times the blood concentration at equilibrium. If one mol of NH_4^+ were excreted daily in one liter of urine, the equilibrium concentration of NH_4^+ in blood would be about 1 mM. Thus a relatively small concentration gradient (maintained, for example, by active secretion) would suffice to hold the blood ammonium concentration at acceptable levels. It seems unlikely that the need to dispose of NH_4^+ could have provided the selective pressure for development of urea synthesis.

In accord with these considerations, the experimental results referred to in the preceding section suggest that the rate of ureagenesis is regulated primarily in response to the need to dispose of HCO_3^-. This type of control might have been predicted by analogy with the regulation of respiration. Breathing serves two essential functions: disposal of CO_2 and acquisition of oxygen. It has long been recognized that respiration is controlled primarily in response to the need to eliminate CO_2. That control pattern is easily rationalized, since small variations in the concentration of CO_2 would affect pH and have much more serious consequences than small variations in the concentration of oxygen. Similarly, small changes in the concentration of HCO_3^- would be more deleterious than small variations in the level of NH_4^+. Maintenance of pH homeostasis is among the most fundamental and most serious problems faced by an organism, and it is not surprising that in the evolution of air-breathing vertebrates the rates of disposal of CO_2 and HCO_3^- should have come to be controlled by pH, and to have regulatory priority, under ordinary conditions, over their respective concomitant functions, the oxygenation of blood and the elimination of NH_4^+.

References

1 Atkinson, D. E. and Camien, M. N. (1982) *Curr. Top. Cell. Regulation* 21, 261–302
2 Halperin, M. L. and Jungas, R. L. (1983) *Kidney International* 24, 709–713

3 Walser, M. (1980) *Kidney International* 17, 709–721

4 Mossberg, S. M. (1967) *Amer. J. Physiol.* 213, 1327–1330

5 Bourke, E. (1977) *Irish J. Med. Sci.* 146, 119–129

6 Oliver, J., Koelz, A. M., Costello, J. and Bourke, E. (1977) *Eur. J. Clin. Invest.* 7, 445–449

7 Häussinger, D., Akerboom, T. P. M. and Sies, H. (1980) *Hoppe-Seylers Z. Physiol. Chem.* 361, 995–1001

8 Lueck, J. D. and Miller, L. L. (1970) *J. Biol. Chem.* 245, 5491–5497

9 Fine, A., Carlyle, J. E. and Bourke, E. (1977) *Eur. J. Clin. Invest.* 7, 587–589

10 Oliver, J. and Bourke, E. (1975) *Clin. Sci. Mol. Med.* 48, 515–520

11 Bean, E. S. and Atkinson, D. E. (1984) *J. Biol. Chem.* 259, 1552–1559

12 Häussinger, D. (1983) *Eur. J. Biochem.* 133, 269–275

13 Hills, A. G. (1973) *Acid–Base Balance*, Williams and Wilkins

Daniel E. Atkinson is at the Department of Chemistry and Biochemistry, University of California, Los Angeles, CA 90024, USA and Edmund Bourke is at the Department of Medicine, Emory University School of Medicine, Atlanta, GA 30303, USA.

Hepatic role in pH regulation:

role of the intercellular glutamine cycle

Dieter Häussinger, Wolfgang Gerok and Helmut Sies

Hepatic urea formation removes bicarbonate (not CO_2), arising from the breakdown of the α-carboxylates of amino acids, in amounts stoichiometric with NH_4^+. Excess NH_4^+ is transported via the bloodstream to the kidney in the form of glutamine, there to be degraded by renal glutaminase and excreted via the tubules. By intricate intercellular compartmentation in the liver of a more periportal localization of urea synthesis and glutaminase, the regulation of hepatic glutaminase provides a major point of pH control in the organism. In acidosis, both these processes are shut off, decreasing bicarbonate removal, favoring hepatic glutamine formation by the perivenously located glutamine synthetase, and causing increased renal excretion of NH_4^+ instead of urea. The converse holds in alkalosis. Thus, a hepatic intercellular glutamine cycle between periportal and perivenous cells of the lobule serves a regulatory function in the pH homeostasis of the organism.

Maintenance of pH homeostasis in higher organisms requires mechanisms to stabilize the HCO_3^-/CO_2 ratio in the blood. While CO_2 and water are the only products of the complete oxidation of carbohydrates and fat, it is important to note that the oxidation of amino acids at physiological pH will also yield HCO_3^- and NH_4^+. Air-breathing animals can excrete volatile CO_2 from their lungs, but not HCO_3^-. The kidney, with a limited volume of urine, cannot remove a daily HCO_3^- production of about one mol (in a man metabolizing 100 g of dietary protein per day). As pointed out by Bourke and co-workers[1,2] and by Atkinson and Camien[3], the major pathway for disposal of HCO_3^- is hepatic urea synthesis which consumes two mol of HCO_3^- and two mol of NH_4^+ per mol urea formed:

$$HCO_3^- + 2\,NH_4^+ \rightarrow H_2NCONH_2 + H^+ + 2\,H_2O$$
$$HCO_3^- + H^+ \rightleftharpoons H_2O + CO_2$$

$$2\,HCO_3^- + 2\,NH_4^+ \rightarrow H_2NCONH_2 + CO_2 + 3\,H_2O$$

Whereas NH_4^+ removal by urea synthesis thus implies the stoichiometric utilization of HCO_3^-, the removal of NH_4^+ by glutamine synthesis does not, and such NH_4^+ would be excreted under the influence of renal glutaminase. Therefore, regulatory means which determine the route of NH_4^+ fixation by synthesis of either urea or glutamine are required, and the problem of pH regulation focuses on bicarbonate removal rather than acid removal.

Intercellular glutamine cycle

Recent studies on the interactions of the NH_4^+, urea and glutamine in the functionally and structurally intact perfused rat liver, revealed the periportal localization of glutaminase and urea synthesis and the perivenous localization of glutamine synthesis in the liver lobule[4]. This is in agreement with the immunohistochemical localization of carbamoyl-phosphate synthetase[5] and glutamine synthetase[6]. Further, an intercellular glutamine cycle, resulting from the simultaneous operation of periportal glutamine degradation and perivenous glutamine synthesis, has been demonstrated[4]. With physiological concentrations of portal glutamine and NH_4^+ of 0.6 mM and 0.3 mM, respectively, the rate of this

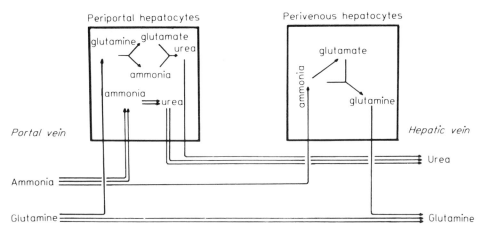

Fig. 1. Role of intercellular glutamine cycle during ureogenesis from portal NH_4^+. The intercellular cycle is seen as a sequence of reactions that take place in distinct cell populations, leading to the regeneration of the initial substrate, glutamine (compare left and right of the Fig.). From Ref. 4.

cycle is 0.15 μmol g^{-1} min^{-1}; this rate is controlled by hormones and pH[7,8]. The role of this intercellular glutamine cycle for almost complete conversion of NH_4^+ is schematically depicted in Fig. 1. Because the removal of NH_4^+ by urea synthesis is restricted to concentrations above 50 μM[4], the glutaminase reaction in the same periportal location feeds in additional substrate for urea synthesis, whereas glutamine is resynthesized in the perivenous area of the liver lobule from NH_4^+ that escaped urea formation. Such a mechanism of complete conversion of portal NH_4^+ into urea, without an accompanying *net* glutamine production by means of intercellular glutamine cycling, reflects the situation obtaining at physiological pH values.

During acidosis, however, which can be induced experimentally simply by infusing HCl, there is a decreased rate of urea formation and increased net glutamine production (Fig. 2a; see also Ref. 2). Such a system should favor pH homeostasis by sparing the HCO_3^- used in urea synthesis. NH_4^+ fixation by glutamine synthesis will then increase, and NH_4^+ will be excreted under the influence of renal glutaminase. This is in line with the finding, in acidosis *in vivo* of an

increased urinary NH_4^+ excretion paralleled by a commensurate fall in urea excretion[9]. Conversely, during metabolic

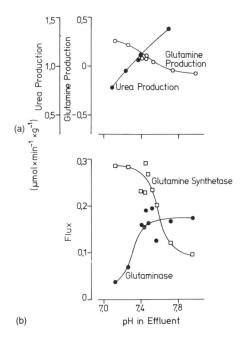

Fig. 2. pH effects on urea and glutamine production (a) and on flux through glutaminase and glutamine synthetase (b) in isolated perfused rat liver. Data points reflect steady state conditions. From Refs 8 and 17.

alkalosis the removal of HCO_3^- is increased by urea formation not only from portal NH_4^+, but also from glutamate and NH_4^+ derived from the portal glutaminase reaction (Fig. 2a), with a consequent decreased net glutamine production which can even become a net uptake.

Switching of glutaminase and glutamine synthetase

The switching of NH_4^+ removal from urea formation to glutamine synthesis in acidosis and, conversely, the increased utilization of portal glutamine for urea formation in alkalosis, is performed by regulation of the intercellular glutamine cycle. There is a strong decrease in glutaminase flux and a simultaneous increase in glutamine synthetase flux in acidosis (Fig. 2b), and vice versa in alkalosis. Thus, the acid–base-induced alterations in urea formation are predominantly due to regulation of the glutaminase reaction which is localized in the same hepatocellular compartment of the liver. However, other factors will also contribute to the decrease in urea formation during acidosis. For example, there are alterations in NH_4^+ distribution between cellular and extracellular compartments as a function of altered pH gradients. Further, in view of the comparatively high $K_m(HCO_3^-)$ of 5.3 mM for carbamoylphosphate synthetase[10], HCO_3^- may become rate-limiting in severe metabolic acidosis[11]. On the other hand, this effect on the rate-limiting enzyme in urea formation is alleviated in part by the slightly acid pH optimum of carbamoylphosphate synthetase[12]. Inhibition of glutaminase during acidosis[8,13,14] is due to an increased $K_a(NH_4^+)$ for glutaminase[15], whereas the simultaneous increase in glutamine synthetase flux might simply be due to an increased NH_4^+ supply as a consequence of the decreased utilization by urea synthesis.

Liver and kidney as a team

This mechanism influencing pH homeostasis by way of NH_4^+ disposal is operational not only during metabolic but also during respiratory pH derangements, because it is the HCO_3^-/CO_2 ratio (via pH) which adjusts the set-point of flux of NH_4^+ into urea or glutamine. This hepatic partitioning also governs the route of final excretion in the kidney. Renal acid excretion by the so-called glutamine mechanism, i.e. the passive diffusion of NH_3 into the tubular lumen and fixation of a proton yielding NH_4^+ has been questioned, because the renal glutaminase reaction produces NH_4^+ instead of NH_3 (Ref. 3). Therefore, the enhancement of renal glutaminase activity in acidosis represents only an adaptation to another route of excess nitrogen excretion, whereas the regulatory decision in pH homeostasis is made in the liver by the control of bicarbonate removal.

The pathogenesis of alkalosis seen in liver disease is explained by the role of the liver in maintaining pH: impaired urea synthesis leads to the accumulation of HCO_3^-. This concept also explains the development of acidosis in animals even after infusion of alkaline ammonium salts[16]: NH_4^+ stimulates urea synthesis and increases the rate of removal of HCO_3^-.

References

1 Oliver, J. and Bourke, E. (1975) Clin. Sci. Mol. Med. 48, 515–520
2 Oliver, J., Koelz, A. M., Costello, J. and Bourke, E. (1977) Eur. J. Clin. Invest. 7, 445–449
3 Atkinson, D. E. and Camien, M. N. (1982) Curr. Top. Cell Regul. 21, 261–302
4 Häussinger, D. (1983) Eur. J. Biochem. 133, 269–275
5 Gaasbeek Janzen, J. W., Moorman, A. F. M., Lamers, W. H., Los, J. A. and Charles, R. (1981) Biochem. Soc. Trans. 9, 279P
6 Gebhardt, R. and Mecke, D. (1983) Embo J. 2, 567–570
7 Häussinger, D. and Sies, H. (1979) Eur. J. Biochem. 101, 179–184
8 Häussinger, D., Gerok, W. and Sies, H. (1983) Biochim. Biophys. Acta 755, 272–278
9 Fine, A., Carlyle, E. and Bourke, E. (1975) Kidney Int. 8, 338–339
10 Guthörlein, G. and Knappe, J. (1969) Eur. J.

Biochem. 8, 207–214

11 Häussinger, D., Weiss, L. and Sies, H. (1975) *Eur. J. Biochem.* 52, 421–431

12 Lusty, C. (1978) *Eur. J. Biochem.* 85, 373–383

13 Lueck, J. D. and Miller, L. L. (1970) *J. Biol. Chem.* 245, 5491–5497

14 Häussinger, D., Akerboom, T. P. M. and Sies, H. (1980) *Hoppe-Seylers Z. Physiol. Chem.* 361, 995–1001

15 Verhoeven, A. J., Van Iwaarden, J. F., Joseph, S. K. and Meijer, A. J. (1983) *Eur. J. Biochem.* 133, 241–244

16 Eiseman, B. and Clark, G. M. (1958) *Surgery* 43, 476–485

17 Sies, H. and Häussinger, D. (1984) in *Glutamine Metabolism in Mammalian Tissues* (Häussinger, D. and Sies, H., eds), pp. 78–97, Springer-Verlag

D. Häussinger and W. Gerok are at the Medizinische Universitätsklinik, Freiburg, FRG. H. Sies is at Institut für Physiologische Chemie I, Universität Düsseldorf, FRG.

Protein kinases in signal transduction

Yasutomi Nishizuka

The biochemical basis of signal transduction across the cell membrane has long been a subject of great interest. The current excitement on protein kinases is focused on a wide variety of extracellular signals which induce phosphorylation of many cellular proteins.

The covalent attachment of phosphate to either seryl or threonyl residues of proteins was first identified by F. Lipmann and P. A. Levene in 1932. The importance of such modifications of proteins in cellular regulation was recognized as early as the 1950s by a series of studies developed by many investigators such as E. W. Sutherland, E. G. Krebs, E. Fischer and J. Larner who clarified the role of reversible phosphorylation in the control of several key enzymes in glycogen metabolism. In the late 1960s E. G. Krebs[1] discovered cAMP-dependent protein kinase (protein kinase A) and its definitive role in signal transduction. Around 1976, when the first issue of *TIBS* was published, several important investigations on protein kinases were started. In April 1978 R. L. Erickson[2] announced from Denver that the *src* gene product is a protein kinase; this was subsequently identified as a tyrosine-specific protein kinase by T. Hunter (1980)[3].

In parallel with these investigations, the studies on inositol phospholipids and receptor functions were initiated by M. R. Hokin and L. E. Hokin in the early 1950s. When inositol phospholipids are degraded, Ca^{2+} is mobilized simultaneously. In 1975, R. H. Michell postulated that this phospholipid breakdown might open the Ca^{2+} gate. At that time, it was becoming clearer from work carried out in Brussels and Nashville that Ca^{2+} is an even more important intracellular mediator in hormone actions

such as hepatic glycogenolysis by α-agonists, angiotensin II and vasopressin (H. G. Hers, 1977; H. de Wulf, 1977; J. H. Exton, 1977). Incidentally, myosin light chain kinase (K. Yagi, 1977; D. J. Hartshorne, 1977), phosphorylase kinase (P. Cohen, 1978) and a species of brain protein kinase (P. Greengard, 1978) were found to be calmodulin-enzymes. These enzymes were previously known to require Ca^{2+}, but the idea that several protein kinases are regulated by a common protein, calmodulin, had been missed for many years (for a review, see Ref. 4).

In 1977, when protein kinase C was first demonstrated in our laboratory as an undefined protein kinase present in many mammalian tissues, the enzyme was activated only by Ca^{2+}-dependent thiol protease and had no obvious role in signal transduction. Later, it was found that the enzyme could also be activated, without proteolysis, by a reversible association with phospholipid in the presence of Ca^{2+}. During the analysis of this protein kinase activation we noticed that the phospholipid prepared from erythrocyte ghosts required Ca^{2+}, while that prepared from brain membranes did not. This difference came from the diacylglycerol that contaminated the brain phospholipid. A small amount of diacylglycerol, one of the primary products of inositol phospholipid breakdown, increased the apparent affinity of protein kinase C for Ca^{2+} dramatically to the 10^{-7} M range, and thereby activated this enzyme without further addition of this divalent cation (Fig. 1). A ubiquitous distribution of this protein kinase in mammalian and other animal tissues was soon confirmed by J. F. Kuo (1980) in Atlanta.

To identify further diacylglycerol as a 'go-between' of protein phosphorylation (American school) and inositol phospholipid turnover (European school), we developed a procedure to activate protein kinase C by applying synthetic diacylglycerols directly to intact cells. Diacylglycerols that have two long-chain fatty acids – such as diolein – could not be readily intercalated into the intact cell membrane. However, by replacing one of the fatty acids with acetyl group, the resulting diacylglycerols such as 1-oleoyl-2-acetyl-glycerol obtained some detergent-like properties, and could be dispersed easily into the phospholipid bilayer to activate protein kinase C directly. In the summer of 1981, we

discussed a possible action of tumour-promoting phorbol esters for protein kinase C, since the tumour promoters have a structure in their molecule very similar to the diacylglycerol we employed. Before long we found that the phorbol esters could activate the enzyme directly as a substitute for diacylglycerol both *in vitro* and *in vivo*. The idea that a protein kinase C–phospholipid complex is the receptor of tumour promoters was presented first at Squaw Valley in March of 1982 (see Ref. 5). This proposal was immediately supported by a number of investigators such as J. E. Niedel (1983) and P. M. Blumberg (1983) who co-purified the phorbol receptor and protein kinase C. Our experiments suggested that, for each molecule of tumour promoters intercalated into the membrane to modify the phospholipid micro-environment, one molecule of protein kinase C moved to it and then produced a quaternary complex of phospholipid,

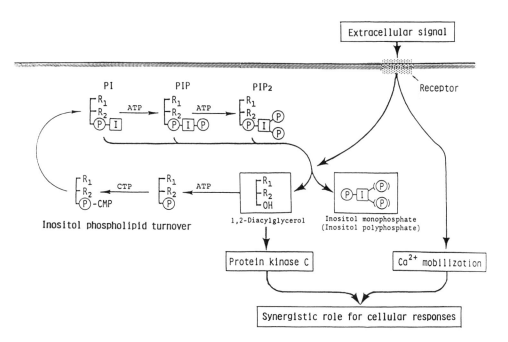

Fig. 1. Synergistic role of Ca^{2+} and protein kinase C for activation of cellular functions and proliferation. PI = phosphatidylinositol; PIP = phosphatidylinositol 4-phosphate; PIP_2 = phosphatidylinositol 4,5-bisphosphate; I = inositol; P = phosphoryl group; R_1 and R_2 = fatty acyl groups.

Ca^{2+}, tumour promoter and protein kinase C, which was fully active for protein phosphorylation (a new concept of the 'mobile receptor')[6]. Indeed, in tissues such as brain, the amount of the phorbol receptor roughly matches the amount of protein kinase C. In physiological processes, it may be that one molecule of diacylglycerol produced from inositol phospholipids in membrane activates one molecule of protein kinase C. If so, four molecules of ATP should be consumed for one molecule of the enzyme activated (Fig. 1). Today, we obviously need new techniques to detect such a tiny change in the membrane, and to measure the precise hydrophobic interactions of lipid and protein.

Although both synthetic diacylglycerol and phorbol ester could fully activate protein kinase C, the release of serotonin from platelets was always incomplete. This raised the question of the relative importance of Ca^{2+} mobilization and protein kinase C activation, both of which are evoked by an extracellular signal such as thrombin. We already knew that, for physiological activation, protein kinase C was dependent on diacylglycerol but not on Ca^{2+}. Thus, we know that these two routes, by which information flows from the cell surface into the cell interior, can be opened selectively by a Ca^{2+} ionophore such as A-23187 and synthetic diacylglycerol or tumour promoter (Fig. 2).

On the way back from a Gordon Conference on Hormone Action in August 1982, I found myself seated next to H. Rasmussen on a non-stop PANAM flight from New York to Tokyo. Perhaps, it was the longest conversation on Ca^{2+} in my life! We were both extremely excited about 'calcium sensitivity modulation'; the sensitivity of platelet serotonin secretion to Ca^{2+} was greatly increased by the activation of protein kinase C. At the Royal Society meeting in London, organized by S. V. Perry and P. Cohen in December of 1982, we presented a synergistic role of Ca^{2+} and protein kinase C for the activation of cellular functions[7]. These two routes may exert differential control over different processes within a single activated cell. It is known for platelets, for instance, that the release reactions from different granules show different sensitivities to thrombin, even though all the release reactions show a similar sensitivity to Ca^{2+} concentrations (D. E. Knight and M. C. Scrutton, 1982). The synergistic role of the two routes was not confined to platelets, but also extended to mast cells and neutrophils for their exocytosis[7]. This proposal was soon supported by D. E. Knight and P. F. Baker (1983)[8] in London for catecholamine release from adrenal medullary cells, and by H. Rasmussen (1983)[9,10] in New Haven for aldosterone secretion from adrenal glomerulosa cells as well as for insulin release from pancreatic islets. By using an intracellular Ca^{2+}-indicator, quin-2, T. J. Rink (1983)[11] in Cambridge later confirmed that serotonin could be released partly from platelets without significant increase of Ca^{2+} when protein kinase C was activated. The synergistic role of the two routes is supported also by J. C. Garrison (1984)[12] in Charlottesville and subsequently by J. N. Fain (1984)[13] in Rhode Island by demonstrating that hepatic glycogenolysis can be provoked by simultaneous addition of Ca^{2+}-ionophore and phorbol ester. J. C. Garrison finds that the opening of these two routes in this way causes the phosphorylation of a full set of the polypeptides that can be phosphorylated by a single extracellular signal such as angiotensin II or vasopressin. The 'synergistic role of Ca^{2+} and protein kinase C' or 'Ca^{2+} sensitivity modulation' is important also for cell proliferation. Using macrophage-depleted lymphocytes treated with phytohemagglutinin, we can show that Ca^{2+} mobilization and protein kinase C activation act synergistically for their growth response[14].

The mechanism of increase in intracellular Ca^{2+} remains unclear. Originally, phosphatidylinositol was regarded as a prime target, but it now becomes clearer that phosphatidylinositol bisphosphate is degraded immediately after stimulation of the receptor (for a review, Ref. 15). In the meetings at Zeist in September of 1983 and at Dallas in January of 1984, M. J. Berridge in Cambridge elicited a discussion on a possible role of inositol 1,4,5-trisphosphate, the other product of the phospholipid breakdown (J. N. Hawthorne, 1977), for the mobilization of Ca^{2+} from its intracellular reservoir (see Ref. 16). This exciting possibility is currently examined further by many investigators, such as H. Streb in Frankfurt, J. Putney in Richmond, J. Williamson in Philadelphia and J. H. Exton in Nashville. On the other hand, the rise of diacylglycerol concentration in membranes is only transient, and this signal mediator disappears within a minute. It is attractive to imagine that the uncontrollable production of an active form of protein kinase C, of either cellular or viral origin, may promote oncogenesis just like tumour-promoting phorbol esters do. The tumour promoters cause the permanent activation of this protein kinase, since they are metabolized only slowly. We need to establish the time sequence and turnover rate of each biochemical event successively occurring after stimulation of receptor.

Although there are dramatic heterogeneities and variations in receptor functions, most tissues possess at least two major classes of receptors (Fig. 2). One class triggers cAMP formation, while the other provokes inositol phospholipid turnover, mobilizes Ca^{2+}, releases arachidonic acid and produces cGMP. Arachidonic acid is derived from inositol phospholipids, but in most tissues this fatty acid is released from other phospholipids as well. Some arachidonic acid metabolites such as prostaglandin endoperoxide may serve as activators for guanylate cyclase. Cyclic GMP-dependent protein kinase (protein kinase G), was first found by P. Greengard in 1970[17]. Because of their very similar properties it has been proposed that protein kinases A and G originated from a single ancestral protein (J. D. Corbin, 1977). We have postulated that, in intact platelets, cGMP may constitute an intracellular feedback control that prevents over-response (Refs. 5–7; also R. J. Haslam, 1980). Conversely, in the platelets permeabilized for low molecular substances, cGMP has been proposed to increase their

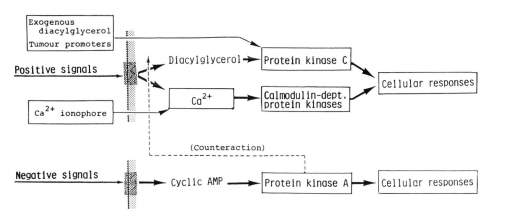

Fig. 2. Transmembrane control of protein kinases in signal transduction.

sensitivity to Ca^{2+} (D. E. Knight and M. C. Scrutton, 1984)[18]. Still, it is possible that one of the functions of cyclic GMP is to decrease intracellular Ca^{2+} concentrations in a manner analogous to cAMP. Nevertheless, we still lack crucial information on the role of cGMP and protein kinase G.

The pleiotropic actions of protein kinase A are now firmly established (see Ref. 19). However, a major role of this protein kinase may be 'counteraction' of the signal-induced activation of cellular functions and proliferation. In some mammalian tissues such as liver, adipose tissue and some endocrine cells (*monodirectional control system*), the two classes of receptors mentioned above appear to function in similar directions. In contrast, in most tissues such as platelets, lymphocytes and some neuronal cells (*bidirectional control system*), cAMP acts 'negatively' rather than 'positively'. The primary target of cAMP appears to be localized in the membrane. It is clear in these tissues that each of receptor-linked events such as inositol phospholipid breakdown, protein kinase C activation, Ca^{2+} mobilization, and arachidonic acid release is all blocked concurrently by an extracellular signal that increases cAMP[5-7]. The molecular basis of this 'counteraction' remains totally unknown. We suspect that this process is not due simply to the direct inhibition of phospholipases by protein kinase A.

An exciting problem is obviously the interaction or cascade of various protein kinases including tyrosine-specific enzymes. This class of enzymes are well known to be associated with the receptors of insulin and other growth-promoting factors such as EGF, PDGF and somatomedin C, and also with certain retroviral oncogene products. Unfortunately, however, no definite information is available as to any function of these protein kinases. At the Cold Spring Harbor meeting on 'The Cancer Cell' in September 1983, a possible cascade from protein kinase C to tyrosine-specific protein kinase was discussed. When cells were stimulated by phorbol ester or diacylglycerol, the amount of cellular phosphoryltyrosine was considerably increased within minutes (M. J. Weber, 1983; G. S. Martin, 1983) (see Ref. 20). However, it was recently suggested that protein kinase C phosphorylates the EGF receptor with a concomitant decrease in its both tyrosine-phosphorylating and EGF-binding activities (T. Hunter, 1984; M. R. Rosner, 1984)[21,22]. Phorbal ester was also shown, in intact cells, to stimulate the phosphorylation of insulin receptor (P. Cuatrecasas, 1983), that has a tyrosine-specific protein kinase activity (C. R. Kahn, 1982). It seems possible on one hand that protein kinase C is involved, directly or indirectly, in 'down-regulation' or 'desensitization' of various receptors, although in a manner as yet uncertain. On the other hand, it is worth noting that tumour promoter and growth factor generally act in concert and synergistically enhance cell proliferation in long term. In fact, the synergistic role of protein kinase C and tyrosine-specific protein kinase is a problem of immediate interest. For insulin, which does not provoke inositol phospholipid turnover, considerable progress has been made on the characterization of its soluble mediators (J. Larner, 1976; L. Jarett, 1979; M. P. Czeck, 1980 – see Ref. 23). However, more information is needed about the transmembrane control of various protein kinases whose intracellular mediators are not elucidated.

We are still far from full understanding of the physiological meaning of an extremely rapid turnover of the phosphate that is covalently linked to protein. However, we do realize that the protein kinases briefly outlined above are on the cross-over point of various pathways for exploring the roles of Ca^{2+}, cAMP, cGMP, diacylglycerol, arachidonic acid and prostaglandins, which all serve as indispensable mediators for signal transduction.

References

1 Walsh, D. A., Perkins, J. P. and Krebs, E. G. (1968) *J. Biol. Chem.* 243, 3763–3765
2 Collett, M. S., and Erickson, R. L. (1978) *Proc. Natl Acad. Sci. USA* 75, 2021–2024
3 Hunter, T. and Sefton, B. M. (1980) *Proc. Natl Acad. Sci USA* 77. 1311–1314
4 Cohen, P. (1982) *Nature* 296, 613–620
5 Nishizuka, Y. (1983) in *Evolution of Hormone-Receptor Systems* (Bradshaw, R. A. and Gill, G. N., eds), pp. 425–439, Alan R. Liss Inc. New York
6 Nishizuka, Y. (1984) *Nature* 308, 693–697
7 Nishizuka, Y. (1983) *Phil. Trans. R. Soc. Lond.* B 302, 101–112
8 Knight, D. E. and Baker, P. E. (1983) *FEBS Lett.* 160, 98–100
9 Kojima, I., Lippes, H., Kojima, K. and Rasmussen, H. (1983) *Biochem. Biophys. Res. Commun.* 116, 555–562
10 Zwalich, W., Brown, C. and Rasmussen, H. (1983) *Biochem. Biophys. Res. Commun.* 117, 448–455
11 Rink, T. J., Sanchez, A. and Hallam, T. J. (1983) *Nature* 305, 317–319
12 Garrison, J. C., Johnsen, D. E. and Campanile, C. P. (1984) *J. Biol. Chem.* 259, 3283–3292
13 Fain, J. N., Li, S.-Y., Litosch, I. and Wallace, M. (1984) *Biochem. Biophys. Res. Commun.* 119, 88–94
14 Kaibuchi, K., Sawamura, M., Katakami, Y., Kikkawa, U., Takai, Y. and Nishizuka, Y. (1985) in *Inositol and Phosphoinositides* (Bleasdale, J. E., Eichberg, J. and Hauser, J., eds) Humana Press
15 Downes, P. and Michell, R. H. (1982) *Cell Calcium* 3, 467–502
16 Streb, H. D., Irvine, R. F., Berridge, M. J. and Schulz, I. (1983) *Nature* 306, 67–69
17 Kuo, J. F. and Greengard, P. (1970) *J. Biol. Chem.* 245, 2493–2498
18 Knight, D. E. and Scrutton, M. C. (1984) *Nature* 309, 66–68
19 Rosen, O. M. and Krebs, E. G., eds (1981) *Protein Phosphorylation, Cold Spring Harbor Conf. Cell Prolif. Vol. 8*, Cold Spring Harbor Laboratory
20 Levine, A. J., Topp, W. C., Vande Woude, G. F. and Watson, J. D. eds (1984) *The Cancer Cell, Cold Spring Harbor Conf. Cell Prolif. Vol. 11*, Cold Spring Harbor Laboratory
21 Cochet, C. C., Gill, G. N., Meisenhelder, J., Cooper, J. A. and Hunter, T. (1984) *J. Biol. Chem.* 259, 2553–2558
22 Friedman, B., Frackelton, A. R., Ross, A. H., Connors, J. M., Fujiki, H., Sugimura, T. and Rosner, M. R. (1984) *Proc. Natl Acad. Sci. USA* 81, 3034–3038
23 Larner, J., Cheng, K., Schwartz, C., Kikuchi, K., Tamura, S., Creacy, S., Dubler, R., Galasko, G., Pullin, C. and Katz, M. (1982) *Fed. Proc.* 41, 2724–2729

Yasutomi Nishizuka is at the Department of Biochemistry, Kobe University School of Medicine, Kobe 650, and Department of Cell Biology, National Institute for Basic Biology, Okazaki 444, Japan.

cAMP-dependent protein kinases: conformational changes during activation

Jürgen Hoppe

cAMP-dependent protein kinases are activated by dissociation of the inactive holo-enzyme into two dissimilar subunits. Structural and conformational changes in the nucleotide binding sites located on the regulatory subunit and the catalytic subunit are reviewed here.

When certain hydrophilic hormones such as adrenaline or glucagon make contact with the receptor on the surface of their target cells, adenylate cyclase is activated to catalyse the formation of the 'second messenger' cAMP within the cell. It is generally assumed that in higher organisms cAMP exerts its action solely by activating protein kinases, enzymes which are able to catalyse the transfer of the γ-phosphoryl from ATP to hydroxyl groups of serine, threonine or tyrosine in proteins or peptides (for review see Refs 1 and 2).

Stoichiometry and cooperativity in the activation process

There are two principal classes of iso-enzymes, called type I and type II on the basis of their elution from DEAE-cellulose. Both isoenzymes are tetrameric proteins and cAMP activates the kinase by dissociating the inactive holoenzymes into the dimeric cAMP-binding subunit R_2 and two monomeric catalytic sub-units[1,2]. The catalytic subunits of the two isoenzymes are very similar, as revealed by peptide mapping[3]. The two regulatory subunits, however, are distinct entities[3]. They differ most obviously in their behaviour towards ATP. In the presence of ATP the catalytic subunits transfer one phosphoryl residue from ATP into each monomeric type II regulatory subunit in an intra-molecular reaction. The autophosphorylation site

shown in Fig. 1 reveals striking similarities to sequences of other substrates of the kinase[4].

Type I regulatory subunit is not auto-phosphorylated, but instead the type I holoenzyme binds ATP with an unusually high affinity of about 50 nM. This occurs because (as shown in Fig. 1) the serine residue which is autophos-phorylated in the type II regulatory sub-unit is replaced by an alanine in type II[5].

The activation of both types of kinases may be described by the formula

$$R_2C_2 + 4 \text{ cAMP} \rightleftharpoons R_2(\text{cAMP})_4 + 2C$$

The stoichiometry of four molecules of cAMP bound to one dimeric regulatory subunit (type I or type II) has now been established by many laboratories[6–9]. The definitive proof came from sequence analysis of the type II regulatory subunit which revealed two homologous regions similar to the cAMP-binding site in the catabolite gene-activating protein from *E. coli* (CAP)[4,10].

The affinity of protein kinase for cAMP depends on the concentrations of the enzyme and NaCl concentration. Under physiological conditions (protein kinase concentration of 0.2–0.7 μM) the dissociation constant of cAMP is ~ 10^{-8}M[11,12]. The affinity between the regulatory subunit and the catalytic sub-unit has been reported to be 0.2–0.6 nM. When cAMP binds to the regulatory subunit(s) this high affinity is lowered by a factor of 10 causing complete dissociation of the subunits. Under physiological conditions, protein kinase activation obeys apparent positive cooperativity and is linearly coupled to cAMP binding. Hill coefficients (h) of 1.6–1.8 were found[9,13]. This cooperativity is mediated by cooperative binding of cAMP to the regulatory subunit and apparent cooperative release of the catalytic subunits[12].

Several pieces of evidence have now been gathered which demonstrate that cAMP activates the protein kinase by forming an intermediate ternary complex of nucleotide and holoenzyme before dissociation of the two different subunits. Despite the inherent diffi-culties in the isolation of such a ternary complex, it is clear that the regulatory subunit can interact with the catalytic subunit in the presence of dissociating amounts of cAMP. In the case of type II isoenzyme, the catalytic subunit is still capable of phosphorylating the cAMP regulatory subunit complex[1]. The reactivity of the essential thiol in the catalytic subunit (cysteine-199) is modulated by the regulatory subunit of type II in the presence of 0.5 mM cAMP, indicating an interaction of the two subunits in a ternary complex of R_2C_2 (cAMP)$_n$ (Ref. 14). Such interactions are also indicated by experiments which show that the presence of the C-subunit stimulates the rate of dissociation of ^{3}H-cAMP from

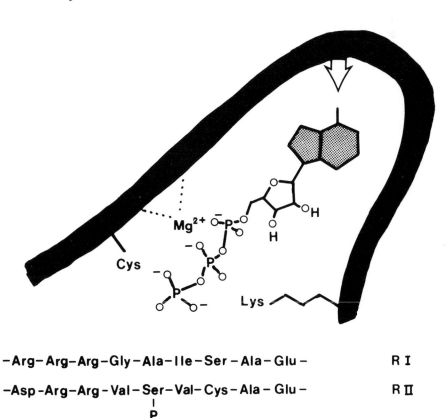

-Arg-Arg-Arg-Gly-Ala-Ile-Ser-Ala-Glu-   R I

-Asp-Arg-Arg-Val-Ser-Val-Cys-Ala-Glu-   R II
                      |
                      P

Fig. 1. A model for the structure of the catalytic site. The arrow indicates a hydrogen bond to the N^6 position of the ATP which is observed in the ATP site of the catalytic subunit as well as in the ATP site of the holoenzyme[25]. Lys-72 and Cys-199 were identified by affinity labeling techniques[26,30]. The two sequences are the hinge regions of type I or type II regulatory subunits interacting with the catalytic subunit[4,5].

the regulatory subunit[15]. Perhaps the most convincing evidence for such a mechanism came from studies on the dissociation and reassociation kinetics of the two subunits from the bovine skeletal muscle type I isoenzyme. The dissociation rate of the catalytic subunit in the absence of cAMP is extremely slow (0.5/h) as compared to the almost immediate activation of the kinase by saturating concentration of cAMP[12]. For a complete dissociation, all four cAMP binding sites must be occupied and all the sites in a dimeric regulatory subunit must interact with each other to generate the high positive cooperativity ($h = 1.8$)[9,12,13]. Interaction of only two sites in a homologous fashion (site 1–site 2) or in a heterologous fashion (site 1–site 1') cannot account for this high cooperativity[16].

cAMP binding domain

A major step in our understanding of the structure and function of cAMP-dependent protein kinase came from the determination of the amino acid sequence of the type II regulatory subunit[4]. Fortunately, at the same time, the crystal structure and amino acid sequence of another cAMP-binding protein (the CAP protein) were determined[10]. There is a clear homology in the sequences of the CAP-protein and two repeated sequences in the regulatory subunit. Fig. 2 shows the basic features of the amino acid sequence of the regulatory subunit. The hydropathy profile (see caption to Fig. 2) indicates similar folding of the two cAMP sites (site 1 and site 2) in the regulatory subunit and the CAP-protein. Note the coincidence of turns in the two sequences. Many residues in contact with cAMP are conserved. These residues interact mainly with the ribose-phosphate moiety of cAMP and are buried in the interior of the protein. Most remarkably, an arginine residue that forms a salt bridge with the negatively charged oxygen of

the phosphate group is conserved. If there are non-conserved residues in contact with cAMP they may be responsible for the different binding specificity of the different sites. For example, in the long α-helix which may interact with cAMP as revealed by its labeling with 8-N$_3$-cAMP[17] in the regulatory subunit type II (Fig. 3) there are no homologous residues between CAP and the regulatory subunit cAMP sites.

In the dimeric structure of the CAP protein the adenine base of cAMP interacts with the long α-helices of both monomers. Even this structural element seems to be preserved in the regulatory subunit type I since the photoaffinity label, 8-N$_3$-cAMP, which bound (non-covalently) only to site 1 upon illumination, crosslinked with peptides of both cAMP sites[18].

Studies with cAMP analogues have shed some light on the specificity and the involvement in the activation process of the two different cAMP sites. The two sites differ dramatically in the exchange rate of bound nucleotides. The dissociation rate for ^{3}H-cAMP is approximately 0.025–0.050/min for site 1 and 0.23–0.26/min for site 2[1]. When bound to the slowly exchanging site 1, cAMP is retained under standard assay conditions using nitrocellulose filtration. However, to detect binding to site 2, histone or excess catalytic subunit must be included in the assay mixture, or an ammonium sulfate precipitation must be carried out. Site 1 has some specificity towards derivatives modified in position C-8 while site 2 tolerates better modifications at the N^6-position[19,20]. Both sites interact with each other but there seems to be a sequential occupation of the sites; site 1 is probably the first occupied[9,21].

Structural changes in the cyclic nucleotide-binding region have been detected by the use of the two diastereoisomers Sp and Rp adenosine cyclic 3',5' phosphorothioate[22]. In these derivatives the negative charge at the phosphoryl group is fixed either in equatorial (Sp) or axial position (Rp). Rp(S)cAMP binds to the regulatory subunit but does not dissociate the holoenzyme, thereby acting as an inhibitor[23]. Sp(S)cAMP binds and activates at concentrations similar to cAMP. It was postulated that cAMP is first recognized by hydrogen bonds to the 5'oxygen, 3'oxygen and 2'hydroxy group. This binding may represent the postulated ternary complexes $R_2C_2(cAMP)_n$ formed prior to the dissociation of the kinase. In a second step, a salt bridge between the equatorial, exocyclic, nega-

tively charged oxygen may be formed with a positively charged amino acid side chain. It is possible that the conserved arginine, which in the case of the CAP protein binds to the phosphoryl group, is this decisive residue. This two-step mechanism may explain the conformational changes in the regulatory ·subunit leading to the dissociation of the catalytic subunit.

Catalytic .domains

Cyclic AMP-dependent protein kinases have a requirement for basic residues at the NH_2-terminal side of the

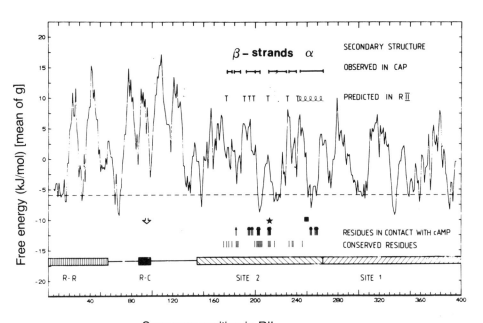

Fig. 2. Properties of the type II regulatory subunit derived from its sequence. The central curve represents a hydropath plot. Hydrophobic constants for the individual amino acid residues are averaged over a segment of nine consecutive residues. Averaged values are then plotted along the amino acid sequence of the protein. Maxima indicate the location of the respective peptide segment at the surface of the protein. Minima indicate segments buried in the interior of the protein. Note the similar profile for the segments site 1 and site 2. There is a general agreement in the folding pattern observed in the CAP protein and predicted for the two cAMP sites in the regulatory subunit. Residues in contact with cAMP in the CAP protein are indicated, as well as conserved residues in these two proteins. For the sake of clarity the analysis is drawn only once for site 2. ★ = position of the invariant arginine residue which binds the cyclophosphate moiety of cAMP; ■ = homologous position of the Tyr-381 which is modified in site 1 by 8-N₃-cAMP; and ⇔ = phosphorylation site in the contact area between regulatory and catalytic subunits.

target serine residue. The sequence around the autophosphorylation site in type II regulatory subunit clearly shows that the regulatory subunit acts as a 'dead-end' substrate[4], i.e. because of its high affinity it remains bound to the active-site of the enzyme. For the type I regulatory subunit, a similar contact region has been determined[5]. Interestingly enough, in this homologous segment the target serine residue is replaced by an alanine, which explains the lack of autophosphorylation in type I regulatory subunit (Fig. 1).

As mentioned above a high-affinity ATP-binding site is generated in the catalytically inactive holoenzyme type I. Affinity labeling with $\gamma[^{32}P]8N_3$-ATP showed this site to be located in the catalytic subunit[24]. The extent of binding was correlated with inhibition of enzyme activity, indicating that the high-affinity ATP-binding site and the ATP-binding site in the catalytic subunit share common binding domains in the catalytic subunit. When the two ATP sites were mapped with a set of different ATP analogues, the adenine binding sites appeared to be identical[25].

The activation process, i.e. conformational changes in the catalytic domain, has been extensively monitored by determining the reactivity of the thiol of cysteine-199 which appears to be located in the active site[26,27]. In the isolated catalytic subunit this thiol is partially protected from the reaction with thiol-modifying reagents by ATP but not by AMP which suggests that it is proximal to the γ-phosphoryl group of ATP. The regulatory subunit provides considerable protection of this residue; complete protection is achieved when ATP and the regulatory subunit are present[28,29].

The following mechanism for inhibition of catalytic activity has now been generally accepted. The hinge regions of the regulatory subunits directly impede the active site of the catalytic subunit.

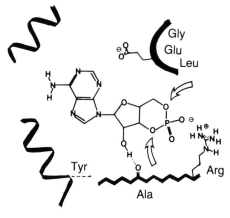

Fig. 3. Possible conformation of the cAMP binding site(s) in type II regulatory subunit. Residues probably in contact with cAMP are indicated by their three-letter codes. Besides Tyr-381 these residues are conserved in the CAP protein (modified from Ref. 10).

For type I this segment provides additional binding residues for interaction with the ribose and phosphate moieties of ATP bound to the catalytic domain; as a consequence the interaction between the subunits is enhanced.

References

1 Flockhart, D. A. and Corbin, J. D. (1982) *Critical Reviews in Biochemistry* 133–186
2 Hoppe, J. and Wagner, K. G. (1979) *Trends Biochem. Sci.* 4, 282–285
3 Zoller, M. J., Kerlavage, A. R. and Taylor, S. S. (1979) *J. Biol. Chem.* 254, 2408–2412
4 Takio, K., Smith, S. B., Krebs, E. G., Walsh, K. A. and Titani, K. (1982) *Proc. Natl Acad. Sci. USA* 79, 2544–2548
5 Potter, R. L. and Taylor, S. S. (1979) *J. Biol. Chem.* 254, 2413–2418
6 Corbin, J. D., Sugden, P. H., West, L., Flockhart, D. A., Lincoln, T. M. and McCarthy, D. (1978) *J. Biol. Chem.* 253, 3997–4003
7 Weber, W. and Hilz, H. (1979) *Biochem. Biophys. Res. Commun.* 90, 1073–1081
8 Builder, S. E., Beavo, J. A. and Krebs, E. G. (1980) *J. Biol. Chem.* 255, 2350–2354
9 deWit, R. J. W. and Hoppe, J. (1981) *FEBS Lett.* 127, 9–12
10 Weber, I. T., Takio, K. and Steitz, T. A. (1982) *Proc. Natl Acad. Sci. USA.* 79, 7679–7683
11 Hofmann, F. (1980) *J. Biol. Chem.* 255, 1559–1564

12 Builder, S. E., Beavo, J. A. and Krebs, E. G. (1980) *J. Biol. Chem.* 255, 3514–3519

13 Øgreid, D. and Døskeland, S. O. (1982) *FEBS Lett.* 150, 161–166

14 Armstrong, R. N. and Kaiser, E. T. (1978) *Biochemistry* 17, 2840–2845

15 Chau, V., Huang, L. C., Romero, G., Biltonen, R. L. and Huang, C, (1980) *Biochemistry* 19, 924–928

16 Swillens, S. (1983) *Eur. J. Biochem.* 137, 581–587

17 Kerlavage, A. R. and Taylor, S. S. (1980) *J. Biol. Chem.* 255, 8483–8488

18 Bubis, J. and Taylor, S. S. (1984) *Fed. Proc.* 43, 1947

19 Robinson-Steiner, A. M. and Corbin, J. D. (1983) *J. Biol. Chem.* 258, 1032–1040

20 Øgreid, D., Døskeland, S. O. and Miller, J. P. (1983) *J. Biol. Chem.* 258, 1041–1049

21 Øgreid, D. and Døskeland, S. O. (1981) *FEBS Lett.* 129, 282–286

22 deWit, R. J. W., Hoppe, J., Stec, W. J., Baraniak, J. and Jastorff, B. (1982) *Eur. J. Biochem.* 122, 95–99

23 Rothermel, J. D., Stec, W. J., Baraniak, J., Jastorff, B. and Botelho, L. H. (1983) *J. Biol. Chem.* 258, 12125–12128

24 Hoppe, J. and Freist, W. (1979) *Eur. J. Biochem.* 93, 141–146

25 Hoppe, J., Friest W., Marutzky, R. and Shaltiel, S. (1978) *Eur. J. Biochem.* 90, 427–432

26 Bramson, H. N., Thomas, N., Matsueda, R., Nelson, N. C., Taylor, S. S. and Kaiser, E. T. (1982) *J. Biol. Chem.* 257, 10575–10581

27 Shoji, S., Ericsson, L. H., Walsh, K. A., Fisher, E. H. and Titani, K. (1983) *Biochemistry* 22, 3702–3909

28 Jiménez, J. S., Kupfer, A., Gani, V. and Shaltiel, S. (1982) *Biochemistry* 21, 1623–1630

29 Kupfer, A., Jiménez, J. S., Gottlieb, P. and Shaltiel, S. (1982) *Biochemistry* 21, 1631–1637

30 Zoller, M. J. and Taylor, S. S. (1979) *J. Biol. Chem.* 254, 8363–8368

J. Hoppe is at the Dept of Cytogenetics, Gesellschaft für Biotechnologische Forschung mbH., Mascheroder Weg 1, D-3300 Braunschweig, FRG.

Renewed interest in the polyphosphoinositides

Stephen K. Fisher, Lucio A. A. Van Rooijen and
Bernard W. Agranoff

The significance of the enhanced cellular phosphatidate and phosphatidylinositol turnover which occurs in response to specific extracellular messengers has been the subject of much interest and speculation. Until recently, much less attention has been paid to the presence of two quantitatively minor phosphorylated derivatives of phosphatidylinositol, known collectively as the polyphosphoinositides. These lipids have an extremely rapid ^{32}P turnover rate and are presumed to be localized predominantly in the plasma membranes. Their turnover now appears to be linked with that of phosphatidate and phosphatidylinositol, and is discussed here in relation to the consequences of ligand–receptor interactions.

Polyphosphoinositides as cell membrane components

Phosphatidylinositol (PhI), as well as two phosphorylated derivatives, phosphatidylinositol 4-phosphate (PhIP) and phosphatidylinositol 4,5-bisphosphate (PhIP$_2$), are found in eukaryotic membranes (see Fig. 1). Because of the highly polar nature of these lipids, their quantitative extraction from tissues usually requires conditions of acidity or high ionic strength, and special thin layer chromatographic procedures are needed for their separation. These two factors may explain much of the past neglect of ligand-stimulated turnover of the polyphosphoinositides. An even more important factor is their rapid resynthesis, such that lipid breakdown can go unnoticed if it is not measured within seconds of ligand addition.

Subcellular distribution and metabolism

PhIP and PhIP$_2$ are synthesized from endogenous PhI via sequential phosphorylation by ATP at the D-4 and D-5 positions of the *myo*-inositol moiety, under the action of specific kinases. In turn, phosphomonoesterases can dephosphorylate PhIP$_2$ to PhIP and PhIP to PhI. The combined effects of the kinases

and monoesterases result in the rapid equilibration of radioactivity in the gamma position of ATP with that of the inositide monoester functions. Alternatively, the entire headgroup of the polyphosphoinositides can be removed via phosphodiesteratic cleavage of the phospholipase C variety to yield the apolar product, diacylglycerol (DAG), together with inositol bis- or trisphosphate from PhIP or PhIP$_2$, respectively. Available information from subcellular fractionation studies suggests that most of the relevant enzymes of polyphosphoinositide metabolism are present in both the plasma membrane and in the cytosol[2]. The ability to form labeled PhIP$_2$ from endogenous PhIP and [γ-^{32}P] ATP is a convenient measure of PhIP kinase, and has been demonstrated in purified plasma membrane preparations, as well as in plasma membrane-enriched tissues, e.g. brain, kidney, polymorphonuclear leukocytes and erythyrocytes[2]. However, PhI kinase and/or PhIP kinase activity has also been documented in adrenal chromaffin granules, mitochondria, lysosomes, Golgi preparations and the nuclear envelope. PhI and PhIP kinases are Mg^{2+}-dependent, while the effects of Mg^{2+}

and Ca^{2+} on the lipid phosphomono-esterase activities appear to vary with the tissue source of the enzyme. There is general agreement that Ca^{2+} ions at millimolar concentrations selectively activate the phosphodiesterase(s), although the optimal concentration appears to depend upon the assay conditions employed. The enzymatic potential for degradation of the polyphosphoinositides in brain exceeds that of synthesis by one or two orders of magnitude, the most active being an apparent 'phospholipase C' phosphodiesteratic activity. Other possible pathways for polyphosphoinositide degradation, for example via phospholipase D or A_2 activity, are minor. It thus appears that the breakdown of polyphosphoinositides via a type C phosphodiesteratic cleavage is likely to be of most physiological significance.

Receptors coupled to polyphosphoinositide turnover

The Hokins first demonstrated that activation of certain receptors (e.g. muscarinic cholinergic or α_1-adrenergic) resulted in increased incorporation of added $^{32}P_i$ into phosphatidate (PhA) and PhI. It was subsequently reported that there was a net loss of PhI upon stimulation with the accumulation of an approximately equivalent amount of PhA[3]. This was thought to arise from an initial phosphodiesteratic breakdown of PhI, liberating DAG which was in turn rapidly rephosphorylated in the presence of $[^{32}P]$ATP to yield $[^{32}P]$PhA. The PhA was then proposed to be converted to PhI via (CDP–DAG)*, completing a 'phosphatidate–phosphatidylinositol cycle' (Fig. 2). The vast number of studies on stimulated incorporation of $^{32}P_i$ into PhA and PhI or of $[^3H]$inositol into PhI are thus several steps away from the presumed site of receptor–ligand action, i.e. phosphodiesteratic cleavage. In an early study, Durell *et*

*CDP–DAG = cytidine diphosphodiacyl glycerol.

al.[4] noted a possible increased production of inositol bisphosphate, under conditions of stimulation of brain homogenate with acetylcholine. Despite this observation, and the known metabolic interrelationships between the inositol lipids, a direct effect of receptor activation on PhIP and PhIP$_2$ turnover was not proposed or examined further until 1977, when Abdel-Latif and colleagues demon-

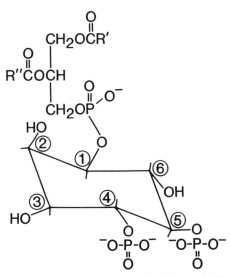

Fig. 1. The structure of phosphatidylinositol 4,5-bisphosphate (PhIP$_2$). Phosphatidylinositol (PhI) is phosphodiesterified at D-1 of myo-inositol, and has no phosphomonoester substituents, while phosphatidylinositol 4-phosphate (PhIP) is phosphorylated only at the D-4 position. PhI, PhIP and PhIP$_2$ are also commonly abbreviated as MPI, DPI and TPI (for mono-, di- and triphosphoinositide). The IUB–IUPAC recommended abbreviations are, respectively, PtdIns, PtdIns4P and PtdIns(4,5)P$_2$. These latter abbreviations, however, have been the subject of some confusion related to their correct structural assignments[1]. In each of the three inositides, the phosphodiesteratically-linked 1,2-diacyl-sn-glycero-3-phosphate is enriched in the 1-stearoyl, 2-arachidonoyl species. The possibility that the inositol lipids serve as a reservoir of arachidonate for prostanoid synthesis has been proposed, although it is not yet clear which inositide or inositide-related lipid is the donor. In this paper, myo-inositol D-1-phosphate, myo-inositol-D-1,4-bisphosphate and myo-inositol-D-1,4,5-trisphosphate are referred to as IP$_1$, IP$_2$ and IP$_3$.

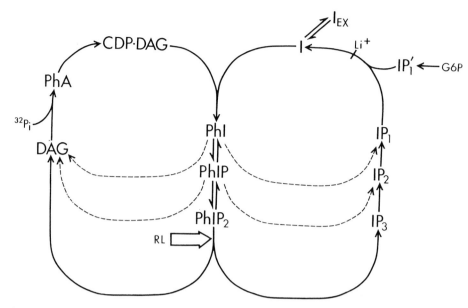

Fig. 2. *Cyclic turnover of inositol lipids. The originally proposed cycle (upper left) of PhI -> DAG -> PhA -> CDP-DAG -> PhI is now extended to include the polyphosphoinositides. While phosphodiesteratic cleavage of PhIP is indicated, there is better evidence for stimulated PhIP$_2$ breakdown following receptor–ligand (RL) activation. The cycle on the right demonstrates the sequential breakdown of IP$_3$ to inositol. The breakdown of IP$_1$ is blocked by Li$^+$. Cellular inositol is supplied exogenously (I$_{ex}$) or produced by degradation of L-myo-inositol phosphate (IP$_i'$) formed via cyclization of glucose-6-phosphate (G6P).*

strated that exposure of the iris smooth muscle to acetylcholine resulted in increased breakdown of ^{32}P-prelabeled PhIP$_2$ (Ref. 5). These experiments, as well as a number of other indirect indications, led to intensified efforts to identify changes in polyphosphoinositides associated with receptor activation. There are by now numerous documented examples of receptor–ligand interaction linked to polyphosphoinositide turnover (Table I). In most instances, this has been measured by loss of polyphosphoinositide radioactivity from [^{3}H]inositol or ^{32}P-prelabeled cells. Such studies indicate that radiolabeled PhIP$_2$, and in some instances PhIP as well, is rapidly diminished following addition of a specific ligand. For example, 20% or more of label in PhIP$_2$ is lost within 5–30 s of exposure of platelets to thrombin, of hepatocytes to vasopressin, or of parotid

gland slices to methacholine. There is evidence in the iris smooth muscle, in platelets, and in blowfly salivary gland for the simultaneous release of inositol trisphosphate, a result consistent with the phosphodiesteratic cleavage of PhIP$_2$ following receptor activation. The rapidity with which the lipid breaks down following ligand addition suggests that the cleavage of PhIP$_2$ rather than of PhI constitutes the initial event following receptor activation and that the disappearance of PhI is a secondary response which reflects the process of replenishment of the depleted polyphosphoinositide pool.

Of potential relevance are recent studies with isolated synaptic membranes. Gispen and colleagues have shown that the addition of adrenocorticotropin (ACTH) to these preparations results in an increase in polyphosphoinositide

Table I. Receptors coupled to polyphosphoinositide turnover in target tissues

Tissue	Receptor	Refs
Iris smooth muscle	Muscarinic cholinergic, α_1-adrenergic	6
Hepatocytes	Vasopressin, angiotensin	7, 8
Parotid gland	Muscarinic cholinergic, α_1-adrenergic, substance P	9, 10
Platelets	Thrombin, ADP, platelet activating factor	11–14
Brain (nerve ending preparations or slices)	Muscarinic cholinergic, ACTH	10, 15, 16
Avian salt gland	Muscarinic cholinergic	17
Blowfly salivary gland	5-HT$_1$	10
Adrenal gland	ACTH	18
Pancreas	Muscarinic cholinergic, caerulein	19

labeling[15]. The effects are interpreted to reflect increased phosphorylation of PhIP to PhIP$_2$. The presumed mechanism is inhibition by ACTH of the phosphorylation of a membrane protein of about M_r 48 000 ('B50') whose phosphorylated form inhibits PhIP kinase. The B50 kinase is thought to be similar or perhaps identical to protein kinase C, found commonly in the cytosol of a number of tissues, particularly brain. While the protein kinase C is isolated from the cytosol and the B50 kinase is membrane-bound, free and bound forms of protein kinase C have been found in cultured cells, and their ratio is reportedly altered by the presence of phorbol esters[20]. ACTH administration, both *in vivo* and *in vitro*, results in a rapid increase in the chemical amounts of both PhIP and PhIP$_2$ in the adrenal, with a time course similar to that reported for corticosterone production[18]. Direct additions of PhIP and PhIP$_2$ to adrenal mitochondria are reported to increase the rate of side chain cleavage of cholesterol to form pregnenolone, a result suggesting that the polyphosphoinositides play a significant role in steroidogenesis.

Calcium and the polyphosphoinositides

Since many receptor–ligand actions that affect polyphosphoinositide turnover exert their physiological effects by increasing intracellular Ca^{2+}, it is not surprising that a direct role for Ca^{2+} in the metabolism of these phospholipids has also been proposed. Central to this issue is the question of whether the increased lipid turnover either (1) is the consequence of an increase in cytosolic Ca^{2+}, (2) mediates the increase in Ca^{2+} permeability, or (3) parallels, but is independent of, Ca^{2+} mobilization. In support of the first possibility is the finding that the breakdown of PhIP$_2$ in iris smooth muscle stimulated by muscarinic cholinergic or α_1-adrenergic receptor activation requires added Ca^{2+}, is abolished in the presence of EGTA or inhibitors of CA^{2+} translocation, and can be induced by the addition of Ca^{2+} ionophores[6]. In hepatocytes, vasopressin stimulation of PhIP$_2$ breakdown is abolished in the presence of EGTA[7]. Furthermore, the introduction of Ca^{2+} into a nerve ending preparation with the divalent cation ionophore A23187 stimulates the breakdown of PhIP and PhIP$_2$, under conditions in which inositol phosphates accumulate[21]. On the other hand, the stimulated breakdown of PhIP$_2$ in the parotid gland, platelet and pancreas appears insensitive to Ca^{2+} depletion, or is at least less so than the attendant physiological responses. This latter result supports the second possibility, namely that PhIP$_2$ breakdown reflects a molecular mechanism whereby cells gate Ca^{2+}, so that increased turnover of PhIP$_2$ is not regulated by the increase in intracellular Ca^{2+}. An alternative explanation is that these cells are not easily depleted of Ca^{2+} in the presence of extracellular EGTA. The various results, taken together, are compatible with the interpretation that polyphosphoinositide turnover is Ca^{2+}-dependent, but may not be Ca^{2+}-regulated.

Because of the known high affinity of polyphosphoinositides for binding Ca^{2+} ions, their plasma membrane localization and potential for rapid degradation upon receptor activation, these lipids have been considered as a possible reservoir of cell Ca^{2+}. It has been demonstrated that the Ca^{2+}-binding activity of erythrocytes increases directly with the state of inositide phosphorylation[22]. Similarly, phosphorylation of renal brush border membrane vesicles results in stimulation of Ca^{2+} intake, with increased phosphoinositide and PhA content[23]. It is less certain, however, that the chemical amounts of Ca^{2+} bound to polyphosphoinositides suffice to account for the increase in cytosolic Ca^{2+} resulting from receptor activation. Calculations of amounts of Ca^{2+} released from PhIP$_2$ in hormone-stimulated hepatocytes indicate that only a small fraction of the measured Ca^{2+} released from these cells could be derived from the polyphosphoinositide pool. In the case of platelets, the calculated amounts of Ca^{2+} released from PhIP$_2$ following ADP addition could, however, account for an increase in intracellular Ca^{2+} by 10 μM[13]. These observations must be tempered by considerations of conditions *in vivo*. For example, these various calculations assume that Ca^{2+} is the sole cation present. Although cytosolic Mg^{2+} is in fact present at greater concentration than Ca^{2+} and binds to the polyphosphoinositides with similar affinity, Mg^{2+}

or Ca^{2+} salts of the polyphosphoinositides probably have different affinities for the enzymes for which they are substrates.

It is alternatively possible that products of phosphoinositide turnover trigger the rise in cell Ca^{2+}. For example, phosphatidate has been shown to have Ca^{2+} ionophore activity, as have arachidonate metabolites. Another candidate is IP$_3$, a product of PhIP$_2$ degradation. Preliminary reports indicate that IP$_3$ can increase Ca^{2+} efflux from cells under specified conditions[24]. In platelets, the physiological response resulting from a rise in intracellular Ca^{2+} can be mimicked by accumulation of DAG, this effect being mediated through activation of protein kinase C (Ref. 25). Thus, the production of both DAG and IP$_3$ may be necessary for expression of a full response. In fact, experimentally-induced increases in intracellular Ca^{2+} and DAG elicit synergistic rather than additive cell responses in the platelet[26].

Inositide turnover in the nervous system

While much of our present knowledge of the polyphosphoinositides has been obtained with non-neural preparations, it is likely that the role of these lipids in the central nervous system will come under increasing scrutiny. Brain contains high concentrations of polyphosphoinositides localized to two distinct pools: a metabolically stable pool associated with myelin and a more labile pool present in neuronal or glial plasma membranes[27]. Nerve ending preparations support a muscarinic cholinergic stimulation of PhA and PhI labeling, which has been localized post-synaptically[28]. Membranes from nerve ending preparations contain Ca^{2+}-activated phosphodiesterase, capable of the rapid degradation of endogenous PhIP$_2$ and PhIP[29]. Although there is evidence for a neurotransmitter-linked effect on PhIP and PhIP$_2$ turnover, direct stimulation of inositol lipid breakdown in the CNS and corresponding release of inositol phosphates is difficult to demonstrate. However, the observation by Allison *et al.*[30] that lithium administration to rats results in an intracerebral accumulation of IP_1, has been successfully exploited *in vitro*. A stimulated release of IP_1 can be detected following the addition of a number of neurohormones to brain slices incubated in the presence of Li^+ (Ref. 31). This effect of Li^+ is believed to be due to an inhibition of the phosphatase that degrades IP_1 (Fig. 2). The increase in IP_1 could result from the phosphodiesteratic cleavage of PhI, but recent evidence favors an initial release of IP_3 (Ref. 10), followed by degradation to IP_1 by phosphatases. Whether this effect of Li^+ can be related to its known psychotherapeutic effects remains an open question. However, its use as an experimental tool can be expected to provide much new information, both in the identification of new neurotransmitter systems which exert their effects through inositol lipid turnover and in the elucidation of the role of polyphosphoinositides in cell–cell communication in the brain.

References

1 Agranoff, B. W. (1978) *Trends Biochem. Sci.* 3, N283–285

2 Michell, R. H. (1975) *Biochim. Biophys. Acta* 415, 81–147

3 Hokin-Neaverson, M. R. (1974) *Biochem. Biophys. Res. Commun.* 58, 763–768

4 Durell, J., Sodd, M. A., Friedel, R. O. (1968) *Life Sci.* 7, 363–368

5 Abdel-Latif, A. A., Akhtar, R. A. and Hawthorne, J. N. (1977) *Biochem. J.* 162, 61–73

6 Abdel-Latif, A. A. (1983) in *Handbook of Neurochemistry*, 2nd Ed., Vol. 3 (Lajtha, A., ed.), pp. 91–131, Plenum Press

7 Rhodes, D., Prpic, V., Exton, J. H. and Blackmore, P. F. (1983) *J. Biol. Chem.* 258, 2770–2773

8 Creba, J. A., Downes, C. P., Hawkins, P. T., Brewster, G., Michell, R. H. and Kirk, C. J. (1983) *Biochem. J.* 212, 733–747

9 Weiss, S. J., McKinney, J. S. and Putney, J. W., Jr (1982) *Biochem. J.* 206, 555–560

10 Berridge, M. J., Dawson, R. M. C., Downes, C. P., Heslop, J. P. and Irvine, R. F. (1983) *Biochem. J.* 212, 473–482

11 Agranoff, B. W., Murthy, P. and Seguin, E. B. (1983) *J. Biol. Chem.* 258, 2076–2078

12 Billah, M. M. and Lapetina, E. G. (1982) *Biochem. Biophys. Res. Commun.* 109, 217–222

13 Vickers, J. D., Kinlough-Rathbone, R. L. and Mustard, J. F. (1982) *Blood* 60, 1247–1249

14 Billah, M. M. and Lapetina, E. G. (1983) *Proc. Natl Acad. Sci.* 80, 965–968

15 Jolles, J., Zwiers, H., Dekker, A., Wirtz, K. W. A. and Gispen, W. H. (1981) *Biochem. J.* 194, 283–291

16 Fisher, S. K. and Agranoff, B. W. (1981) *J. Neurochem.* 37, 968–977

17 Fisher, S. K., Hootman, S. R., Heacock, A. M., Ernst, S. A. and Agranoff, B. W. (1983) *FEBS Lett.* 155, 43–46

18 Farese, R. V., Sabir, A. M., Vandor, S. L. and Larson, R. E. (1980) *J. Biol. Chem.* 255, 5728–5734

19 Putney, J. W., Burgess, G. M., Halenda, S. P., McKinney, J. S. and Rubin, R. P. (1983) *Biochem. J.* 212, 483–488

20 Kraft, A. S. and Anderson, W. B. (1983) *Nature* 301, 621–623

21 Griffin, H. D. and Hawthorne, J. N. (1978) *Biochem. J.* 176, 541–552

22 Buckley, J. T. and Hawthorne, J. N. (1972) *J. Biol. Chem.* 247, 7218–7223

23 Hruska, K. A., Mills, S. C., Khalifa, S. and Hammerman, M. R. (1983) *J. Biol. Chem.* 258, 2501–2507

24 Streb, H., Irvine, R. F., Berridge, M. J. and Schulz, I. *Nature* 306, 67–69

25 Nishizuka, Y. (1983) *Trends Biochem. Sci.* 8, 13–16

26 Michell, R. H. (1983) *Trends Biochem. Sci.* 8, 263–265

27 Eichberg, J. and Hauser, G. (1967) *Biochim. Biophys. Acta* 144, 415–422

28 Agranoff, B. W. (1983) *Life Sci.* 32, 2047–2054

29 Van Rooijen, L. A. A., Seguin, E. B. and Agranoff, B. W. (1983) *Biochem. Biophys. Res. Commun.* 112, 919–926

30 Allison, J. H., Blisner, M. E., Holland, W. H., Hipps, P. P. and Sherman, W. R. (1976) *Biochem. Biophys. Res. Commun.* 71, 664–670

31 Berridge, M. J., Downes, C. P. and Hanley, M. R. (1982) *Biochem. J.* 206, 587–595

The authors are at the Neuroscience Laboratory Building, University of Michigan, Ann Arbor, MI 48109, USA. The present address of S. K. Fisher is: Department of CNS Research, Medical Research Division of American Cyanamid Company, Lederle Laboratories, Pearl River, NY 10965, USA.

Addendum

The role of IP_3 and diacylglycerol as intracellular second messengers which initiate a signal cascade in many cells, has attracted considerable interest. The observation of Streb *et al.*[5] that the addition of micromolar concentrations of IP_3 to 'leaky' pancreatic acinar cells stimulates the efflux of intracellular calcium has been replicated in permeabilized hepatocytes by measuring $^{45}Ca^{2+}$ release or increased fluorescence of the intracellular Ca^{2+}-indicator quin-2[32,33]. Whereas IP_3 releases intracellular Ca^{2+}, inositol, IP_1 and IP_2 are ineffective. An assertion that *non*-mitochondrial stores of Ca^{2+} are mobilized by adding IP_3 has received direct support from experiments showing release of Ca^{2+} following addition of IP_3 to microsomal, but not to mitochondrial, fractions of rat insulinoma. These results strongly suggest that IP_3 plays the role of a second messenger in the mobilization of intracellular Ca^{2+}.

Polyphosphoinositides have also been implicated in the proliferative response that many cultured cells undergo following the addition of mitogens. Addition of platelet-derived growth factor to Swiss 3T3-fibroblasts is reported to increase the breakdown of PIP_2 to IP_3, and results in a release of Ca^{2+} from intracellular stores[35]. Mitogenic stimuli exert their effects by means of alterations in both Ca^{2+} permeability and activation of a neutral Na^+/H^+ exchange carrier. It is thus of additional interest that DAG, formed together with IP_3 during $PhIP_2$ breakdown, has been implicated in the regulation of Na^+ entry and H^+ extrusion via activation of protein kinase C (Ref. 35). Of potentially great significance is the observation that certain oncogene products (e.g. tyrosine kinases coded by the *src* oncogene of Rous sarcoma virus and the *ros* oncogene of the avian sarcoma virus, UR2) may also act as inositol lipid kinases and thus increase the concentrations of polyphosphoinositides in infected cells[36,37]. By increasing the formation of a pool of polyphosphoinositides ' susceptible to receptor-mediated breakdown, the oncogenes may serve to elevate concentrations of IP_3 and DAG, which in turn may be instrumental in the initiation of tumorogenesis.

At the Chilton Conference on 'Inositol and Phosphoinositides' held in Dallas in January 1984, it was recommended that the following abbreviations be adopted in the interests of consistency: PI, PIP and PIP_2 for phosphatidylinositol, phosphatidylinositol 4-phosphate and phosphatidylinositol 4,5-bisphosphate, respectively. IP_1, IP_2 and IP_3 refer to D-*myo*-inositol 1-phosphate, 1,4-bisphosphate and 1,4,5-trisphosphate, respectively[38].

References

32 Burgess, G. M., Godfrey, P. P., McKinney, J. S., Berridge, M. J., Irvine, R. F. and Putney, J. W., Jr (1984) *Nature* 309, 63–66
33 Thomas, A. P., Alexander, J. and Williamson, J. R. (1984) *J. Biol. Chem.* 259, 5574–5584
34 Prentki, M., Biden, T. J., Janjic, D., Irvine, R. F., Berridge, M. J. and Wollheim, C. B. (1984) *Nature* 309, 562–564
35 Berridge, M. J. (1984) *Biochem. J.* 220, 345–

360

36 Sugimoto, Y., Whitman, M., Cantley, L. C. and Erikson, R. L. (1984) *Proc. Natl Acad. Sci. USA* 81, 2117–2121

37 Macara, I. G., Marinetti, G. V. and Balduzzi, P. C. (1984) *Proc. Natl Acad. Sci. USA* 81,

2728–2732

38 Agranoff, B. W., Eisenberg, F., Jr, Hauser, G., Hawthorne, J. N. and Michell, R. H. (1985) in *Inositol and Phosphoinositides* (Bleasdale, J., Hauser, G. and Eichberg, J., eds)

Enzyme translocation in the regulation of phosphatidylcholine biosynthesis

Dennis E. Vance and Steven L. Pelech

Phosphatidylcholine biosynthesis is regulated by translocation of the rate-limiting enzyme (CTP:phosphocholine cytidylyltransferase) from the cytosol, where it is inactive, to the endoplasmic reticulum (microsomes) where it is activated. The process is regulated by reversible protein phosphorylation and by fatty acids.

Phosphatidylcholine (PC) is the major phospholipid present in mammalian cells but is notably absent from *E. coli* and most other bacteria (exceptions include *Clostridium beijerinickii*, *Agrobacterium tumefaciens* and *Rhodopseudomonas spheroides*). The lipid has a primarily structural function in biological membranes, as well as in lipoproteins and bile. PC is also a critically important component of lung surfactant. PC serves as a donor of the fatty acyl moiety for the synthesis of cholesterol ester in plasma in a reaction catalysed by lecithin–cholesterol acyltransferase. In addition, PC donates arachidonic acid for the synthesis of prostaglandins, leukotrienes, thromboxanes and related compounds. Recently, a particular molecular species of PC (1-alkyl-2-acetyl-PC) has been identified as a potent biological agent (active at 10^{-10} M) which causes platelet aggregation and is a potent vasodepressor compound. The primary importance of PC is underscored by the lack of any known diseases related to its metabolism, suggesting that any such defects may be lethal at an early stage of development.

The major pathway for PC biosynthesis was described in the 1950s and involves the sequential conversion of choline to choline-phosphate, CDP-choline and PC[1]. Towards the end of the 1970s, it was recognized that the rate of PC biosynthesis was usually determined by the activity of the enzyme which synthesizes CDP-choline (CTP: phosphocholine cytidylyltransferase)[2]. At that time, most studies concentrated on the activity of the cytosolic cytidylyltransferase and the microsomal activity was not emphasized. Recent studies have made it clear that the microsomal, rather than the cytosolic, cytidylyltransferase governs the rate of PC biosynthesis in a variety of systems. The enzyme in cytosol appears to be relatively inactive and is stored in reserve.

Evidence for a regulatory role of enzyme translocation

The conclusion that enzyme translocation governs the rate of PC biosynthesis arises largely from correlation experiments (Table I). In particular, the experiments with cultured rat hepatocytes and established cell lines have been the most convincing.

Cyclic AMP and its stable analogues have been known to inhibit glycogen synthesis for several decades and more recently fatty acid and cholesterol synthesis[3]. Thus, the discovery that cAMP analogues mediate a partial inhibition of PC biosynthesis[4] fits into the general scheme of cAMP action, which is an inhibitor of biosynthetic reactions. The decreased rate of PC biosynthesis correlated with a decrease in microsomal cytidylyltransferase activity[4].

Opposite effects were obtained when rat hepatocytes were incubated with various fatty acids[5]. All long chain fatty acids tested caused a two- to three-fold increase in the rate of PC biosynthesis and a corresponding translocation of cytidylyltransferase from the cytosol to the microsomes, increasing the specific activity of the enzyme by a factor of 1.8 (Ref. 5). Fatty acids were also able to reverse the cAMP-mediated inhibition of PC biosynthesis[6].

The conversion of phosphatidylethanolamine to PC via the methylation pathway is also an important source of PC in liver[7]. Experiments with rat hepatocytes have shown that an analogue of adenosine, 3-deazaadenosine was a potent inhibitor of this methylation pathway[8]. Treatment of hepatocytes with this compound doubles the rate of the CDP-choline pathway[8]. Translocation of the cytidylyltransferase from cytosol to microsomes resulted in a two-fold increase in this microsomal enzymatic activity. Taken together, the experiments in the rat hepatocytes indicate a strong correlation between the rate of PC synthesis and localization of the cytidylyltransferase on the microsomes.

In a different approach, cultured chick embryonic myoblasts and CHO cells were depleted of PC by treatment with phospholipase C (Refs 9 and 11). Subsequently, the rate of PC synthesis was increased three-fold and a similar increase in the microsomal activity was observed. Treatment of the myoblasts for 3 h with cycloheximide did not alter the cellular response to phospholipase C treatment[9]. Thus, protein synthesis was required neither for translocation of the cytidylyltransferase nor for the concomitant increase in PC biosynthesis. Moreover, 6 h after removal of the phospholipase C its effect on choline incorporation in CHO cells was fully reversed[11]. However, a correlation between the reversal of choline incorporation and binding of the cytidylyltransferase to microsomes was not reported[11].

Verification of the translocation theory in cultured cells

The above experiments strongly indicate the regulatory importance of translocation of the cytidylyltransferase. However, a firm conclusion from this data cannot be made for two reasons. First, although the changes were statistically significant, the magnitude of the effects (two- to three-fold changes) were not large. Secondly, experiments have shown that phospholipase C treatment of cultured cells[9-11] or supplementation of hepatocytes with fatty acids[6,7], increase the amount of diacylglycerol. *In vitro* this lipid promotes aggregation of the cytidylyltransferase[12] and might enhance the binding of the enzyme to microsomes. Hence, the presence of increased diacylglycerol in the cell may have caused the increased binding of cytidylyltransferase to membranes during the homogenization procedure and, therefore, be responsible for the increased enzyme activity. However, recent experiments with HeLa cells and digitonin have discounted these two reservations[6,13].

In one set of experiments, treatment of HeLa cells with 1 mM oleic acid produced a twenty-fold stimulation of the rate of PC biosynthesis within 15 min[13]. Such a large stimulation of PC biosynthesis had never been observed before (in other systems, the change was only two- to three-fold; see Table I). This unprecedented increase in PC biosynthesis had important implications for the translocation theory. If the proposal were correct, this increase in PC synthesis should be the result of virtually complete translocation of the cytidylyltransferase to microsomes. Whereas under normal conditions, 65% of the enzyme is recovered from HeLa cell

Table I. Correlation between microsomal cytidylyltransferase activity and the rate of phosphatidylcholine biosynthesis

System	Change in PC synthesis	Change in activity of microsomal cytidylyl-transferase	Refs
cAMP analogues/rat hepatocytes	↓ 35%	↓ 34%	4
Fatty acids/rat hepatocytes	↑ 2-fold	↑ 1.8-fold	5,6
3-Deazaadenosine/rat hepatocytes	↑ 2–3-fold	↑ 1.9-fold	8
Fatty acids/HeLa cells	↑ 20-fold	↑ 4-fold	13
Phospholipase C/myoblasts, CHO cells, LM cells	↑ 3-fold	↑ 2–4-fold	9,10
Cholesterol-cholate/rat liver	↑ 3.5-fold	↑ 1.9–4.8-fold	17
Premature delivery/rat lung	↑ 2-fold	↑ 2–3-fold	15
Development/rat liver	↑ 3–4-fold	↑ 3–4-fold	16

cytosol, treatment with 1 mM oleate caused greater than 95% of the enzyme to become associated with the microsomes[13]; the concentration of diacylglycerol in the cells treated with fatty acid was not increased.

Digitonin is known to release cytosolic enzymes from cultured cells more rapidly than membrane-associated enzymes[14]. Thus, after treatment of cells with digitonin, the microsomal-associated cytidylyltransferase would be released more slowly than the cytosolic enzyme. In fatty acid supplemented hepatocytes and HeLa cells, where an increased association of enzyme with microsomes occurs[5,6,13], a reduced rate of cytidylyltransferase release would be expected from digitonin-treated cells. Indeed, a marked inhibition of enzyme release was observed after digitonin treatment of fatty acid supplemented cells[6,13]. Thus, the evidence that *active* cytidylyltransferase is membrane-bound is most convincing.

Evidence for translocation theory in intact animals

There are now several animal systems in which an increase in microsomal cytidylyltransferase activity has been correlated with a similarly increased rate of PC synthesis. Fetal rats were delivered prematurely after either 20 or 21 days gestation[15]. The incorporation of choline into PC was evaluated in lung slices at the time of delivery or 3 h after incubation of the fetus in a special chamber. During the 3 h period, there was an apparent two-fold stimulation of PC synthesis[15]. During this same period, there was a two- to three-fold redistribution of enzyme from cytosol to the microsomes[15]. Correspondingly, immediately after birth, the rate of PC synthesis tripled in rat liver and this correlated with translocation of the enzyme to microsomes[16]. More recently, a three-fold increase in PC synthesis has been induced in the livers of young rats fed a diet enriched in cholesterol and cholate[17]. Once again, a correlation between increased enzyme activity and its translocation to the microsomes was demonstrated. Taken together, the combined evidence from various cell cultures and animal studies make a strong case for regulation of the rate of PC biosynthesis by a reversible translocation of cytidylyltransferase between the cytosol and endoplasmic reticulum. The cytidylyltransferase fits well into the class of enzymes originally described as 'ambiquitous'[18].

A final point relates to the requirements of the cytidylyltransferase for certain phospholipids (phosphatidylserine, phosphatidylinositol, phospha-

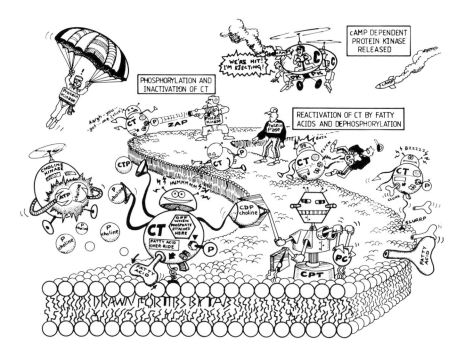

tidylglycerol and lyso-phosphatidyl-ethanolamine) for maximal activity of the enzyme[2]. It seems unlikely that the cytosolic species of the enzyme would be the active species in the cell since phospholipids are usually found exclusively in the membranes.

Mechanism for subcellular movement of the cytidylyltransferase

How does the cell control the location of this enzyme which appears to regulate PC biosynthesis? There is evidence for two different modes of regulation. One involves reversible phosphorylation of the cytidylyltransferase (or possibly of an activator and/or inhibitor protein). Cyclic AMP analogues cause a decrease in the cytidylyltransferase activity associated with microsomes[4]. The activity of this enzyme is regulated in rat liver by cAMP-dependent protein kinases and protein phosphatases[19]. Thus, it appears that cAMP-dependent protein kinase causes a decrease in the enzyme activity associated with microsomes, whereas dephosphorylation promotes the binding of the enzyme to microsomes where it is activated.

A second mechanism involves the apparently direct effect of long chain fatty acids or acyl-CoAs on the enzyme[5,6,13,20]. The fatty acids do not directly stimulate the enzyme activity. Instead, they appear to increase the affinity of the enzyme for membranes which contain phospholipids which in turn activate the cytidylyltransferase. The fatty acid can apparently reverse the phosphorylation-mediated decrease in cytidylyltransferase activity associated with microsomes[6].

A third possible mechanism which has been suggested is that a depletion of PC in the membranes causes increased binding of the enzyme to microsomes[10,11]. This proposal seems unlikely since even in systems in which the concentration of PC increases in membranes[5,8,13,15–17], there is an increased amount of cytidylyltransferase bound to microsomes. An alternative explanation for the above proposal[10,11] is that a higher concentration of diacylglycerol[5,9,10,17], rather than a depletion of PC, caused the enzyme to bind to microsomes. Moreover, it is known that diacylglycerol causes soluble cytidylyltransferase to aggregate and bind to membranes[12]. An additional possibility which should be considered is that fatty acid concentrations are also increased concomitantly with diacylglycerol by the action of diacylglycerol lipase. It should also be noted that high levels of diacylglycerol are not an absolute requirement for translocation since, in HeLa cells exposed to fatty acids, there was a marked translocation of the cytidylyltransferase to microsomes even though the diacylglycerol content in these cells had decreased[13].

Future directions

The evidence summarized in this paper strongly supports the theory that PC biosynthesis is regulated by a reversible translocation of the cytidylyltransferase between cytosol and endoplasmic reticulum. The cell can control this process by either reversible phosphorylation or by modulation of the level of fatty acid (or fatty acyl-CoA). With this reasonably good understanding of the events responsible for enzyme translocation, we can now address our efforts toward the determination, at the molecular level, of the mechanisms involved. Future experiments should involve reconstitution of pure cytidylyltransferase with artificial membranes of known lipid composition. The application of pure protein kinases and phosphatases should enable us to demonstrate whether or not the cytidylyltransferase is indeed phosphorylated and how this modulation affects its affinity for membranes. Similarly, the mechanism by which fatty acids enhance binding of the enzyme to membranes could be studied. It should also be feasible to see if physiological concentrations of diacylglycerol in model membranes will promote the binding of the pure enzyme.

Acknowledgement

We are grateful to the Medical Research Council of Canada and the B.C. Heart Foundation for support of the research from our laboratory. We thank Dr Jean Vance and Dr Dave Brindley for their helpful comments on this manuscript.

References
1 Kennedy, E. P. (1962) *Harvey Lect.* 57, 143–171
2 Vance, D. E. and Choy, P. C. (1979) *Trends Biochem. Sci.* 4, 145–148
3 Geelen, M. J. H., Harris, R. A., Beynen, A. C. and McCune, S. A. (1980) *Diabetes* 29, 1006–1022
4 Pelech, S. L., Pritchard, P. H. and Vance, D. E. (1981) *J. Biol. Chem.* 256, 8283–8286
5 Pelech, S. L., Pritchard, P. H., Brindley, D. N. and Vance, D. E. (1983) *J. Biol. Chem.* 258, 6782–6788
6 Pelech, S. L., Pritchard, P. H., Brindley, D. N. and Vance, D. E. (1983) *Biochem. J.* 216, 129–136
7 Sundler, R. and Åkesson, B. (1975) *J. Biol. Chem.* 250, 3359–3367
8 Pritchard, P. H., Chiang, P. K., Cantoni, G. L. and Vance, D. E. (1983) *J. Biol. Chem.* 257, 6362–6367
9 Sleight, R. and Kent, C. (1980) *J. Biol. Chem.* 255, 10644–10650
10 Sleight, R. and Kent, C. (1983) *J. Biol. Chem.* 258, 824–830
11 Sleight, R. and Kent, C. (1983) *J. Biol. Chem.* 258, 831–835
12 Choy, P. C., Farren, S. B. and Vance, D. E. (1979) *Can. J. Biochem.* 57, 605–612
13 Pelech, S. L., Cook, H. W., Paddon, H. B. and Vance, D. E. *Biochim. Biophys. Acta* (in press)
14 Mackall, J., Meredith, M. and Lane, M. D. (1979) *Anal. Biochem.* 95, 270–274
15 Weinhold, P. A., Feldman, D. A., Quade, M. M., Miller, J. C. and Brooks, R. L. (1981) *Biochim. Biophys. Acta* 665, 134–144
16 Pelech, S. L., Power, E. and Vance, D. E. (1983) *Can. J. Biochem. Cell Biol.* 61, 1147–1152
17 Lim, P. H., Pritchard, P. H., Paddon, H. B. and Vance, D. E. (1983) *Biochim. Biophys. Acta* 753, 74–82
18 Wilson, J. E. (1978) *Trends Biochem. Sci.* 3, 124–125
19 Pelech, S. L. and Vance, D. E. (1982) *J. Biol. Chem.* 257, 14198–14202
20 Feldman, D. A., Brubaker, P. G. and Weinhold, P. A. (1981) *Biochim. Biophys. Acta* 665, 53–59

Dennis E. Vance and Steven L. Pelech are at the Department of Biochemistry, University of British Columbia, Vancouver, British Columbia V6T 1W5, Canada.

Control of *Escherichia coli* isocitrate dehydrogenase: an example of protein phosphorylation in a prokaryote

H. G. Nimmo

In micro-organisms growing on acetate, isocitrate can be metabolized either by the tricarboxylic acid cycle or by the glyoxylate bypass. In Escherichia coli this branch-point is controlled by reversible phosphorylation and inactivation of isocitrate dehydrogenase. Both phosphorylation and dephosphorylation are catalysed by a single bifunctional kinase/phosphatase. The properties of this enzyme suggest that phosphorylation of isocitrate dehydrogenase is controlled by the concentrations of several central metabolites, including isocitrate, the adenine nucleotides and phosphoenolpyruvate.

Over the last six years the existence of protein kinases and phosphatases in prokaryotes has been well established[1]. However, in only one case are the physiological role and the molecular details of a prokaryotic phosphorylation system understood at a level comparable to that achieved for many such systems in eukaryotes; this is the control of isocitrate dehydrogenase (ICDH) in *E. coli*. The purpose of this article is to summarize recent advances in our understanding of this system.

Control of the branch-point at isocitrate

The ICDH of *E. coli*, an NADP-linked enzyme, is a dimer of identical subunits of M_r 45 000 (Ref. 2); the enzyme is not subject to allosteric control by adenine nucleotides or, so far as is known, any other effectors. There is no reason to believe that ICDH plays a significant role in regulating flux through the tricarboxylic acid (TCA) cycle under most growth conditions. However, during growth on acetate, the glyoxylate bypass must be used to generate the precursors necessary for biosynthesis[3] (Fig. 1). These conditions induce isocitrate lyase (ICL) and malate synthase and ICDH

and ICL compete for the available isocitrate.

The mechanisms involved in the regulation of this metabolic branch-point were first studied by Bennett and Holms in Glasgow[4,5]. They found that the ICDH of *E. coli* ML308 became partially inactivated during adaptation to growth on acetate. However, the ICDH activity in cells growing on acetate could be increased rapidly in several ways. For example, addition of pyruvate caused a 4-fold increase in the specific activity of ICDH and an increase in growth rate; these changes were reversed after exhaustion of the pyruvate[5]. The activity changes were independent of protein synthesis and Bennett and Holms[5] concluded that one possible mechanism was a reversible covalent modification of ICDH. They suggested that the role of inactivation of ICDH was to restrict the flow of carbon round the TCA cycle and to favour operation of the glyoxylate bypass[4].

The first evidence implicating phosphorylation in the control of ICDH came from Reeves' group[6,7]. Acetate was added to a culture of *E. coli* K12 grown to stationary phase and then

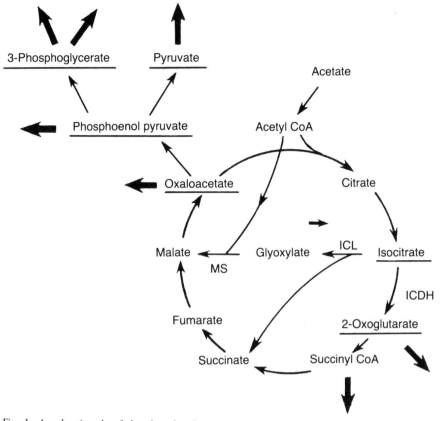

Fig. 1. Anaplerotic role of the glyoxylate bypass. Filled arrows (➤) represent biosynthetic routes. Intermediates that activate ICDH phosphatase and inhibit ICDH kinase are underlined. The abbreviations are: ICDH, isocitrate dehydrogenase; ICL, isocitrate lyase; and MS, malate synthase.

incubated with $^{32}P_i$; this caused partial inactivation of ICDH[6]. A phosphorylated form of ICDH, containing ^{32}P as phosphoserine, was isolated from the culture[6,7]. These reports constituted the first proof that ICDH could be phosphorylated *in vivo*. However, detailed analysis of the effects of phosphorylation and dephosphorylation on the activity of ICDH came only after isolation of the kinase and phosphatase involved.

A bifunctional ICDH kinase/phosphatase

LaPorte and Koshland[8] made the fascinating discovery that *E. coli* contains a bifunctional ICDH kinase/phosphatase. They purified the protein by fractionation with $(NH_4)_2SO_4$, ion-exchange chromatography and chroma-

tography on immobilized ICDH. The two activities were co-eluted from the ion-exchange and affinity columns, and the purified enzyme gave a single band (M_r 66 000) on SDS-gel electrophoresis. We have confirmed these results[9] and our data also suggest that the native form of the kinase/phosphatase is a dimer and that no separate monofunctional kinase or phosphatase exists.

The reactions catalysed by ICDH kinase/phosphatase have now been characterized. The kinase transfers the γ-phosphoryl group of ATP to a serine residue in ICDH[9] with a stoichiometry of one per subunit[9,10]. This causes almost complete loss of enzyme activity, measured under V_{max} conditions[9,10]. In agreement with this, we have isolated an essentially inactive, phosphate-containing form of ICDH from *E. coli* ML308 grown on acetate[2]. The phosphorylated and unphosphorylated forms of ICDH can be separated by nondenaturing gel electrophoresis; they differ in charge but not in size[2,9]. The sequence around the phosphorylation site in the ICDH has now been reported[11,12]. It is unlike most of the sequences phosphorylated by cyclic AMP dependent protein kinase[13]; not surprisingly, ICDH is not phosphorylated by the latter enzyme[11].

ICDH phosphatase requires a divalent metal ion and either ADP or ATP for activity[8,9]. The enzyme catalyses the release of P_i from phosphorylated ICDH[9]. The effects on the activity of ICDH depend on the incubation conditions[9]. When ATP is used to activate the phosphatase, $^{32}P_i$ is released from ^{32}P-phosphorylated ICDH but little reactivation of the enzyme occurs because the kinase and phosphatase are both active under these conditions. On the other hand, in the presence of ADP, or ATP plus an inhibitor of the kinase, the phosphatase catalyses full reactivation of ICDH[9].

ICDH kinase and ICDH phosphatase activities are clearly associated with a single protein. However it is not yet clear whether this protein contains only a single type of polypeptide chain or whether it is a heterodimer of two subunits that have very similar M_r values. If the former is correct and a bifunctional polypeptide does exist, this species could contain a single bifunctional active site or two spatially distinct sites. LaPorte and Koshland[8] speculated that the phosphatase may have evolved from the kinase by gene duplication and, perhaps, fusion. This hypothesis might explain the adenine nucleotide requirement of the phosphatase.

At least two other bifunctional regulatory enzymes that catalyse opposing reactions are known to exist; one catalyses both adenylation and deadenylation of *E. coli* glutamine synthetase[14] and the other catalyses both the formation and the hydrolysis of fructose 2,6-bisphosphate[15]. We do not yet know what the advantages are, if any, of localizing opposing regulatory activities on a single protein. Clearly many fascinating questions concerning the structure, organization, function and evolution of ICDH kinase/phosphatase remain to be answered. Since the purified protein is available only in small amounts at the moment, a combination of gene cloning and sequencing, the construction of over-expressing strains and then experiments at the level of the protein will probably be required to answer these questions.

Phosphorylation of ICDH in intact cells

An important part of the investigation of any phosphorylation system is a study of the occurrence and significance of phosphorylation *in vivo*[13]. The reversible activation of ICDH caused by the addition of pyruvate to *E. coli* ML308 growing on acetate (see above) affords a simple experimental system for such studies. By labelling cells with $^{32}P_i$ we have recently shown that the phosphorylation state of ICDH *in vivo* is inversely related to its activity and that the reversible activation/deactivation of the enzyme results entirely from dephosphorylation and rephosphorylation[16].

Cells grown on acetate contain a mixture of totally inactive and active forms of ICDH[2]. The two forms of the enzyme can be separated because the inactive species is unable to bind to Procion Red-Sepharose[2]. We have used this to purify ICDH that had been phosphorylated *in vivo*. Isolation and analysis of the phosphopeptide from this enzyme allowed us to show unambiguously that the only residue phosphorylated in ICDH *in vivo* is identical to the serine residue phosphorylated by the kinase/phosphate *in vitro*[16]. This work rigorously establishes the importance of the reversible phosphorylation catalysed by ICDH kinase/phosphatase in the control of ICDH activity *in vivo*.

Molecular mechanism of the inactivation of ICDH

Many of the eukaryotic enzymes regulated by phosphorylation are allosteric proteins and phosphorylation frequently results in changes in the affinity of the target enzyme for a substrate or an allosteric effector rather than changes in V_{max}. ICDH clearly does not fit into this general pattern; it is not an allosteric protein and the phosphorylated form is almost totally inactive. This led us to consider the molecular mechanism by which phosphorylation inactivates ICDH[17].

Inactive ICDH does not bind to Procion Red-Sepharose, whereas active ICDH does bind and can be eluted by $NADP^+$. This observation prompted us to suggest that phosphorylated ICDH is inactive precisely because it cannot bind coenzyme[2]. This idea was supported by the results of fluorescence titration experiments with NADPH. These showed that, while NADPH bound stoichiometrically to active ICDH, it did not bind to inactive enzyme. We also found that either phosphorylation or binding of $NADP^+$ to active ICDH induce similar conformational changes as judged by sensitivity to limited proteolysis[17].

One attractive explanation of these results is that the phosphorylation of active ICDH may occur close to, or at, its NADP-binding site[17]. The introduction of a negatively charged phosphate group near the coenzyme-binding site could prevent binding of NADP by charge repulsion and could also trigger a conformational change similar to that induced by binding of the negatively charged coenzyme (Fig. 2). This hypothesis would also explain why phos-

phorylated ICDH cannot be reactivated by proteolytic removal of the phosphorylation site[17] and why both $NADP^+$ and NADPH inhibit the phosphorylation of ICDH[18]. The serine residue phosphorylated in ICDH is that in the sequence Arg–Ser–Leu–Asn[11]. An identical sequence is found close to the NADP-binding site of chicken liver dihydrofolate reductase[19]; this lends further support to our hypothesis. If our idea is correct, phosphorylation inactivates ICDH by a mechanism quite different from those involved in most other phosphorylation systems.

Control of the phosphorylation state of ICDH

ICDH kinase and ICDH phosphatase can be active simultaneously both *in vitro*[9] and in intact cells[16] so that the phosphorylation state of the enzyme *in vivo* must represent the steady-state balance between the two activities. We have carefully examined the regulatory properties of the two activities *in vitro* and the results led us to propose a hypothesis for the control of the phosphorylation of ICDH *in vivo*[18].

As is shown in Fig. 3, several metabolites both inhibit ICDH kinase and activate ICDH phosphatase[10,18]. Isocitrate gives sigmoid inhibition of the kinase but the other effects are hyperbolic[18]. In addition, the phosphatase is strongly inhibited by NADPH but not by other nicotinamide nucleotides[18]. Since several metabolites have opposite effects on the activities of the two enzymes, the system should show great sensitivity in responding to small changes in the intracellular concentrations of these metabolites. The sensitivity of the system may also be enhanced by the operation of 'zero-order sensitivity'[10]. Consideration of the probable intracellular concentrations of metabolites led us to suggest that the effectors most likely to be significant *in vivo* are isocitrate, phosphoenolpyruvate, AMP,

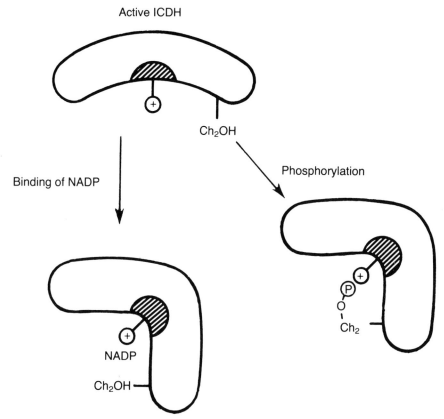

Fig. 2. *Hypothetical scheme for the inactivation of ICDH by phosphorylation. The hatched area represents the coenzyme binding site and the CH₂OH group is the side-chain of the phosphorylatable serine residue. The positive sign at the surface of the enzyme represents a positively charged group (or groups) that interact with the negatively charged phosphate groups of NADP.*

ADP and NADPH[18].

Bennett and Holms[4,5] proposed that the role of the inactivation of ICDH was to allow ICL to compete successfully for the available isocitrate. We can now suggest in more detail how this might occur. Apparently the kinase/phosphatase is induced during growth on acetate[5,9] and therefore the following discussion refers to this situation. The K_m of ICDH for isocitrate is 1–2 μM[18] whereas that of ICL is 3 mM[20], considerably greater than the likely intracellular concentration of isocitrate (Ref. 21 and El-Mansi, E. M. T., Holms, W. H. and Nimmo, H. G., unpublished results). We believe that the role of the phosphorylation of ICDH is to render it rate-limiting in the TCA cycle during growth on acetate;

this would cause an increase in the level of isocitrate compared to growth on other carbon sources, and facilitate flux through ICL. In agreement with this idea, the intracellular level of isocitrate is low in cells grown on glucose or glycerol but much higher in cells grown on acetate (Ref. 21 and El-Mansi *et al.*, unpublished results).

In this context, it becomes clear that isocitrate could play a central role in controlling the phosphorylation state of ICDH *in vivo*. Any change in conditions that causes an increase in the concentration of isocitrate, for example addition of another carbon source, would increase the flux through ICL, the activity of ICDH, the rate of ATP generation and consequently the growth rate[18]. Addition of pyruvate to cells growing on acetate does indeed cause increases in the activity of ICDH and the growth rate[5] and we have recently shown that it also causes a transient doubling of the concentration of isocitrate (El-Mansi *et al.*, unpublished results).

The other effectors of the kinase and phosphatase fall into three categories and in most cases their effects are easy to rationalize in terms of metabolic control. Phosphoenolpyruvate, pyruvate, 2-oxoglutarate, oxaloacetate and 3-phosphoglycerate are all precursors for biosynthesis (Fig. 1). One would expect high levels of such compounds to favour flux through the TCA cycle at the expense of the glyoxylate bypass, and all these metabolites do, indeed, activate ICDH phosphatase and inhibit ICDH kinase. Of the functions of adenine nucleotides, the effect of ATP in activating the phosphatase seems anomalous in terms of metabolic regulation; perhaps it is best viewed in terms of the evolution of the phosphatase (see above) rather than of its control. The effects of AMP and ADP are more easily understood since a decrease in the energy charge would lead to activation of ICDH, mediated by the effects of these compounds on the kinase/phosphatase, and thus an increase in the rate of flux through the TCA cycle. Anaerobiosis causes activation of ICDH in *E.*

coli grown on acetate (El-Mansi *et al.*, unpublished results) and changes in the energy charge may be responsible for this. Finally, inhibition of ICDH phosphatase by NADPH could be viewed as a case of feedback inhibition of the TCA cycle by one of its end products.

The ICDH system is thus capable of integrating a wide variety of metabolic information because the kinase/phosphatase can respond to a large number of metabolites. The observation that phosphorylation of ICDH can occur in mutants devoid of a functional glyoxylate bypass[22] is not incompatible with our views of the role and control of the phosphorylation; the system responds to the levels of many metabolites rather than to the rate of flux through the bypass. It will, of course, be difficult to assess the relative contributions made by the different regulators in different circumstances. The ICDH system bears some resemblance to the regulation of *E. coli* glutamine synthetase by adenylation/deadenylation[23]; in both cases the converter enzymes respond to intermediates in mainstream metabolic pathways rather than to 'signal' molecules such as cyclic AMP or fructose 2,6-bisphosphate.

Conclusions

There have been major advances in our understanding of the phosphorylation of *E. coli* ICDH over the last two

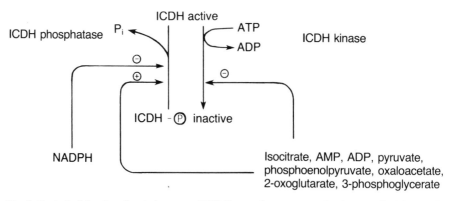

Fig. 3. Control of the phosphorylation state of ICDH. + and − represent stimulatory and inhibitory effects respectively.

years. There is now a wealth of information on the regulatory properties of kinase/phosphatase and the operation of the control system *in vivo*. Krebs and Beavo[13] set out stringent criteria by which the physiological significance of phosphorylation systems should be assessed and all of these have now been met for ICDH. There are, of course, a number of fascinating questions that remain to be answered, particularly with regard to the properties of ICDH kinase/phosphatase.

The phosphorylation of ICDH is very unusual in that it can cause total inactivation of the enzyme (see above); consideration of the evolutionary origin of the system may throw some light on this. *E. coli* can extract energy from acetate only by oxidizing it in the TCA cycle. It probably evolved the capacity to grow on acetate at a relatively late stage, after the TCA cycle itself had evolved. There is no reason to believe that ICDH is a regulatory enzyme on carbon sources other than acetate or compounds that can be converted solely to acetyl CoA. Thus development of the ability to grow on acetate would have necessitated development of the ability to reduce the activity of ICDH and thus to make it rate-limiting in the TCA cycle.

The mechanism that has been selected to do this in *E. coli* is the phosphorylation and inactivation of ICDH. In this context it is understandable that phosphorylation affects V_{max} and that it seems to be directed towards the active site. Thus the molecular details of the ICDH system seem pleasingly compatible with our current views of its evolution and its physiological role.

Acknowledgements

I wish to thank all my colleagues who have contributed to this work and in particular Drs W. H. Holms and G. A. Nimmo for many valuable discussions. Work from this laboratory was supported by a grant from the Science and Engineering Research Council, London.

References

1 Cozzone, A. J. (1984) *Trends Biochem. Sci.* 9, 400–403
2 Borthwick, A. C., Holms, W. H. and Nimmo, H. G. (1984) *Eur. J. Biochem.* 141, 393–400
3 Kornberg, H. L. (1966) *Essays Biochem.* 2, 1–31
4 Holms, W. H. and Bennett, P. M. (1971) *J. Gen. Microbiol.* 65, 57–68
5 Bennett, P. M. and Holms, W. H. (1975) *J. Gen. Microbiol.* 87, 37–51
6 Garnak, M. and Reeves, H. C. (1979) *Science* 203, 1111–1112
7 Garnak, M. and Reeves, H. C. (1979) *J. Biol. Chem.* 254, 7915–7920
8 LaPorte, D. C. and Koshland, D. E. Jr, (1982) *Nature* 300, 458–460
9 Nimmo, G. A., Borthwick, A. C., Holms, W. H. and Nimmo, H. G. (1984) *Eur. J. Biochem.* 141, 401–408
10 LaPorte, D. C. and Koshland, D. E. Jr, (1983) *Nature* 305, 286–290
11 Borthwick, A. C., Holms, W. H. and Nimmo, H. G. (1984) *FEBS Lett.* 174, 112–115
12 Malloy, P. J., Reeves, H. C. and Spiess, J. *Curr. Microb.* (in press)
13 Krebs, E. G. and Beavo, J. A. (1979) *Annu. Rev. Biochem.* 48, 923–959
14 Caban, C. and Ginsburg, A. (1976) *Biochemistry* 15, 1569–1580
15 El-Maghrabi, M. R., Claus, T. H., Pilkis, J., Fox, E. and Pilkis, S. J. (1982) *J. Biol. Chem.* 257, 7603–7607
16 Borthwick, A. C., Holms, W. H. and Nimmo, H. G. (1984) *Biochem. J.* 222, 797–804
17 Garland, D. and Nimmo, H. G. (1984) *FEBS Lett.* 165, 259–264
18 Nimmo, G. A. and Nimmo, H. G. (1984) *Eur. J. Biochem.* 141, 409–414
19 Volz, K. W., Matthews, D. A., Alden, R. A., Freer, S. T., Hansch, C., Kaufman, B. T. and Kraut, J. (1982) *J. Biol. Chem.* 257, 2528–2536
20 Bautista, J., Satrustegui., J. and Machado, A. (1979) *FEBS Lett.* 105, 333–336
21 Lowry, O. H., Carter, J., Ward, J. B. and Glaser, L. (1971) *J. Biol. Chem.* 246, 6511–6521
22 Reeves, H. C. and Malloy, P. J. (1983) *FEBS Lett.* 158, 239–242
23 Stadtman, E. R., Chock, P. B. and Adler, S. P. (1976) in *Metabolic Interconversion of Enzymes, 1975* (Shaltiel, S., ed.), pp. 142–149, Springer-Verlag, Heidelberg.

H. G. Nimmo is at the Department of Biochemistry, University of Glasgow, Glasgow G12 8QQ, UK.

Fructose 2,6-bisphosphate

Henri-Géry Hers, Louis Hue and Emile Van Schaftingen

Fructose 2,6-bisphosphate present in animal tissues, higher plants and fungi, is a potent stimulator of phosphofructokinase and an inhibitor of fructose 1,6-bisphosphatase. It also stimulates plant PPi-fructose 6-phosphate phosphotransferase. It is formed from fructose 6-phosphate in the liver by a specific 6-phosphofructo 2-kinase and converted back to fructose 6-phosphate by a specific fructose 2,6-bisphosphatase. These two enzymes are controlled by the concentration of various metabolites and also through phosphorylation by cyclic AMP-dependent protein kinase. Fructose 2,6-bisphosphate is an intracellular signal which signifies that glucose is abundant; in this respect, its action is opposed to that of cyclic AMP.

Fructose 2,6-bisphosphate was discovered in 1980[1] as a low-molecular-weight stimulator of phosphofructokinase (PFK), which was formed in the liver after a glucose load and was destroyed after glucagon treatment. The interest in this compound grew very rapidly because it shares with cyclic AMP the property of being an intracellular signal present in much of the living world including yeast, higher plants and animals. Fructose 2,6-bisphosphate has been the subject of two recent reviews[2,3] in which additional information and references to the original publications can be found.

Fructose 2,6-bisphosphate, a low-molecular-weight stimulator of liver PFK

In the liver, glucagon inhibits glycolysis and stimulates gluconeogenesis. Recently, this effect has been associated with a change in the kinetic properties of PFK which is considered to be a major regulatory enzyme of glycolysis in most tissues, including liver. The activity of PFK is controlled by the concentration of its two substrates, ATP and fructose 6-phosphate and of a large series of effectors. ATP acts as a negative allosteric effector, which induces co-operativity for fructose 6-phosphate, whereas fructose 6-phosphate relieves the inhibition by ATP. Positive effectors, like fructose 1,6-bisphosphate, the product of the reaction, and AMP, reinforce the effects of fructose 6-phosphate, whereas negative effectors, such as citrate and H^+, act synergistically with ATP.

Treating isolated hepatocytes with glucagon reduces the affinity of PFK for fructose 6-phosphate and it also increases its sensitivity to inhibition by ATP. These changes were first believed to result from a phosphorylation of the enzyme by cyclic AMP-dependent protein kinase. However, it appeared that they could also be obtained by gel filtration of an extract from control hepatocytes and could therefore be attributed to the removal of a low-molecular-weight positive effector of PFK. This effector, which was neither fructose 1,6-bisphosphate nor AMP, was characterized and isolated. It was recognized as an extremely acid-labile, non-nucleotidic phosphoric ester with a molecular weight similar to that of fructose 1,6-bisphosphate. Limited acid hydrolysis of the partially purified stimulator yielded equimolar amounts of fructose 6-phosphate, P_i and of a reducing group. This led to the conclusion that in the native structure, phosphate was linked to fructose 6-phosphate by its anomeric carbon, as in fructose 2,6-bisphosphate. Furthermore, a stimulator of PFK which had all the chemical and biochemical properties of the natural one could be synthesized by reversal of the acid hydrolysis during incubation of phosphoric acid with fructose 6-phosphoric acid. This was proof that the stimulator was indeed fructose 2,6-bisphosphate since it was made of fructose 6-phosphate and phosphate only. Later on, fructose 2,6-bisphosphate could be formed on a millimole scale by conversion of fructose 1,6-bisphosphate into its 1,2 cyclic phosphodiester and alkaline hydrolysis of the latter. By this method, fructose 2,6-bisphosphate became available in large quantities for chemical and metabolic studies. NMR analysis revealed that this osyl-phosphate had the β configuration.

Fructose 2,6-bisphosphate now appears to be the most potent known positive effector of liver PFK, acting at concentrations 1000-fold smaller than fructose 1,6-bisphosphate. Its action is remarkably synergistic with that of AMP. The dose-response curve of the enzyme for fructose 2,6-bisphosphate is, however, highly dependent upon the concentration of substrates and of other effectors. The K_a is presumably in the micromolar range under physiological conditions. The action of fructose 2,6-bisphosphate on PFK is not limited to the liver enzyme but also applies to all mammalian PFKs that were tested as well as to PFKs of *Xenopus* oocytes, yeasts and other fungi, and to the plastid PFK from higher plants; no effect was detected on PFKs from plant cytosol or *Escherichia coli*[2-5].

An inhibitor of fructose 1,6-bisphosphatase

In gluconeogenic cells, such as hepatocytes and yeast cells grown in the absence of glucose, the action of PFK is antagonized by the hydrolysis of fructose 1,6-bisphosphate into fructose 6-phosphate and P_i by a specific fructose 1,6-bisphosphatase. The main kinetic properties of that enzyme are its absolute dependence on Mg^{2+}, its high affinity for its substrate ($K_m = 3$–$5\ \mu M$) and its sensitivity to AMP which acts as an allosteric noncompetitive inhibitor. Fructose 2,6-bisphosphate, at micromolar concentrations, is a potent inhibitor of liver fructose 1,6-bisphosphatase. The main characteris-

tics of this inhibition are that: (1) it is much stronger at low than at high substrate concentrations; (2) it is markedly synergistic with the action of AMP; and (3) it changes the substrate saturation curve from hyperbolic to sigmoidal. Fructose 1,6-bisphosphatase from skeletal muscle, yeast and higher plants was also strongly inhibited by fructose 2,6-bisphosphate.

A stimulator of plant PPi-PFK

A PPi:Fru-6-P phosphotransferase (PPi-PFK), the activity of which is greatly increased by fructose 2,6-bisphosphate is widespread in higher plants. The reaction catalyzed by that enzyme is easily reversible and its direction depends on the relative concentration of substrates and products. However, the fact that fructose 6-phosphate increases and that P_i decreases the positive effect of fructose 2,6-bisphosphate[6] favors the glycolytic function of the enzyme at low fructose 2,6-bisphosphate concentrations. The respective role of ATP-PFK and of PPi-PFK in plant glycolysis is unknown as are the conditions that affect the concentration of fructose 2,6-bisphosphate in plants.

Fructose 2,6-bisphosphate had no effect on PPi-PFK from *Entamoeba histolytica* and from *Propionibacterium shermanii*[6].

Biosynthesis and biodegradation of fructose 2,6-bisphosphate

The mechanism by which fructose 2,6-bisphosphate is formed and degraded in the liver and its control by hormones and metabolites is shown in Fig. 1. Fructose 2,6-bisphosphate is synthesized from fructose 6-phosphate and ATP by an enzyme called PFK 2 and it is hydrolyzed into fructose 6-phosphate and P_i by a specific fructose 2,6-bisphosphatase also called FBPase 2. The activity of both enzymes is affected by the concentration of various metabolites, an important one being fructose 6-phosphate which favors the formation of fructose 2,6-bisphosphate and strongly inhibits FBPase 2. Conversely, metabolites beyond PFK, such as glycerophosphate, dihydroxyacetone phosphate, P-enolpyru-

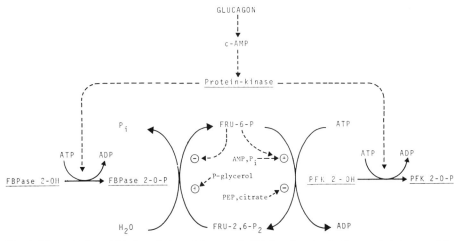

Fig. 1. Biosynthesis and biodegradation of fructose 2,6-biphosphate in the liver and their control by glucagon and metabolites; (PEP = P-enolpyruvate)[3].

vate and citrate decrease the activity of PFK 2 or favor that of FBPase 2. Furthermore, PFK 2 is inactivated and FBPase 2 is activated by cyclic AMP dependent protein kinase and this effect explains the fact that glucagon causes the disappearance of fructose 2,6-bisphosphate from isolated hepatocytes.

It is interesting to note that PFK 2 and FBPase 2 copurified in the course of all fractionation procedures, suggesting that the two catalytic properties belong to a single protein[7–9]. This would be the first example of a multifunctional enzyme which is modified by phosphorylation and dephosphorylation.

Presence of fructose 2,6-bisphosphate in various cells

Fructose 2,6-bisphosphate can be assayed by its ability to stimulate mammalian PFK or plant PPi-PFK. It can also be measured after separation from fructose 6-phosphate by the amount of fructose 6-phosphate formed upon acid hydrolysis. The PPi-PFK procedure is the most sensitive and convenient one[6].

In the liver, the concentration of fructose 2,6-bisphosphate is in the micromolar range. This concentration depends on the nutritional state. It reaches 15–20 μM after a glucose load and is decreased to very low values during fasting, after glucagon treatment and in diabetes. It tends to decrease in hepatocytes incubated with gluconeogenic precursors such as lactate and glycerol. It is also decreased under anoxic conditions. Fructose 2,6-bisphosphate has also been found in brain, heart, skeletal muscle, lung, kidney, epididymal fat, pancreatic islets and in hepatoma tumor cells. It is not detectable in erythrocytes[4]. Its concentration in perfused muscle is increased by insulin and epinephrine but decreased after electrical stimulation.

Fructose 2,6-bisphosphate has also been found in higher plants, including mung beans and spinach leaves, as well as in yeast and other fungi. It is not measurable in *Saccharomyces cerevisiae* grown in the absence of glucose but appears within 1 min of the addition of glucose to the medium. It was not detected in *E. coli*[4].

Role of fructose 2,6-bisphosphate in the control of glycolysis and gluconeogenesis

Because of its action on both phosphofructokinase and fructose 1,6-bisphosphatase, the most obvious role of fructose 2,6-bisphosphate is to control glycolysis and gluconeogenesis. This role is of particular importance in the liver, in which both pathways can operate. Gluconeogenesis is stimulated by glucagon and predominates during fasting and diabetes, whereas glycolysis becomes operative in plethoric conditions as well as in anoxia. Are these large changes in metabolic fluxes mediated by fructose 2,6-bisphosphate or by some other effector?

All the available evidence indicates that fructose 2,6-bisphosphate plays a major role in the hormonal and nutritional control of phosphofructokinase and fructose 1,6-bisphosphatase activity. The rate of glycolytic flux can be correlated with the concentration of fructose 2,6-bisphosphate in the liver under these circumstances, but not with those of ATP, AMP or citrate[10]. As mentioned above, two major effectors control the concentration of fructose 2,6-bisphosphate in the liver: fructose 6-phosphate, which favours synthesis and

prevents degradation; and cyclic AMP, which has the opposite effect. Glucagon, which has a cyclic AMP-mediated glycogenolytic action, increases the concentration of both effectors but apparently the negative effect of cyclic AMP predominates over the positive effect of fructose 6-phosphate. The overall action of glucagon is thus to cause the disappearance of fructose 2,6-bisphosphate and to favor gluconeogenesis. In contrast, other glycogenolytic agents, like vasopressin and phenylephrine, the actions of which are not mediated by cyclic AMP, increase the concentration of fructose 2,6-bisphosphate and the rate of glycolysis, secondarily to an increased concentration of hexose 6-phosphates. A high level of glycaemia has a similar effect.

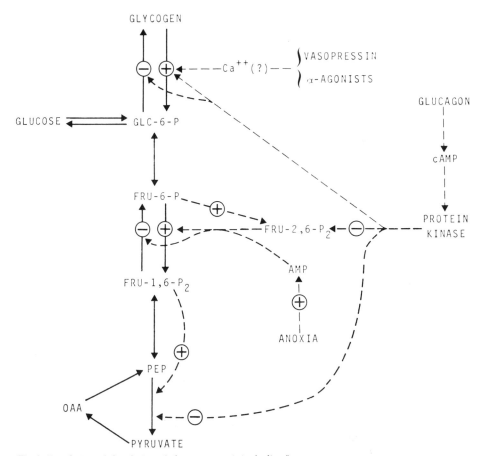

Fig. 2. Regulation of glycolysis and gluconeogenesis in the liver[3].

It is important to recall that glucagon can also stimulate gluconeogenesis through inactivation of pyruvate kinase by cyclic AMP-dependent protein kinase. The hormone also favors the carboxylation of pyruvate through a poorly understood effect on mitochondria[11].

Despite the fact that fructose 2,6-bisphosphate is a potent inhibitor of fructose 1,6-bisphosphatase, there is good experimental evidence that this inhibition is not complete. Indeed, in livers of fed animals, there is a recycling of metabolites between fructose 6-phosphate and fructose 1,6-bisphosphate, indicating that PFK and fructose 1,6-bisphosphatase operate simultaneously. The concentration of fructose 1,6-bisphosphate is then nearly 10-fold greater than in the fasting state, and this increased concentration of its substrate appears then to overcome part of the inhibition of fructose 1,6-bisphosphatase by fructose 2,6-bisphosphate. The advantage of this mechanism seems to be the prevention of an excessive accumulation of fructose 1,6-bisphosphate in the liver. Because fructose 1,6-bisphosphate is a potent activator of pyruvate kinase, it seems probable that the activity of the latter enzyme is also increased under these circumstances. These mechanisms are illustrated in Fig. 2.

In the liver, lipogenesis and ketogenesis are largely controlled by the availability of pyruvate, and the antagonistic effects of glucose and of glucagon on these processes appear to be mediated by changes in the activity of PFK and, therefore, in the concentration of fructose 2,6-bisphosphate. In pancreatic islets, the stimulation of glycolysis might be related to the control of insulin secretion. In skeletal muscle, fructose 2,6-bisphosphate may play a role in the stimulation of glycolysis brought about by adrenalin and insulin. Its function and the mechanisms that control its concentration in other tissues, including brain and heart muscle, remain to be defined.

The presently available data do not indicate that fructose 2,6-bisphosphate plays a major role in the Pasteur effect nor is it responsible for the high glycolytic rate occurring in cancer cells. Anoxia increases the concentration of AMP, the action of which both on PFK and on fructose 1,6-bisphosphatase is remarkably synergistic with that of fructose 2,6-bisphosphate. Other effectors, such as ATP, P_i and citrate may also play a role.

Fructose 2,6-bisphosphate versus cyclic AMP

Fructose 2,6-bisphosphate and cyclic AMP are both regulatory molecules with a long evolutionary history. Both act as signals, in the sense defined by Stryer[12]. Indeed, 'although they are formed from ubiquitous molecules which are at the center of metabolic transformations, they are themselves not part of a major metabolic pathway. They are used only as integrators of metabolism, not as biosynthetic precursors or intermediates in energy production. Hence, their concentration can be independently controlled'. Cyclic AMP has been called a hunger signal, which signifies the absence of glucose[12]. In contrast, fructose 2,6-bisphosphate is the signal which signifies that glucose is abundant and can be freely used and that gluconeogenesis can be stopped.

Trends in fructose 2,6-bisphosphate research

Several approaches can be used when looking for new effects of fructose 2,6-bisphosphate on various biological mechanisms. Firstly, as explained in the preceding section, fructose 2,6-bisphosphate can be considered as a signal for glucose and could therefore play a role in any biological effect of that sugar. This might be the case for insulin secretion and also for various effects of glucose on protein synthesis and degradation, as for instance in the catabolite inactivation of fructose 1,6-bisphosphatase in yeast. Secondly, the concentration of fructose 2,6-bisphosphate is greatly decreased by the presence of glucagon and, as stated above, the effects of that hormone on glycolysis, gluconeogenesis and lipogenesis can be, at least in part, explained on this basis; other effects of the hormone could, therefore, be explained in a similar way. Thirdly, fructose 2,6-bisphosphate, as a structural analogue of fructose 1,6-bisphosphate, might have effects previously recognized for its isomer. It is by this kind of approach that Sabularse and Anderson[13] discovered the effect of fructose 2,6-bisphosphate on plant PP$_i$-PFK. Fourthly, because of the presumably large energy content of the fructofuranosylphosphate linkage, fructose 2,6-bisphosphate is a potential donor of either a phosphoryl or a 6-phosphofructosyl group, but no indication of this action has yet been obtained.

References

1 Van Schaftingen, E., Hue, L. and Hers, H. G. (1980) *Biochem. J.* 192, 897–901

2 Pilkis, S. J., El-Maghrabi, M. R., McGrane, M., Pilkis, J., Fox, E. and Claus, T. H. (1982) *Mol. Cell Endocrinol.* 25, 245–266

3 Hers, H. G. and Van Schaftingen, E. (1982) *Biochem. J.* 206, 1–12

4 Hers, H. G., Hue, L. and Van Schaftingen, E. (unpublished data)

5 Miernyk, J. A. and Dennis, D. T. (1982) *Biochem. Biophys. Res. Commun.* 105, 793–798

6 Van Schaftingen, E., Lederer, B., Bartrons R. and Hers, H. G. (1982) *Eur. J. Biochem.* 129, 191–195

7 Van Schaftingen, E., Davies, D. R. and Hers, H. G. (1981) *Biochem. Biophys. Res. Commun.* 103, 362–368

8 Van Schaftingen, E., Davies, D. R. and Hers, H. G. (1982) *Eur. J. Biochem.* 124, 143–149

9 El-Maghrabi, M. R., Fox, E., Pilkis, J. and Pilkis, S. J. (1982) *Biochem. Biophys. Res. Commun.* 106, 794–802

10 Hue, L. (1982) *Biochem. J.* 206, 359–365

11 Siess, E. A., Fahimi, F. M. and Wieland, O. H. (1981) *Hoppe-Seyler's Z. Physiol. Chem.* 362, 1643–1651

12 Stryer, L. (1981) *Biochemistry*, 949 pp., W. H. Freeman and Co.

13 Sabularse, D. C. and Anderson, R. L. (1981) *Biochem. Biophys. Res. Commun.* 103, 848–855

Henri-Géry Hers, Louis Hue and Emile Van Schaftingen are at the Laboratoire de Chimie Physiologique, Université de Louvain and International Institute of Cellular and Molecular Pathology, UCL 75.39, 75 Avenue Hippocrate B-1200 Bruxelles, Belgium.

Addendum

During the last two years, evidence has accumulated that liver PFK 2 and FBPase 2 are actually part of a single bifunctional protein, made of two subunits, each of which has two active sites and one phosphorylatable site[14,15,16]. In isolated hepatocytes, the same concentration of glucagon causes the phosphorylation of this protein, of glycogen phosphorylase and of pyruvate kinase. However, the phosphorylation of PFK 2/FBPase 2 is several times slower than that of the two other enzymes[17]. In isolated pancreatic islets, as well as in purified B cells, the concentration of fructose 2,6-bisphosphate increased up to 15-fold in the presence of glucose but was not decreased by glucagon[18].

Fructose 2,6-bisphosphate is formed in the liver and also in *Saccharomyces cerevisiae* in the presence of high concentrations of glucose. In the liver, this glucose effect is believed to be mediated by the formation of fructose 6-phosphate, which is a substrate for PFK 2 and a potent inhibitor of FBPase 2. A very different mechanism is now known to operate in *S. cerevisiae*[26]. In these cells, glucose causes an increase in cyclic AMP concentration, an effect which is in marked contrast with the idea that cyclic AMP is a signal for the lack of glucose. Cyclic AMP-dependent protein kinase then catalyses the phosphorylation of PFK 2 (which is simultaneously activated instead of being inactivated, as in the liver) and of fructose-1,6-bisphosphatase (which is partially inactivated). Also, the cyclic AMP-dependent phosphorylation of fructose-1,6-bisphosphatase is greatly accelerated by fructose 2,6-bisphosphate[19].

A puzzling observation made in several lower eukaryotic organisms is the dramatic (up to 250-fold) increase in fructose 2,6-bisphosphate concentration under various conditions which have in common a resumption of metabolic activity after some kind of dormancy (this term being taken in a very broad sense); this was observed in spores of *Phycomyces blakesleeanus* and of other fungi after breaking of dormancy by a heat shock or other means[20], in slices of Jerusalem artichoke tubers incubated at 25°C[21] and in seeds after imbibition[22]. Fructose 2,6-bisphosphate also appears to play a role in regulating carbon flow in higher plants. It could be a signal in the leaf cell for catabolism of sugars and inhibition of sucrose synthesis[23]. However, we were unable to confirm the claim[24] that potato tuber contains a uridine diphosphate glucose (UDPG) phosphorylase, the activity of which would be greatly stimulated by fructose 2,6-bisphosphate.

Escherichia coli fructose-1,6-bisphosphatase was reported[25] to be inhibited by fructose 2,6-bisphosphate, making it the first prokaryotic enzyme known to be affected by this regulator. So far, fructose 2,6-bisphosphate has not been found in bacteria.

References

14 Hers, H. G. and Van Schaftingen, E. (1984) *Adv. Cycl. Nucl. Prot. Phosphoryl. Res.* 17, 343–349

15 Claus, T. H., El-Maghrabi, M. R., Regen, D. M., Stewart, H. B., McGrane, M., Kountz, P. D., Nyfeler, F., Pilkis, J. and Pilkis, S. J. (1984) *Curr. Top. Cell. Regul.* 23, 57–86

16 Pilkis, S. J., Regen, D. M., Stewart, H. B., Pilkis, J., Pate, T. M. and El-Maghrabi, M. R. (1984) *J. Biol. Chem.* 259, 949–958

17 Bartrons, R., Hue, L., Van Schaftingen, E. and Hers, H. G. (1983) *Biochem. J.* 214, 829–837

18 Sener, A., Van Schaftingen, E., Van de Winkel, M., Pipeleers, D. G., Malaisse-Lagae, F., Malaisse, W. J. and Hers, H. G. (1984) *Biochem. J.* 221, 759–764

19 Gancedo, J. M., Mazon, M. J. and Gancedo, C. (1983) *J. Biol. Chem.* 258, 5998–5999

20 Van Laere, A., Van Schaftingen, E. and Hers, H. G. (1983) *Proc. Natl Acad. Sci. USA* 80, 6601–6605

21 Van Schaftingen, E. and Hers, H. G. (1983) *FEBS Lett.* 164, 195–200

22 Hers, H. G. (1984) *Biochem. Soc. Trans.* 12, 729–735

23 Preiss, J. (1984) *Trends Biochem. Sci.* 9, 24–27

24 Gibson, D. M. and Shine, W. E. (1983) *Proc. Natl Acad. Sci. USA* 80, 2491–2494

25 Marcus, F., Edelstein, I. and Rittenhouse, J. (1984) *Biochem. Biophys. Res. Commun.* 119, 1103–1108

26 François, J., Van Schaftingen, E. and Hers, H. G. (1984) *Eur. J. Biochem.* 145, 187–193

2,3-Bisphosphoglycerate in erythroid cells

Ryuzo Sasaki, Koji Ikura, Hiroshi Narita, Shin-ichi Yanagawa and Hideo Chiba

2,3-Bisphosphoglycerate accumulates in erythrocytes where it facilitates the supply of oxygen to the tissues by binding to hemoglobin. The concentration of 2,3-bisphosphoglycerate changes in a number of physiological and pathological conditions and during animal ontogeny. During erythroid differentiation in bone marrow the synthesis of 2,3-bisphosphoglycerate is induced. The regulation of 2,3-bisphosphoglycerate metabolism is beginning to be understood.

2,3-Bisphosphoglycerate (2,3-DPG) is a cofactor of the glycolytic enzyme phosphoglyceromutase (Fig. 1). However, the concentration of 2,3-DPG in many mammalian red blood cells is much greater than would be needed for the maximum rate of phosphoglyceromutase. In 1967, it was found that 2,3-DPG binds to hemoglobin (Hb) and has a higher affinity for the deoxy form. The oxygen tension in the lungs is sufficient to ensure at least 95% saturation of arterial blood, but the tension falls as blood travels from the lungs and oxygen is released from HbO_2. The binding of 2,3-DPG to the deoxy Hb displaces the $HbO_2 \rightleftharpoons Hb$ equilibrium to the deoxygenated side, thereby facilitating oxygen transfer from red cells to tissues. This finding prompted many investigations of 2,3-DPG[1,2]. In addition, several other roles for 2,3-DPG in erythroid cells have been presented[2-4]. Here we will deal with the regulatory properties of the enzymes involved in 2,3-DPG metabolism, the mechanism by which 2,3-DPG is accumulated in differentiating erythroid cells, and changes in the intraerythrocytic concentration of 2,3-DPG in the course of animal development.

2,3-Bisphosphoglycerate concentration

In the red cells of most adult mammals there is more 2,3-DPG than any other phosphorylated metabolite; exceptions are the red cells of cats and ruminants which contain small amounts (Table I). Red cells of birds also have very low 2,3-DPG concentrations but they contain large amounts of inositol pentaphosphate which can also bind to Hb and thus substitute for 2,3-DPG. In some mammalian species, however, 2,3-DPG concentrations drop transiently during development, and in ruminants and birds there are developmental stages at which the red cells contain large amounts of 2,3-DPG. Tissue cells contain very little 2,3-DPG, even in those animals which have high concentrations in their red cells[5]. The 2,3-DPG concentration in red cells changes *in vivo* in a number of physiological and pathological conditions; increasing with adaptation to high altitude, hypoxemia, anemia, chronic liver disease, hyperthyroidism, and red cell pyruvate kinase deficiency; and decreasing with severe acidosis[6].

2,3-Bisphosphoglycerate metabolism

For a long time it was believed that the enzymes responsible for 2,3-DPG metabolism, bisphosphoglyceromutase (now designated 2,3-DPG synthase) and 2,3-DPG phosphatase, were different proteins, because the reactions they catalysed were both essentially irreversible (Fig. 1). However, it was found with human[7], pig[8], and rabbit[9] red cells that these two enzyme activities are manifested by one protein and that this protein is always accompanied with phosphoglyceromutase activity. In these red cells there are three isozymes (peaks I, II, and III) which have the three enzyme activities in differing ratios (Table II). The contribution of the activities of each peak to the total in the hemolysates indicates that peak III is responsible for the metabolism of 2,3-DPG and peak I (possibly peak II in human and rabbit) functions as phosphoglyceromutase in glycolysis; the phosphoglyceromutase activity of peak III and the activities of 2,3-DPG synthase and 2,3-DPG phosphatase of peak I are physiologically insignificant. Therefore, peak III is designated 2,3-DPG synthase-phosphatase and peak I can correctly be called phosphoglyceromutase. 2,3-DPG synthase-phosphatase is present in all red cells which have high 2,3-DPG levels [10-12]. The low concentration of 2,3-DPG in cats and ruminants is due to the presence of only small amounts or the absence of 2,3-DPG synthase–phosphatase. Several lines of evidence concerning the human red cell enzyme have shown that both 2,3-DPG synthase and 2,3-DPG phosphatase activities are manifested at a common active site on 2,3-DPG synthase–phosphatase[13]. The mechanism by which the two enzyme activities are displayed at a common active site and the novel implication of this finding for the regulation of 2,3-DPG metabolism have been presented[2]. Briefly, as expected, there are reciprocal effects of substrates and effectors on the synthase and the phosphatase. Glycerate-3-P, which is a substrate of the synthase, is an inhibitor of the phosphatase and 2,3-DPG, which is a substrate of the phosphatase, is an inhibitor of the synthase. Inorganic phosphate, an activator of the phosphatase, is an inhibitor of the synthase. Thus, the effect of a ligand on one of the

Table I. 2,3-Bisphosphoglycerate (2,3-DPG) concentrations in erythrocytes and properties of hemoglobins

Species	2,3-DPG in erythrocyte (mM) Adult	Fetus or newborn		Occurrence of HbF	Oxygen affinity	Response to 2,3-DPG HbA	HbF
Human, Ref. 6,24	5.1	5.4	(newborn)	Yes	HbF = HbA	yes	much less sensitive
Rabbit, Ref. 25	9.6[a]	0.18[a]	(near term)	no	–	yes	–
Rat, Ref. 26	6.4[a]	0.13[a]	(near term)	no	–	yes	–
Dog, Ref. 27	4.4	0.85	(newborn)	no	–	yes	–
Pig, Ref. 28	8.5	2.4	(near term)	no	–	yes	–
Sheep, Ref. 23	0.12	10.5	(newborn)	yes	HbF > HbA	no	no

[a] Calculated from the data in references.

Table II. Properties of the enzymes related to 2,3-bisphosphoglycerate (2,3-DPG) in human erythrocytes[7]

Peak	Activity in the hemolysate (%) Synthase	Phosphatase	Mutase	Specific activity of the purified enzymes Synthase	Phosphatase	Mutase
I (Phosphoglyceromutase)	0.3	0.5	55	1	0.28	763
II	9	7	27	–	–	–
III (2,3-DPG synthase-phosphatase)	90.7	92.5	18	9.8	2.0	9.8

Synthase = 2,3-bisphosphoglycerate synthase; phosphatase = 2,3-bisphosphoglycerate phosphatase; mutase = phosphoglyceromutase.

two enzyme activities can be amplified by exerting the opposite effect on the other. Normally, an irreversible biochemical reaction accompanying the consumption of a high energy bond and its reverse reaction are catalysed by different enzymes (for example, phosphofructokinase and fructose-1,6-P_2 phosphatase). Allosteric transition is the prevailing mechanism for the regulation of these enzymes. The reg-

ulatory mechanism of 2,3-DPG metabolism in red cells is a new type of metabolic regulation achieved by one multifunctional enzyme which is capable of catalysing two irreversible reactions.

Human red cells consume 2–3 μmol of glucose/h/ml of cells. The 2,3-DPG bypass accounts for about 15–25% of the overall flux through glycolysis. From these values, the turnover rate of 2,3-DPG is 0.6–1.5

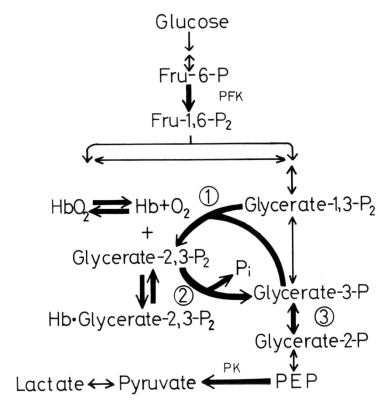

① Glycerate-2,3-P_2 synthase : Glycerate-1,3-P_2 + Glycerate-3-P $\longrightarrow$
  Glycerate-2,3-P_2 + Glycerate-3-P

② Glycerate-2,3-P_2 phosphatase : Glycerate-2,3-P_2 + H_2O $\longrightarrow$
  Glycerate-3-P + Pi

③ Phosphoglyceromutase : Glycerate-2,3-P_2 + Glycerate-3-P $\rightleftharpoons$
  Glycerate-2,3-P_2 + Glycerate-2-P

Fig. 1. 2,3-Bisphosphoglycerate (glycerate-2,3-P_2) cycle in erythrocyte.

μmol/h/ml of cells. From the 2,3-DPG synthase activity in the hemolysate, human red cells can synthesize maximally about 200 μmol of 2,3-DPG/h/ml of cells[7]. The physiological concentration of glycerate-3-P, a substrate of the synthase, is about 100-fold higher then the K_m value; the concentration of the other substrate, glycerate-1,3-P_2, is one-tenth of the K_m value[14]. The synthase, therefore, must be severely inhibited. 2,3-DPG is a competitive inhibitor of glycerate-1,3-P_2 with a K_i of 53 μM[14]. This inhibition is very effective in keeping 2,3-DPG synthase-phosphatase unavailable for 2,3-DPG synthesis. Conditions that lead to an increase in glycerate-1,3-P_2 always elevate the concentration of 2,3-DPG. 2,3-DPG phosphatase has the slowest activity of all the enzymes connected with glycolysis in human red cells. The phosphatase is activated by a number of anions such as Cl^- and P_i and is inhibited by monophosphoglycerates. The rate of 2,3-DPG breakdown in human red cells was calculated to be 0.08 μmol/h/ml of cells on the basis of kinetic data for the phosphatase and physiological concentrations of substrates and effectors[15]. This rate is too low to account for the observed contribution of the 2,3-DPG bypass to the overall glycolytic flux. The presence of glycolate-2-P, a potent activator of the phosphatase, was reported recently[16], and this may explain the discrepancy.

2,3-Bisphosphoglycerate in differentiating erythroid cells

After a multipotent hematopoietic stem cell has become committed to the erythroid lineage and subsequent differentiation into erythroid progenitor cells, the cells further differentiate into morphologically distinguishable erythroid cells, proerythroblasts, basophilic erythroblasts, polychromatic erythroblasts, orthochromatic erythroblasts, and reticulocytes, in order of increasing maturity. The bone marrow reticulocytes go into the blood and become mature erythrocytes. Hb is synthesized in erythroblasts and reticulocytes and the nucleus is lost at the orthochromatic stage. In birds, erythrocytes mature without loosing their nuclei. Although all blood cells (erythrocyte, granulocyte, and megakaryocyte) are derived from common multipotent stem cells, 2,3-DPG accumulates greatly only in erythroid cells. When and how is this compound accumulated in erythroid cells? Is the accumulation co-ordinated with that of Hb?

Rabbits were made anemic to different extents by phenylhydrazine injections so as to vary the differentiation stages of the erythroid cells in their peripheral blood and bone marrow[17]. The more severe the anemia, the lower the concentration of 2,3-DPG in the bone marrow cells and in the circulating erythroid cells. The 2,3-DPG concentration rose linearly during erythroid differentiation with the Hb level. The bone marrow cells were fractionated according to size (i.e. cell maturity) and the enzyme activities in the cells measured. The accumulation of 2,3-DPG was primarily attributable to the increase in 2,3-DPG synthase activity. The 2,3-DPG phosphatase concentration also increased as the cells matured because both synthase and phosphatase activities reside in one protein. Since the synthase activity of this protein is much higher than the phosphatase activity, an increase in the amount of this protein results in an increased 2,3-DPG concentration. In addition, pyruvate kinase concentration decreased steeply as the cells matured, while that of phosphofructokinase increased slightly. Such changes in the key enzymes of glycolysis would lead to an increased concentration of glycerate 1,3-P_2 by stimulating the flux of hexose phosphates into triose phosphates and by reducing the conversion of glycerate 3-P to pyruvate (Fig. 1). The increase in glycerate 1,3-P_2 favors 2,3-DPG synthesis by relieving 2,3-DPG synthase from product inhibition. Then the question arises whether the increase in 2,3-DPG synthase activity is due to an increase in the specific activity of the enzyme by post-translational modification or to accumulation of the enzyme. Antibody-binding studies showed that the increased activity is achieved solely through an increase in the amount of enzyme[18]. It was shown that 2,3-DPG synthase was synthesized in nucleated erythroid precursor cells and also in anucleated reticulocytes. The mRNA of this protein appears to be fairly stable in reticulocytes. Because Hb and 2,3-DPG are present at almost equimolar amounts in red cells and together they ensure a supply of oxygen to the tissues. It would be interesting to find out how globin and 2,3-DPG synthase are produced synchronously in differentiating erythroid cells. Friend erythroleukemia cells are mouse spleen cells transformed by the Friend virus complex. These cells can be induced to form erythroid cells by a variety of compounds. Coordinate expression of Hb and 2,3-DPG synthase was found during dimethylsulfoxide-induced differentiation of Friend cells[19]. 2,3-DPG concentrations rose concomitantly.

A working hypothesis to account for the increased 2,3-DPG synthase activity was that phosphoglyceromutase (peak I) might be converted to the synthase by a post-translational modification, because of the similarity in several physicochemical and enzymatic properties of the two enzymes[20,21]. In fact, phosphoglyceromutase activity declines drastically during erythroid cell differentiation[17]. Yeast phosphoglyceromutase also has the three enzyme activities and their ratios change through limited proteolysis[22]. However, the following two results have made this hypothesis very unlikely: (1) no immunoreaction was observed between anti-erythrocyte 2,3-DPG synthase antibody and phosphoglyceromutase (peak I)[20], and (2) 2,3-DPG synthase protein is synthesized *de novo* in erythroid cells[18]. However, we still believe that there is a relationship between the two enzymes. Our present hypothesis is that the synthesis of 2,3-DPG synthase involves either rearrangement of the phosphoglyceromutase gene or differential processing of a common nuclear RNA precursor.

2,3-Bisphosphoglycerate in animal development

Almost universally in mammals, fetal red cells have a higher oxygen affinity than do maternal red cells. This enhances the transport of oxygen across the placenta. How is this higher oxygen affinity of fetal red cells obtained? 2,3-DPG concentrations in red cells change during ontogeny. Does 2,3-DPG assist in providing the higher oxygen affinity in fetal cells? In most species, red cells in the early embryo contain an Hb which is structurally distinct from the adult type. Embryonic Hb has higher oxygen affinity. In primates and ruminants, embryonic Hb is succeeded by a specific fetal Hb (HbF) during middle and late fetal development, and by an adult Hb (HbA) in near term and after birth. In many other species there is a direct transition from embryonic to adult Hb. Three different mechanisms are used to increase the oxygen affinity of fetal red cells (Table I). In ruminants (1), HbF has higher oxygen affinity than its adult counterpart. 2,3-DPG has no influence on the oxygen affinity of either HbF or HbA. Nevertheless, 2,3-DPG concentrations do increase transiently in the red cells of new born sheep[23]. It is claimed that accumulation of this compound reduces the intracellular pH, and the lower pH reduces the oxygen affinity by the Bohr effect. This transient increase in 2,3-DPG keeps a low oxygen affinity of the red cells during replacement of HbF by HbA. In primates (2), the hemoglobins of fetus and adult are similar in oxygen affinity, but quite different in their response to 2,3-DPG[6,24]. The HbF is much less sensitive to 2,3-DPG. Thus, higher oxygen affinity of fetal red cells can be achieved without the need to change the 2,3-DPG concentrations during development. Many mammals (3) which lack a specific HbF acquire higher oxygen affinity of their fetal red cells by reducing the concentration of 2,3-DPG[25-28]. In the near term fetus of rabbit there is very little 2,3-DPG, but the concentration rises very rapidly after birth[25]. The low 2,3-DPG concentration in the fetal stage has been attributed to a high pyruvate kinase activity[29]. By contrast 2,3-DPG synthase activity in the red cells decreases moderately throughout development. In the rat fetus no 2,3-DPG synthase can be detected and this is presumably responsible for the low 2,3-DPG[26]. A postnatal increase in 2,3-DPG is caused by the appearance of 2,3-DPG synthase and a concomitant decrease in pyruvate kinase. 2,3-DPG accumulates in red cells of avian embryos to the extent of 4–5 mM[12]. This accumulation is due to a high concentration of 2,3-DPG synthase. The physiological function of 2,3-DPG in avian embryos is unclear.

References

1 Benesch, R. E. and Benesch, R. (1974) in *Adv. Protein Chem.* (Anfinsen, C. B., Edsall, J. T. and Richard, F. M., eds), Vol. 28, pp. 211–237, Academic Press

2 Chiba, H. and Sasaki, R. (1978) in *Current Topics in Cellular Regulation* (Horecker, B. L. and Stadtman, E. R., eds), Vol. 14, pp. 75–116, Academic Press

3 Sasaki, R., Ikura, K., Katsura, S. and Chiba, H. (1976) *Agric. Biol. Chem.* 40, 1797–1803

4 Narita, H., Ikura, K., Sasaki, R. and Chiba, H. (1979) *Biochem. Biophys. Res. Commun.* 86, 755–761

5 Sasaki, R., Ikura, K., Sugimoto, E. and Chiba, H. (1974) *Anal. Biochem.* 61, 43–47

6 Oski, F. A. and Delivoria-Papadopoulos, M. (1970) *J. Pediat.* 77, 941–956

7 Sasaki, R., Ikura, K., Sugimoto, E. and Chiba, H. (1975) *Eur. J. Biochem.* 50, 581–593

8 Sasaki, R., Ikura, K., Narita, H. and Chiba, H. (1976) *Agric. Biol. Chem.* 40, 2213–2221

9 Narita, H., Utsumi, S., Ikura, K., Sasaki, R. and Chiba, H. (1979) *Int. J. Biochem.* 10, 25–38

10 Rosa, R., Audit, I. and Rosa, J. (1975) *Biochimie.* 57, 1059–1063

11 Rose, Z. B. and Dube S. (1976) *Arch. Biochem. Biophys.* 117, 284–292

12 Harkness, D. R., Isaacks, R. E. and Roth, S. C. (1977) *Eur. J. Biochem.* 78, 343–351

13 Ikura, K., Sasaki, R., Narita, H., Sugimoto, E. and Chiba, H. (1976) *Eur. J. Biochem.* 66, 515–522

14 Rose, Z. B. (1973) *Arch. Biochem. Biophys.* 158, 903–910

15 Rose, Z. B. and Liebowitz, J. (1970) *J. Biol. Chem.* 245, 3232–3241

16 Rose, Z. B. and Salon, J. (1979) *Biochem. Biophys. Res. Commun.* 87, 869–875

17 Narita, H., Ikura, K., Yanagawa, S., Sasaki, R., Chiba, H., Saimyoji, H. and Kumagai, N. (1980) *J. Biol. Chem.* 255, 5230–5235

18 Narita, H., Yanagawa, S., Sasaki, R. and Chiba, H. (1981) *J. Biol. Chem.* 256, 7059–7063

19 Narita, H., Yanagawa, S., Sasaki, R. and Chiba, H. (1981) *Biochem. Biophys. Res. Commun.* 103, 90–96

20 Ikura, K., Narita, H., Sasaki, R. and Chiba, H. (1978) *Eur. J. Biochem.* 89, 23–31

21 Hass, L. F., Kappel, W. K., Miller, K. B. and Engle, R. L. (1978) *J. Biol. Chem.* 253, 77–81

22 Sasaki, R., Utsumi, S., Sugimoto, E. and Chiba, H. (1976) *Eur. J. Biochem.* 66, 523–533

23 Baumann, R., Bauer, C. H. and Rathschlag-Schaefer, A. M. (1972) *Respir. Physiol.* 15, 151–158

24 Tyuma, I. and Shimizu, K. (1969) *Arch. Biochem. Biophys.* 129, 404–405

25 Jelkmann, W. and Bauer, C. (1977) *Pflügers Archiv.* 372, 149–156

26 Jelkmann, W. and Bauer, C. (1980) *Pflügers Archiv.* 389, 61–68

27 Dhindsa, D. S., Hoversland, A. S. and Templeton, J. W. (1972) *Biol. Neonate* 20, 226–235

28 Baumann, R., Teischel, F., Zoch, R. and Bartels, H. (1973) *Respir. Physiol.* 19, 153–161

29 Jelkmann, W. and Bauer, C. (1978) *Pflügers Archiv.* 375, 189–195

Ryuzo Sasaki, Koji Ikura, Hiroshi Narita, Shin-ichi Yanagawa and Hideo Chiba are at the Department of Food Science and Technology, Faculty of Agriculture, Kyoto University, Kyoto 606, Japan.

Metabolic regulation: could Mn^{2+} be involved?

Vern L. Schramm

It is possible that Mn^{2+} acts as a regulatory signal in metabolism. Phosphoenolpyruvate carboxykinase, a regulated enzyme of hepatic gluconeogenesis, is considered as a prototypic enzyme for which Mn^{2+} may act as a regulatory ion.

The manganous ion serves an essential role in the metabolism of mammalian liver as a cofactor which binds tightly to enzymes such as pyruvate carboxylase, superoxide dismutase and arginase. Several other enzymes are reported to be activated by Mn^{2+} or to give greater catalytic rates in the presence of Mn^{2+} than with Mg^{2+}. These effects have frequently been invoked as having the potential for metabolic regulation[1]. However, regulation by Mn^{2+} ions has remained speculative owing to the lack of experimental data for intracellular concentrations of free and bound Mn^{2+} and the lack of kinetic constants for the effects of Mn^{2+} on enzymes. Recently, we have developed magnetic resonance techniques which can distinguish free Mn^{2+} from bound Mn^{2+} in intact cells and have determined free and bound Mn^{2+} in rat hepatocytes[2]. With the availability of this information, it is opportune to summarize the factors which are *required* for Mn^{2+} effects in metabolic regulation. The properties of P-enolpyruvate carboxykinase are examined as a model system for considering enzymic regulation by intracellular concentrations of Mn^{2+}.

Necessary conditions for enzymic regulation by Mn^{2+}

Direct regulation of an enzyme by Mn^{2+} requires Mn^{2+} to bind to the target enzyme followed by a metabolically significant response in catalytic activity. This simple tenet, and the knowledge of Mn^{2+} concentrations in the cell allows us to predict the

properties an enzyme must exhibit to be regulated by Mn^{2+} *in vivo*.

To permit interaction between Mn^{2+} and a target enzyme;

(1) *The kinetic constant(s) for the interaction of Mn^{2} must approximate the intracellular free Mn^{2} concentration at physiological substrate concentrations.*

The kinetic constants for Mn^{2+} dissociation can be evaluated by steady-state kinetic methods. Special precautions are required to regulate the concentration of free Mn^{2+} since substrates, especially those which contain pyrophosphates, are avid chelators of divalent cations. The kinetic constants for Mn^{2+} must be determined over a range of substrate concentrations to evaluate the effect of substrates on the interaction of Mn^{2+}. For example, the kinetic constant for Mn^{2+} activation of galactosyltransferase changes from greater than 1 mM to less than 1 μM as a function of substrate and Ca^{2+} concentrations[3]. The kinetic constants for Mn^{2+} should be extrapolated to zero and saturating concentrations of substrate or other effectors in order to estimate the free Mn^{2+} concentration required to alter the enzyme at given metabolite concentrations. Kinetic constants for Mn^{2+} obtained in this manner should be below 5 μM since free Mn^{2+} is in the range 0.2–1 μM in isolated rat hepatocytes[2].

(2) *The binding site(s) for Mn^{2+} must discriminate strongly against Mg^{2+}.*

Enzymes which are regulated by Mn^{2+} must discriminate between Mg^{2+} and Mn^{2+} to a degree which approximates or exceeds the intracellular ratio of free Mg^{2+} to free Mn^{2+}. The similarity of the chelate structures of these ions accounts for the almost universal ability to substitute Mg^{2+} and Mn^{2+}, even though the affinities for the two ions can differ by orders of magnitude in proteins or in model chelating compounds. For example at pH 8, the stability constant for Mn^{2+}-EDTA is 10^5 times greater than that for Mg^{2+}-EDTA. With intracellular free Mg^{2+} of approximately 1 mM[4] and free Mn^{2+} of 0.2–1.0 μM in hepatocytes, a binding site specific for Mn^{2+} must bind Mn^{2+} at least 10^3 times tighter than it binds Mg^{2+}. Steady-state kinetic measurements to determine constants for Mn^{2+} must therefore be performed in the presence of Mg^{2+}. When it is possible to overcome the effects of Mn^{2+} by excess Mg^{2+}, direct inhibition experiments can establish the $K_{Mg^{2+}}/K_{Mn^{2+}}$. This ratio must equal or exceed 1000 for Mn^{2+} specific effects to occur in the presence of physiological concentrations of Mg^{2+}.

(3) *The amount of intracellular, exchangeable Mn^{2+} must approximate or exceed the molarity of target enzymes required for observed metabolic flux.*

Enzymes or other molecules which contain tightly bound Mn^{2+} represent a non-exchangeable pool of Mn^{2+} which cannot participate in rapidly reversible binding to target enzymes. The quantity of enzyme protein which could be affected by the reversible binding of Mn^{2+} is therefore limited by the amount of exchangeable Mn^{2+}. Estimates of exchangeable ions in the extramitochondrial compartment can be made by the addition of digitonin to isolated hepatocytes. Low concentrations of digitonin make the plasma membrane permeable, allowing the release of ions which are freely exchangeable in the cytosolic compartment[5]. Estimation of exchangeable Mn^{2+} by this technique gives approximately 13 μM Mn^{2+} (13 nmol Mn^{2+} per ml of cell H_2O)[6]. If the average cytosolic protein is assumed to be of mol. wt 50 000, 13 μM Mn^{2+} could saturate 650 μg/ml protein, or 10 such proteins which are present at 65 μg/ml of cell H_2O.

(4) *The intracellular free Mn^{2+} must change in response to altered physiological or hormonal states.*

Regulation of enzymes by Mn^{2+} requires changes in the intracellular concentration of the ion. Such changes could result from the active transport of Mn^{2+} into the cell, or from redistribution of Mn^{2+} between subcellular compartments in response to a metabolic change and/or a homonal signal. Changes in the concentration of free Mn^{2+} could also occur in response to the induction of proteins which bind Mn^{2+} or in response to factors which increase the affinity of target proteins for Mn^{2+}. The observed change in Mn^{2+} concentration must be accompanied by a change in the catalytic activity of the target enzymes.

These four conditions are *necessary* to permit Mn^{2+}-mediated regulation of an enzyme. The remainder of this article will consider a specific enzyme, P-enolpyruvate carboxykinase from rat liver cytosol. Each of the four conditions will be evaluated to the extent possible with the experimental evidence currently available.

Could Mn^{2+} regulate P-enolpyruvate carboxykinase?

The activation of P-enolpyruvate carboxykinase by Mn^{2+} was one of the earliest observations of the kinetic properties of the enzyme[7]. The physiological role of Mn^{2+} activation was later discounted because of the relatively low concentration of total cytosolic Mn^{2+} in fractionated rat liver[8]. Recent studies of Mn^{2+} interaction with both mitochondrial and cytosolic P-enolpyruvate carboxykinases[9–11] and the demonstration that Mn^{2+} can be rapidly accumulated by mitochondria[12] suggested that Mn^{2+} requires re-investigation as a potential effector of P-enolpyruvate carboxykinase.

Activation constant for Mn^{2+}

The kinetic constant for activation of P-enolpyruvate carboxykinase by Mn^{2+} is 1.7 μM, using the physiological nucleotide ($MgGTP^{2-}$) and maintaining free Mg^{2+} in excess. P-enolpyruvate carboxykinase can be activated at least 10-fold by Mn^{2+}, and this effect is predominantly a V_{max} effect[9, 10, 13]. Changes in $MgGTP^{2-}$ and oxaloacetate over the concentration ranges thought to exist *in vivo* have no significant effect on the activation constant for Mn^{2+} (Ref. 9).

For Mn^{2+} to affect P-enolpyruvate carboxykinase *in vivo*, the free Mn^{2+} must approximate the activation constant. The free Mn^{2+} of hepatocytes is estimated directly by placing freshly prepared cells in an electron paramagnetic resonance (EPR) instrument. This is a non-destructive technique and the cells remain viable throughout[2]. The Mn^{2+} EPR spectra from such an experiment are shown in Fig. 1. The experiments indicate that free Mn^{2+} is approximately 1.0 μM and 0.2 μM in hepatocytes from fed and fasted rats, respectively[2, 6]. These values are sufficiently near the activation constant of 1.7 μM for Mn^{2+} to permit substantial interaction of Mn^{2+} and P-enolpyruvate carboxykinase at *in vivo* concentrations of Mn^{2+} and the enzyme.

Mn^{2+}/Mg^{2+} discrimination factor

Mg^{2+} is a competitive inhibitor of the Mn^{2+} activation of P-enolpyruvate carboxykinase. This relationship allows a direct comparison of the dissociation constants for Mg^{2+} and Mn^{2+} at the site which leads to activation. The inhibition constant of 5 mM for Mg^{2+} gives a Mn^{2+}/Mg^{2+} discrimination of approximately 3000, sufficient to allow Mn^{2+} interaction with the enzyme in the presence of free Mg^{2+} in the millimolar range[9].

Exchangeable Mn^{2+}

The total Mn^{2+} of rat liver has been reported by a number of investigators to be approximately 35 nmol/ml cell H_2O^2. Treatment of cells with digitonin allows release of 13 nmol Mn^{2+} per ml of cell H_2O (Fig. 1)[6]. These findings indicate that about one-third of the total Mn^{2+} is extramitochondrial and is not tightly bound to protein. The cellular concentrations of

pyruvate carboxylase, arginase and superoxide dismutase can be calculated to be approximately 20 μM, thereby accounting for most of the remaining, non-exchangeable Mn^{2+}. Since the concentration of P-enolpyruvate carboxykinase varies from approximately 3 μM in de-induced liver to 10 μM in induced liver[14], a stoichiometeric quantity of exchangeable Mn^{2+} is available. The catalytic capacity of P-enolpyruvate carboxykinase in induced liver is approximately 10 times greater than the maximum rates of gluconeogenesis. Thus, no more than 10% of the total P-enolpyruvate carboxykinase need be active to account for the observed rates of gluconeogenesis. Approximately 1 μM Mn^{2+} would be required to bind to the enzyme for the observed rates of gluconeogenesis. These considerations are consistent with the postulate that adequate extramitochondrial Mn^{2+} is present to account for Mn^{2+} activation of P-enolpyruvate carboxykinase as well as other enzymes in rat hepatocytes.

Mn^{2+} in metabolic states

The concentration of free Mn^{2+} varies three-fold in hepatocytes depending on whether the rats are fed or fasted[2]. Total Mn^{2+} in these cells shows no significant change under the same conditions. The free Mn^{2+} of rat liver is therefore in dynamic equilibrium with cellular proteins and exhibits sufficient variation to influence target proteins. In the case of P-enolpyruvate carboxykinase, the observed decrease of free Mn^{2+} in hepatocytes from fasted rats could represent an increased affinity of the enzyme for Mn^{2+} thus decreasing the free Mn^{2+} of the cells. The mechanism for the observed change in free Mn^{2+} in response to dietary state is unknown, but could be caused by Mn^{2+} uptake by mitochondria or by induction of molecules which bind Mn^{2+}. Although no direct experimental evidence is yet available to address these possibilities, there is good evidence that P-enolpyruvate carboxykinase can exist in forms with differing

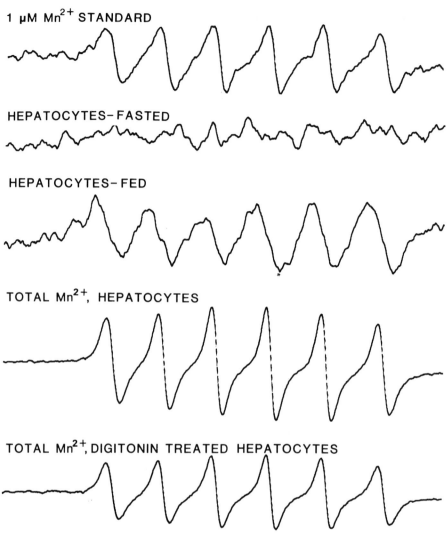

Fig. 1. EPR spectra of Mn^{2+} in hepatocytes and hepatocyte extracts. Instrument gain in the upper three spectra is approximately 10 times greater than for the lower two spectra. Spectra 2 and 3 are the free Mn^{2+} in hepatocytes. Spectra 4 and 5 are perchloric acid extracts of hepatocytes before and after treatment with digitonin (see Ref. 2 for the methods of these determinations).

responses to Mn^{2+} activation[9, 13].

Conclusions

Four conditions are necessary for the regulation of enzyme steps by Mn^{2+}. Determination of Mn^{2+} activation constants for P-enolpyruvate carboxykinase and the concentration of free and bound Mn^{2+} in rat hepatocytes has demonstrated that the necessary conditions have been met for an enzyme–Mn^{2+} interaction. Even though the necessary conditions for Mn^{2+} activation of P-enolpyruvate carboxykinase have been met, additional information is required to determine whether these factors are sufficient for regulation. The relatively large amount of exchangeable Mn^{2+}, compared to that required for activation of P-enolpyruvate carboxykinase, suggests that more than one protein is regulated by Mn^{2+}. Another candidate for such regulation is arginase, the cytosolic enzyme responsible for urea formation. Arginase also appears to contain binding sites for Mn^{2+} which may influence the catalytic activity[15].

Acknowledgement

This work was supported by research grant AM 25551 from the National Institutes of Health.

References

1 Williams, R. J. P. (1982) *FEBS Lett.* 140, 3–10
2 Ash, D. E. and Schramm, V. L. (1982) *J. Biol. Chem.* 257, 9261–9264
3 Morrison, J. F. and Ebner, K. E. (1971) *J. Biol. Chem.* 246, 3977–3984
4 Veloso, D., Guynn, R. W., Oskarsson, M. and Veech, R. L. (1973) *J. Biol. Chem.* 248, 4811–4819
5 Zuurendonk, P. F. and Tager, J. M. (1974) *Biochim. Biophys. Acta* 333, 393–399
6 Schramm, V. L. and Ash, D. E. (1982) *Fed. Proc.* 41, 5060
7 Utter, M. F. and Kolenbrander, H. M. (1972) *Enzymes* 3rd edn, 6 pp, 136–154
8 Foster, D. O., Lardy, H. A., Ray, P. D. and Johnston, J. B. (1967) *Biochemistry* 6, 2120–2128
9 Schramm, V. L., Fullin, F. A. and Zimmerman, M. D. (1981) *J. Biol. Chem.* 256, 10803–10808
10 Colombo, G. and Lardy, H. A. (1981) *Biochemistry* 20, 2758–2767
11 Lee, M. H., Hebda, C. A. and Nowak, T. (1981) *J. Biol. Chem.* 256, 12793–12801
12 Lehninger, A. L., Carafoli, E. and Rossi, C. S. (1967) *Adv. Enzymol.* 29, 259–320
13 Brinkworth, R. I., Hanson, R. W., Fullin, F. A. and Schramm, V. L. (1981) *J. Biol. Chem.* 256, 10795–10802
14 Ballard, F. J. and Hanson, R. W. (1969) *J. Biol. Chem.* 244, 5625–5630
15 Hirsch-Kolb, H., Kolb, H. J. and Greenberg, D. M. (1971) *J. Biol. Chem.* 246, 395–401

Vern L. Schramm is at the Department of Biochemistry, Temple University School of Medicine, Philadelphia, PA 19140, USA.

A family of guanine nucleotide regulatory proteins

Miles D. Houslay

Three distinct guanine nucleotide regulatory (binding) proteins, mediating information exchange across biological membranes, have been identified. These are transducin (T), which allows rhodopsin to stimulate a high affinity cyclic GMP phosphodiesterase upon photoactivation; N_s (also termed variously G/F and G_s) which effects hormonal stimulation of adenylate cyclase; and N_i (or G_i) which mediates hormonal inhibition of adenylate cyclase. Recently a number of important advances have been made which add considerably to our knowledge of these systems. These are the identification and purification of N_i and the ability to separate and reconstitute, in various ways, the subunits of N_s and transducin. Such studies highlight the structural and functional similarities of these proteins.

N_s and N_i contain two non-identical subunits (α,β) and transducin contains three (α,β,γ). Remarkably, the β-subunit associated with all three of these regulatory proteins is apparently an identical species of M_r 35 000, whereas their α-subunits, which provide the guanine nucleotide binding site, are very different[1]. The α-subunit of transducin (T^α) also has a binding site for rhodopsin[2] and it is highly probable that the α-subunits of both N_i (N_i^α) and N_s (N_s^α) will be shown to have complementary sites for interaction with the receptors which trigger their activation.

In both N_s (Ref. 3) and transducin[2], the biological effect results from the release of an activated α-subunit from the regulatory complex, usually by hormone receptor being occupied and photoactivation, respectively. However, activation can also be elicited by non-hydrolysable GTP analogues such as p[NH]ppG, which bind tightly to the α-subunits. It is contended that N_s^α interacts with and activates the catalytic unit of adenylate cyclase by increasing the affinity of the enzyme for Mg^{2+} (Ref. 4), whereas T^α activates cyclic GMP phosphodiesterase by relieving the inhibitory effect[5] exerted by the phosphodiesterase's own γ-subunit. Despite the different molecular weights and different proposed mode of action of the α-subunits of N_s and transducin, it has been claimed that T^α can also activate adenylate cyclase when inserted in various other membrane systems[7], which suggests that there is a close structural analogy between them.

The precise mechanism by which N_i causes inhibition of adenylate cyclase is still the subject of much discussion[8,9]. One argument is that it is solely the release of the β-subunit from N_i that causes inhibition of adenylate cyclase by both promoting the deactivation of N_s^α and inhibiting the release of N_s^α from N_s. Certainly, both of these processes occur in detergent solutions of the purified components where it can be demonstrated quite clearly that the β-subunit is essential for the deactivation of N_s^α to form the dimeric N_s complex[3,9]. It is possible, however, that within the membrane, N_i^α itself could inhibit adenylate cyclase by either exerting a direct effect on the catalytic unit or by competing with N_s^α for its binding site on adenylate cyclase. By analogy with N_s^α and T^α, a functional role might thus be expected for N_i^α. N_s^α has recently been purified when N_i^α can also be obtained in a pure state, these alternatives can be tested.

In all three regulatory proteins, the β-

subunit appears to deactivate the free α-subunit by recombining with it. From observations made with transducin[2], it may well be that the α-subunit is released free and active with GTP bound to it. Termination of its activity (on re-association with the β-subunit) then leads to the concomitant hydrolysis of GTP to GDP, i.e. the β-subunit promotes a GTPase activity inherent in the α-subunit. It is clear however, that further investigations need to be made in order to characterize and quantitate fully the role of GTP hydrolysis in the functioning of these guanine nucleotide regulatory proteins.

The identification of these regulatory proteins, certainly in the case of N_i, owes a lot to the ability of certain toxins to elicit their NAD-dependent, ADP-ribosylation[10]. Cholera toxin acts on both transducin[11] and N_s, whereupon dissociation of the complex occurs, liberating the permanently activated and ribosylated α-subunit. On the other

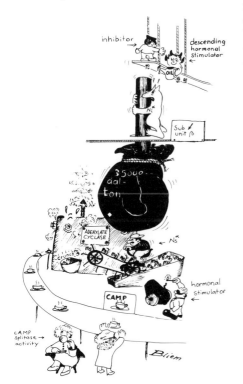

hand a component of pertussis toxin (islet activating protein, IAP) acts specifically on the α-subunit of N_i (and not that of N_s), preventing its dissociation and blocking the action of inhibitory hormones. IAP-mediated ribosylation and various other techniques have all been used recently to demonstrate that a clone of lymphoma cells, deficient in N_s activity (cyc⁻), actually expresses N_i[12,13]. This inhibitory protein allowed somatostatin receptors on cyc⁻ cells to inhibit adenylate cyclase activity and was therefore fully functional[14]. Indeed, two other cell lines (UNC, H21a), which express a malfunctioning N_s, in fact exhibit a functional N_i. Furthermore, the β-subunits present in these cells can be extracted and demonstrated to deactivate N_s^α in a reconstituted system, suggesting that the abnormality apparent in such mutant cells takes the form of a crippled N_s^α subunit[9]. This view is reinforced by the observation[3] that a normal stimulatory (N_s) response could be reconstituted in membranes from these cells merely by the insertion of purified N_s^α. All such experiments indicate that the β-subunit is a separate gene product whose synthesis is controlled separately from that of N_s^α. Indeed, the β-subunit appears in far greater (10-fold) quantities than N_s, being found predominantly as part of the N_i complex[9].

There are still a number of controversial aspects to this system: for example, the precise molecular weights of certain components, the rates of interaction between the subunits and the physiologically relevant mechanism whereby N_i exerts its inhibitory effect. Nevertheless, N_i and N_s provide an example of a structurally- and functionally-related system with distinct homologies to what at first appears to be a very different system, transducin. Is it possible that these are just the first members to be identified of a much wider family of GTP-binding proteins mediating information transfer across biological membranes? Indeed, recently roles for specific guanine nucleotides regulating Ca^{2+} channels in mast cells[15] and mediating certain of insulin's effects[16] have been proposed.

References

1 Manning, D. R. and Gilman, A. G. (1983) *J. Biol. Chem.* 258, 7059–7063

2 Fung, B. K. K. (1983) *J. Biol. Chem.* 258, 10495–10502

3 Northup, J. K., Smigel, M. D., Sternweis, P. C. and Gilman A. G. (1983) *J. Biol. Chem.* 258, 11369–11376

4 Iyengar, R. and Birnbaumer, L. (1982) *Proc. Natl Acad. Sci. USA* 79, 5179–5183

5 Yamazaki, A., Stein, P. J., Chernoff, N. and Bitensky, M. W. (1983) *J. Biol. Chem.* 258, 8188–8194

6 Hurley, J. B. and Stryer, L. (1982) *J. Biol. Chem.* 257, 11094–11099

7 Bitensky, M. W., Wheeler, M. A., Rasenick, M. M., Yamazaki, A., Stein, P. J., Halliday, K. R. and Wheeler, G. L. (1982) *Proc. Natl Acad. Sci. USA* 79, 3408–3412

8 Codina, J., Hildebrandt, J., Iyengar, R., Birnbaumer, L., Sekura, R. D. and Manclark, C. R. (1983) *Proc. Natl Acad. Sci. USA* 80, 4276–4280

9 Northup, J. K., Sternweiss, P. C. and Gilman, A. G. (1983) *J. Biol. Chem.* 258, 11361–11368

10 Bokuch, G. M., Katada, T., Northup, J. K., Hewlett, E. L. and Gilman, A. G. (1983) *J. Biol. Chem.* 258, 2072–2075

11 Abood, M. E., Hurley, J. B., Poppone, M.-C., Bourne, H. R. and Stryer, L. (1982) *J. Biol. Chem.* 257, 10540–10543

12 Hildebrandt, J. D., Hanoune, J. and Birnbaumer, L. (1982) *J. Biol. Chem.* 257, 14723–14725

13 Hildebrandt, J. D., Sekura, R. D., Codina, J., Iyengar, R., Manclark, C. R. and Birnbaumer, L. (1983) *Nature* 302, 706–707

14 Jakobs, K. H. and Schultz, G. (1983) *Proc. Natl Acad. Sci. USA* 80, 3899–3902

15 Gomperts, B. D. (1983) *Nature* 306, 64–66

16 Houslay, M. D. and Heyworth, C. M. (1983) *Trends Biochem. Sci.* 8, 449–452

Miles D. Houslay is at the Department of Biochemistry, UMIST, PO Box 88, Manchester M60 1QD, UK.

Cyclic nucleotides – teaching an old dogma new tricks

David C. Laporte

In eukaryotic systems, many of the effects of extracellular stimulation are mediated inside the cell by 'second messengers'. Perhaps the most extensively studied of the second messengers are the cyclic nucleotides: cAMP and cGMP. It has been generally accepted that, in eukaryotes, cAMP acts exclusively through cAMP-dependent protein kinase[1]. Although the functions of cGMP are not as defined as those of cAMP, it is also thought to act through stimulation of a specific protein kinase. These kinases respond to changes in the cellular level of their cyclic nucleotides by altering the phosphorylation states of key proteins. This view is being challenged by Nelson Goldberg and co-workers, who have suggested that, in some cases, the important parameter may be the rate of cyclic nucleotide turnover, and not its concentration[2]. If this can be established, it would argue that response mechanisms other than the protein kinases must exist.

An essential step in the resolution of this problem is the development of a method to measure the rate of cyclic nucleotide turnover. To accomplish this, Goldberg et al. have taken advantage of the ability of cyclic nucleotide phosphodiesterase to catalyse the incorporation of $(^{18}O)H_2O$ into the α-phosphates of the adenine and guanine nucleotides[2]. Although this is not the only route for labeling the α-phosphate in vivo, it appears to be the principal one. In order to measure the turnover rate, the tissue is immersed in a medium which is highly enriched in $(^{18}O)H_2O$. The rate of appearance of ^{18}O in the α-phosphates of the adenine or guanine nucleotides is then taken as a measure of the turnover rate.

This technique has been used to investigate the behavior of cGMP in the visual system[2]. In the retina, cGMP, guanylate cyclase and cGMP specific phosphodiesterase are largely confined to the outer segments of the photoreceptor cells[3]. Stimulation of the cGMP-specific phosphodiesterase is believed to be a key step in visual reception, possibly leading to the hyperpolarization of the photoreceptor membrane[4,5]. Goldberg et al. have found that exposure of retinas to low level illumination could stimulate cGMP turnover up to 5-fold[2]. In contrast, these levels of illumination had relatively little effect on cGMP concentration, which suggests a parallel activation of guanylate cyclase. These observations appear to rule out the participation of cGMP-dependent protein kinase, since this enzyme can only respond to changes in cGMP concentration.

The nature of the coupling of cGMP turnover to the hyperpolarization of the photoreceptor membrane remains unclear. A number of possibilities can be presented after inspection of the relevant reactions[2]:

$$\text{Metal·GTP}^{2-} \xrightarrow{\substack{\text{guanylate} \\ \text{cyclase}}} \text{cGMP}^{1-} + \text{H}^+ + \text{Metal·PP}_i^{2-}$$

$$\text{H}_2\text{O} + \text{cGMP}^- \xrightarrow{\text{phosphodiesterase}} \text{GMP}^{2-} + \text{H}^+$$

Stimulation of cGMP turnover might yield a significant increase in the concentrations of pyrophosphate or protons. These metabolites could then act to stimulate the next step in the cascade. Alternatively, the free energy released through this cycle might be harnessed, perhaps to drive a calcium pump. Probably the most striking distinction between these models and those which are currently popular is that the cyclic nucleotide is not, itself, the signal. Instead, its role is to provide the metabolic precursor or the energy source from which the signal is produced.

Regardless of the exact mechanism of coupling, the available evidence suggests that cGMP-dependent protein kinase is probably not a participant in this system. This represents a major departure from the conventional wisdom in the field of cyclic nucleotide metabolism. If this proves to be correct, it will require a re-evaluation of other systems in which cyclic nucleotides participate.

References

1 Kuo, J. F. and Greengard, P. (1969) *J. Biol. Chem.* 244, 3417–3419
2 Goldberg, N. D., Ames, A., Gander, J. and Walseth, T. F. (1983) *J. Biol. Chem.* 258, 9213–9219
3 Berger, J. J., DeVries, G. W., Carter, J. G., Schulz, D. W., Passoneau, P. N., Lowry, O. H. and Ferrendelli, J. A. (1980) *J. Biol. Chem.* 255, 3128–3133
4 Keirns, J. J., Miki, N., Bitensky, M. W. and Keirns, M. (1975) *Biochemistry* 14, 2760–2766
5 Fung, B. K.-K. and Stryer, L. (1980) *Proc. Natl Acad. Sci. USA* 77, 2500–2504

David C. Laporte is at the Department of Biochemistry, University of Minnesota, Minneapolis, MN 55455, USA.

Index

The articles in this book have been reprinted
from the monthly review journal

TRENDS IN BIOCHEMICAL SCIENCES

This journal is available on subscription from

Elsevier Publications (Cambridge)
68 Hills Road
Cambridge CB2 1LA
United Kingdom

Write for details of the personal edition and library edition of *Trends in Biochemical Sciences* and our special reduced prices for students.